Prognosis Research
in Healthcare

Prognosis Research in Healthcare
Concepts, Methods, and Impact

Edited by

Richard D Riley

Danielle A van der Windt

Peter Croft

Karel GM Moons

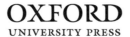

OXFORD
UNIVERSITY PRESS

Great Clarendon Street, Oxford, OX2 6DP,
United Kingdom

Oxford University Press is a department of the University of Oxford.
It furthers the University's objective of excellence in research, scholarship,
and education by publishing worldwide. Oxford is a registered trade mark of
Oxford University Press in the UK and in certain other countries

Published in the United States of America by Oxford University Press
198 Madison Avenue, New York, NY 10016, United States of America

British Library Cataloguing in Publication Data
Data available

Library of Congress Control Number: 2018960772

ISBN 978–0–19–879661–9

Printed and bound by
CPI Group (UK) Ltd, Croydon, CR0 4YY

Oxford University Press makes no representation, express or implied, that the
drug dosages in this book are correct. Readers must therefore always check
the product information and clinical procedures with the most up-to-date
published product information and data sheets provided by the manufacturers
and the most recent codes of conduct and safety regulations. The authors and
the publishers do not accept responsibility or legal liability for any errors in the
text or for the misuse or misapplication of material in this work. Except where
otherwise stated, drug dosages and recommendations are for the non-pregnant
adult who is not breast-feeding

Links to third party websites are provided by Oxford in good faith and
for information only. Oxford disclaims any responsibility for the materials
contained in any third party website referenced in this work.

For Doug, our inspiration to improve prognosis research

We dedicate this book to our families
To Lorna, Sebastian, and Imogen
To Ynze
To Margaret, Louise, and Suzanne
To my sister, Lian, and brother, Michel

Acknowledgements

The editors would like to acknowledge all members of the PROGRESS study group, some of whom are co-authors of chapters in this textbook. The group, which was partly funded by a UK Medical Research Council (MRC) partnership grant, and included journal editors, clinicians, and researchers from a wide range of disciplines, has been the inspiration for this textbook, together with the four original PROGRESS papers authored by the group and published in the *BMJ* and *PLoS Medicine* in 2013. The editors would also like to thank their affiliated institutions and departments: the Research Institute for Primary Care and Health Sciences at Keele University, UK and the Julius Center for Health Sciences and Primary Care at UMC Utrecht, Utrecht University, The Netherlands.

Contents

List of Abbreviations

AIDS	acquired immune deficiency syndrome		EPV	events per variable
			FAB	fear avoidance beliefs
ARR	absolute rate or risk reduction		GRADE	grades of recommendation, assessment, development, and evaluation
ACR	albumin:creatinine ratio			
AI	artificial intelligence		HbA1c	haemoglobin A1c
AIC	Akaike information criterion		HCUP	Health care cost and utilization project
AMI	acute myocardial infarction		HER2	human epidermal growth factor
BIC	Bayesian information criterion		HIV	human immunodeficiency virus
BMD	bone mineral density		HR	hazard ratio
CABG	coronary artery bypass graft		ICU	intensive care unit
CCTA	coronary computed tomographic angiography		IMPACT	International mission for prognosis and analysis of clinical trials
CD4	cluster of differentiation 4			
CEA	carcinoembryonic antigen		IPD	individual participant data
CHD	coronary heart disease		IRR	incidence rate ratio
CONSORT	consolidated standards of reporting trials		LASSO	least absolute shrinkage and selection operator
COPD	chronic obstructive pulmonary disease		LBP	low back pain
			ML	machine learning
CPCSSN	Canadian primary care sentinel surveillance network		NCI-CDP	cancer diagnosis programme of the National Cancer Institute
CPRD	Clinical practice research datalink		NICE	National Institute for Health and Clinical Excellence
CRASH-2	clinical randomization of an antifibrinolytic in significant haemorrhage		NNR	number needed to read
			NNT	number needed to treat
ECG	electrocardiogram		NPI	Nottingham prognostic index
EGFR-TK	epidermal growth factor receptor tyrosine kinase			
EHR	electronic healthcare record		OR	odds ratio
EMA	European Medicines Agency		PBC	primary biliary cirrhosis
			PCI	percutaneous coronary intervention
EPP	events per candidate predictor parameter		PMR	polymyalgia rheumatica

PROGRESS	prognosis research strategy	SHCR	Swedish Skåne county health care register
QoF	quality and outcomes framework	SIDIAP	Information system for the development of research in primary care
QOL	quality of life		
QALYs	quality-adjusted life years		
QUIPS	quality in prognosis studies	SSC	statistical software components
PICO	population, intervention, comparison, and outcome	sST2	soluble growth stimulation expressed gene 2
PROBAST	prediction model risk of bias assessment tool	STRATOS	Strengthening analytical thinking for observational studies
PSA	prostate-specific antigen	TARN	Trauma audit and research network
RBC	red blood cell		
RD	rate or risk difference	THIN	The health improvement network
REMARK	Reporting recommendations for tumour marker prognostic studies	TNM staging	tumour size, nodal status, and metastasis
		ToPs	trees of predictors
ROC	receiver operating characteristic	TRIPOD	transparent reporting of a multivariable prediction model for individual prognosis or diagnosis
RR	risk ratio		
RSS	risk scoring method		
SBP	systolic blood pressure	VAS	visual analogue scale
		VIF	variance inflation factor

List of Contributors

Douglas G Altman
Professor of Statistics in Medicine
Centre for Statistics in Medicine
Nuffield Department of
Orthopaedics, Rheumatology &
Musculoskeletal Sciences
University of Oxford, UK

Gary S Collins
Professor of Medical Statistics
Centre for Statistics in Medicine
Nuffield Department of
Orthopaedics, Rheumatology &
Musculoskeletal Sciences
University of Oxford, UK

Peter Croft
Emeritus Professor of
Epidemiology
Research Institute for Primary
Care and Health Sciences
Keele University, UK

Michael J Crowther
Lecturer in Biostatistics
Biostatistics Research Group
Department of Health Sciences
University of Leicester, UK

Thomas PA Debray
Assistant Professor
Julius Center for Health Sciences and
Primary Care
UMC Utrecht, Utrecht University
Utrecht, The Netherlands

Kate M Dunn
Professor of Epidemiology
Research Institute for Primary Care
and Health Sciences
Keele University, UK

Nadine E Foster
NIHR Professor of Musculoskeletal
Health in Primary Care
Keele Clinical Trials Unit
and
Research Institute for Primary Care
and Health Sciences
Keele University, UK

Jill A Hayden
Associate Professor
Department of Community Health &
Epidemiology
Faculty of Medicine
Dalhousie University, Canada

Harry Hemingway
Professor of Clinical Epidemiology
UCL Institute of Health Informatics
University College London, UK
and
Director, Health Data Research
UK, London

Aroon Hingorani
Professor of Genetic Epidemiology
Director, UCL Institute of
Cardiovascular Science,
University College London, UK

Kelvin P Jordan
Professor of Biostatistics
Centre for Prognosis Research
Research Institute for Primary Care
    and Health Sciences
Keele University, UK

Karel GM Moons
Professor of Clinical Epidemiology
Julius Center for Health Sciences and
    Primary Care
UMC Utrecht, Utrecht University
Utrecht, The Netherlands

Katherine I Morley
Lecturer
National Addiction Centre
Institute of Psychiatry, Psychology,
    and Neuroscience
King's College London, UK

Pablo Perel
Associate Professor
Co-Director Centre for Global
    Chronic Conditions
London School of Hygiene &
    Tropical Medicine, UK

Richard D Riley
Professor of Biostatistics
Centre for Prognosis Research
Research Institute for Primary Care
    and Health Sciences
Keele University, UK

Mark J Rutherford
Lecturer in Biostatistics
Biostatistics Research Group
Department of Health Sciences
University of Leicester, UK

Willi Sauerbrei
Professor in Medical Biometry
Institute for Medical Biometry and
    Statistics
Faculty of Medicine and
    Medical Center
University of Freiburg, Germany

Mihaela van der Schaar
John Humphrey Plummer Professor
    of Machine Learning, Artificial
    Intelligence and Medicine
University of Cambridge, UK
and
Turing Faculty Fellow
The Alan Turing Institute
British Library, London, UK

Kym IE Snell
Research Fellow in Biostatistics
Centre for Prognosis Research
Research Institute for Primary Care
    and Health Sciences
Keele University, UK

Ewout W Steyerberg
Professor of Medical Decision
    Making
Department of Public Health
Erasmus MC,
Rotterdam, The Netherlands
and
Professor of Clinical Biostatistics and
    Medical Decision Making
Chair, Department of Biomedical
    Data Sciences
Leiden University Medical Center,
Leiden, The Netherlands

Adam Timmis
Professor of Clinical Cardiology
Queen Mary University London UK
and
Consultant Cardiologist
Barts Heart Centre
London UK

Danielle A van der Windt
Professor of Primary Care
  Epidemiology
Centre for Prognosis Research
Research Institute for Primary Care
  and Health Sciences
Keele University, UK

A Note on Language and Terminology

Prognosis study reports are generally inconsistent in their language and terminology. This presents a major hurdle for researchers, reviewers, healthcare professionals, and other stakeholders, whether new to the field or not. The lack of a clear taxonomy across publications of prognosis studies inhibits the integration, standardization, and implementation of prognosis research methods and results.

To address this, the editors have tried to harmonize the text across chapters and use consistent language, especially to represent the four key themes: overall prognosis, prognostic factors, prognostic models, and predictors of treatment effect. In particular, we use the terms 'prognostic factor' and 'prognostic model' rather than broader terms such as 'risk factor' or 'prediction model'.

Also, although we tend to use 'outcomes' to describe the consequences of a disease or health condition (in the context of healthcare) for groups and individuals, and 'endpoints' to describe the corresponding study endpoints, we generally use them interchangeably.

'Treatment' and 'intervention' are also used interchangeably. We do not restrict the term 'treatment' to the use of drugs but extend it to any type of therapeutic or self-management intervention to improve outcomes for individuals.

Prologue

'What's going to happen to me?' asks a patient newly diagnosed with a heart attack.
'Once the team have done some more investigations and discussed the best lines of treatment with you, there is every chance you will soon be back at work and living life as normal,' replies the nurse.

The nurse has given a prognosis. *Prognosis* in healthcare is the forecast of future outcomes in people with a particular health condition—for example the probability of recovery from back pain within one month or of an adverse outcome in pregnant women diagnosed with pre-eclampsia. It is fundamental to the practice of health professionals, as it helps them to inform individuals and their families about likely future outcomes, and to identify, in shared decision making, the best medical treatment options. Prognosis is also crucial for patients more generally as they prepare for the future and make choices about everyday behaviours and activities related to health.

An evidence-based prognosis statement depends on findings from high-quality prognosis research studies. *Prognosis research* is the study of future outcomes among people with a particular health condition. The aims and findings from prognosis research studies are broad. They may summarize the average risk of an outcome (e.g. death) or average value of an outcome (e.g. pain score) among people with the health condition of interest in a particular healthcare setting; identify prognostic factors that are associated with better or worse outcomes; predict an individual's outcome risk or mean outcome value using combinations of factors in a prognostic model; or identify how to tailor treatment decisions for individual patients according to who will and will not benefit.

Prognosis research focuses on outcomes relevant or important to the individual, their family, or healthcare and society as a whole. They include death, recovery, recurrence, disability, treatment side effects, quality of life, and capacity to work. They can be binary (e.g. onset of vision loss in patients with diabetes) or continuous (e.g. blood pressure level in patients after a heart attack). The timing of outcome measurement may range from minutes, hours, days, weeks, and months, to years or even a life-time, and concern one point in time or the course of outcomes over a clinically relevant time period.

0.1 Why is this book relevant?

Prognosis research findings are increasingly sought for each health condition encountered in medical practice and healthcare, in order to improve health outcomes for those affected. This includes people with a disease such as type 2 diabetes (e.g. the ten-year risk of developing loss of sight) or breast cancer (e.g. the risk of dying within five years), but also people with a symptom such as back pain (e.g. the risk of work absence), women who are pregnant (e.g. the first trimester risk of pre-eclampsia in the next six months), or babies born prematurely (e.g. the risk of lung dysfunction).

More people are now living with one or more disease or health-impairing condition than ever before. Because of this, politicians and healthcare leaders across the world have become increasingly interested in what happens to people who are treated or managed in their prevailing healthcare systems. They want to ensure that outcomes such as disease-specific survival or return-to-work rates do not lag behind other countries.

As an example, the UK National Health Service (NHS) Commissioning Board in 2013 proposed to spend 80 billion pounds per year on healthcare. The thread of its spending strategy was outcomes. The plan stated that: 'The Government has set out a clear vision for a modernized NHS driven by a new commissioning system focused relentlessly on improving outcomes for patients ... The purpose of the Board will be to use its budget to secure the best possible outcomes for patients' (1).

Prognosis research contributes to an evidence base that is fundamental to achieving the aims of modern healthcare. Its findings help to drive better outcomes and increased effectiveness and efficiency of healthcare delivery. Prognosis research provides the evidence base for patients to receive treatments best matched to their personal situation.

This book provides a comprehensive introduction to the rationale, concepts, and methods for undertaking prognosis research, addressing all aims and types of such research.

0.2 **Why is this book needed?**

'Prognosis is now virtually extinct as a discrete classroom subject in medical schools.' (2)

Results from high-quality prognosis research should be integral to clinical decision making and healthcare policy, and yet prognosis research is far from straightforward and seldom taught. The concepts, methods, and applications of prognosis research are wide-ranging, borrowing expertise from several scientific fields and disciplines, including biology and medicine, population and clinical epidemiology, biostatistics, health services research, health economics, and data sciences. It uses a wide range of study designs and data sources, including randomized trials, observational studies, routinely collected healthcare data and disease registries, and, more recently, data obtained from diverse sources such as social media. This means that, whilst prognosis research has developed as a research field in its own right, it is often pursued in a piecemeal and disjointed way (2).

A series of four papers in 2013 set out to address the lack of a clear unified framework for prognosis research in a field riddled by inconsistent terminology and muddled concepts. The papers appeared as a joint publication between the *BMJ* and *PLOS Medicine* (3–6), and were written by a group of healthcare professionals, researchers, and journal editors called the 'PROGRESS' (PROGnosis RESearch Strategy) partnership. The series developed a framework of four types of prognosis research, each with a specific rationale for studying prognosis. The papers proposed the use of consistent terminology and clear definitions, and made recommendations about optimal study design and statistical analyses for each type of prognosis research.

This book draws heavily on the PROGRESS framework, but goes well beyond the 2013 series of PROGRESS papers by covering core methods, novel approaches, and emerging opportunities in substantial detail. Practical guidance is given about the whole process of undertaking prognosis research, from identifying the research question to design, analysis, reporting, and impact.

A key motivation for this textbook comes from the scientific defects afflicting much published prognosis research (7, 8). Prognosis studies are often done poorly, with evidence of poor methodological standards, inappropriate statistical analyses, and incomplete and selective reporting, such that 'prognosis research studies too often fall a long way short of the high standards required in other fields … such as genetic epidemiology and randomized controlled trials.…with a concerning gap between the potential and actual impact of prognosis research on health' (3). The consequence is that prognosis research findings are often mistrusted and criticized, frequently fail to provide clear recommendations or change behaviour and decision making in policy and practice, and hence are not achieving the objective of improving outcomes at either individual or population levels.

This textbook has been written to help change this situation by providing a systematic guide to understanding and conducting high-quality prognosis research. Box 0.1 reveals the frustration of systematic reviewers of prognosis research, who

Box 0.1 Sample of quotes from authors attempting systematic reviews and meta-analyses of prognosis studies but confronted with the poor state of reporting and conduct of prevailing prognosis research in their field

Bladder cancer

'After ten years of research, evidence is not sufficient to conclude whether changes in P53 act as markers of outcome in patients with bladder cancer ... That a decade of research on P53 and bladder cancer has not placed us in a better position to draw conclusions relevant to the clinical management of patients is frustrating.' (9)

Acute orthopaedic trauma

'There was limited evidence for the role of any factor as a predictor of return to work ... Due to the lack of factors considered in more than one cohort, the results of this review are inconclusive. The review highlights the need for more prospective studies that are methodologically rigorous, have larger sample sizes and consider a comprehensive range of factors.' (10)

Osteosarcoma

'Ninety-three papers were studied in depth, ...Only 7 papers were of sufficient quality to analyze ... Because of heterogeneity of the studies, pooling results is hardly possible. There is a need for standardization of studies and reporting.' (11)

Anxiety disorders

'Overall, the present state of evidence based on the studies included in this review appears to be very heterogeneous: findings point to the presence of a priori selection bias as well as reporting bias that may render interpretation of results limited ... based on this risk of bias assessment we conclude that the present status quo in search of neurobiological markers of treatment response in anxiety disorders is still on a proof-of-concept level.' (12)

Source: data from Riley RD, et al. (2013) Prognosis research strategy (PROGRESS) 2: prognostic factor research. *PLoS Med* 10, e1001380. Copyright © 2013 PLoS MED.

typically conclude that better quality primary studies are needed, even when multiple studies containing hundreds of participants already exist. Such evidence of poor quality may invoke gloom in the reader. But the problems are solvable, and provide us with a stimulus and drive for the content of this book, which is designed to be a practical guide to doing prognosis research and *doing it well*.

0.3 **What does this book cover?**

This book is a practical text about prognosis research for people who are developing, conducting, interpreting, and appraising prognosis studies, from primary research to systematic reviews and meta-analyses, and beyond.

Our book introduces each of the four prognosis research types in the PROGRESS framework: overall prognosis research, prognostic factor research, prognostic model research, and prognosis research for predicting treatment effects. For each type, we provide explicit guidance on the conduct of prognosis studies—from establishing the research question, and planning the study (including participant selection, data collection, data measurement, and the approach to statistical analysis), to clear reporting of study findings, and ensuring impact and implementation of findings in healthcare.

The book covers the use of primary study data, as well as use of aggregate data in systematic reviews and meta-analysis of primary prognosis studies. It addresses more recent developments in using individual participant data from multiple studies and data from routinely collected electronic health records and disease registries, as well as the contribution of information or data science to prognosis research.

0.4 **What is the structure of this book?**

The book is divided into five parts. Throughout all five parts, we aim to:

- Emphasize the scope of prognosis research and how it can be used to improve healthcare research and health outcomes of the targeted individuals.
- Emphasize good research practice and conduct to stimulate an improvement in the quality and usefulness of published prognosis studies.

The specific aims of each part are as follows.

Part 1 provides a background to prognosis and introduces a framework for prognosis research.

- Chapter 1 outlines the role and history of prognosis in healthcare.
- Chapter 2 introduces the purpose of prognosis research and the PROGRESS framework of four different types of prognosis research, each related to different questions about prognosis.

Part 2 details fundamental statistical principles on which the analysis of most prognosis studies is based.

◆ Chapter 3 introduces the main statistical measures and analysis methods used in prognosis research.

◆ Chapter 4 describes ten important principles to improve the current standards of statistical analysis within prognosis research studies.

Part 3 forms the core of the book, detailing the key concepts, methods, applications, and clinical impact of prognosis research.

◆ Chapters 5–8 address each of the four prognosis research types in the PROGRESS framework, describing for each type the rationale, methods, and reporting of primary studies, alongside a range of examples.

◆ Chapter 9 introduces and describes the methods for design, analysis, and reporting of systematic reviews and meta-analysis of published prognosis studies, to synthesize results and summarize the current evidence base from multiple primary studies in each of the four research types.

Part 4 provides, in Chapters 10–12, detailed clinical examples (back pain, coronary heart disease, and traumatic bleeding) of how the results of prognosis research have informed healthcare. These are designed to showcase the importance and impact of prognosis research for targeted individuals or patients, healthcare professionals, and policymakers.

Part 5 introduces novel and growing areas in the field of prognosis research which take advantage of large existing databases ('Big Data'). The areas covered are:

◆ Chapter 13: Individual participant data (IPD) meta-analysis, a technique which extends traditional systematic reviews of aggregate data from published studies, by obtaining and synthesizing the original individual-level data used by those studies.

◆ Chapter 14: Electronic health records, which routinely record data and outcomes from individuals attending health care.

◆ Chapter 15: Novel statistical analysis approaches (such as multi-state models) that take advantage of opportunities (such as the use of prognostic information at multiple time points) afforded by emerging big datasets.

◆ Chapter 16: Data science and machine learning techniques that provide a new perspective on the potential for big datasets to contribute to prognosis research.

The Appendix provides details of our website (http://www.prognosisresearch. com/) and links to other resources, such as guidelines, checklists, and complementary textbooks notably Steyerberg (13) and Harrell (14).

References

1. **NHS England** (2013) *Everyone Counts. Planning for Patients 2014/15–2018/19.* London: NHS England.

2. **Hemingway H** (2006) Prognosis research: why is Dr Lydgate still waiting? *J Clin Epidemiol* **59**(12), 1229–38.

3. **Hemingway H, Croft P, Perel P, Hayden JA, Abrams K, Timmis A**, et al. (2013) Prognosis research strategy (PROGRESS) 1: a framework for researching clinical outcomes. *BMJ* **346**, e5595.

4. **Riley RD, Hayden JA, Steyerberg EW, Moons KG, Abrams K, Kyzas PA**, et al. (2013) Prognosis research strategy (PROGRESS) 2: prognostic factor research. *PLoS Med* **10**(2), e1001380.

5. **Steyerberg EW, Moons KG, van der Windt DA, Hayden JA, Perel P, Schroter S**, et al. (2013) Prognosis research strategy (PROGRESS) 3: prognostic model research. *PLoS Med* **10**(2), e1001381.

6. **Hingorani AD, Windt DA, Riley RD, Abrams K, Moons KG, Steyerberg EW**, et al. (2013) Prognosis research strategy (PROGRESS) 4: stratified medicine research. *BMJ* **346**, e5793.

7. **Collins GS, Reitsma JB, Altman DG**, and **Moons KG** (2015) Transparent Reporting of a multivariable prediction model for Individual Prognosis Or Diagnosis (TRIPOD). *Ann Intern Med* **162**(10), 735–6.

8. **Moons KG, Altman DG, Reitsma JB, Ioannidis JP, Macaskill P, Steyerberg EW**, et al. (2015) Transparent Reporting of a multivariable prediction model for Individual Prognosis Or Diagnosis (TRIPOD): explanation and elaboration. *Ann Intern Med* **162**(1):W1–73.

9. **Malats N, Bustos A, Nascimento CM, Fernandez F, Rivas M, Puente D**, et al. (2005). P53 as a prognostic marker for bladder cancer: a meta-analysis and review. *Lancet Oncol* **6**, 678–86.

10. **Clay FJ, Newstead SV**, and **McClure RJ** (2010) A systematic review of early prognostic factors for return to work following acute orthopaedic trauma. *Injury* **41**, 787–803.

11. **Bramer JA, van Linge JH, Grimer, RJ**, and **Scholten RJ** (2009) Prognostic factors in localized extremity osteosarcoma: a systematic review. *Eur J Surg Oncol* **35**, 1030–6.

12. **Lueken U, Zierhut KC, Hahn T, Straube B, Kircher T, Reif A**, et al. (2016) Neurobiological markers predicting treatment response in anxiety disorders: A systematic review and implications for clinical application. *Neurosci Biobehav Rev* **66**, 143–62.

13. **Steyerberg EW** (2009) *Clinical Prediction Models: a Practical Approach to Development, Validation, and Updating.* New York: Springer.

14. **Harrell FE**, Jr. (2015) *Regression Modeling Strategies: with Applications to Linear Models, Logistic and Ordinal Regression, and Survival Analysis* (second edition). New York: Springer.

Part 1

Introduction to prognosis and prognosis research

Chapter 1

Prognosis in healthcare

Peter Croft, Richard D Riley,
Danielle A van der Windt,
and Karel GM Moons

The word prognosis stems from the Greek word πρόγνωση, meaning fore-knowing, foreseeing, foretelling, or predicting. This chapter explores the role and history of prognosis in healthcare.

1.1 Introduction

In healthcare, prognosis is the forecast of future outcomes in people with a particular disease or health condition. This is expressed as the expected average value of an outcome (e.g. pain score at six months), or the risk of developing a particular outcome (such as death by a particular time point). It may concern outcomes at a single time point in the future (e.g. recovery or death) or their course over a period of time (e.g. average serum cholesterol level over six months after starting cholesterol-lowering treatment). Together with diagnosis of the underlying disease or condition, and treatment and care of the individual, prognosis forms the 'classical triad' and basis of healthcare practice.

Traditionally, prognosis has been part of a doctor's area of expertise in their clinical or medical practice and specifically in their consultations with patients. However, the task of prognosis forms part of the daily work of many other healthcare professionals, and prognosis can also be assessed by individuals themselves. So we have adopted 'healthcare' in this book as a generic term to cover all these settings and possibilities, and not only consider sick or symptomatic individuals as relevant populations for prognosis, but also healthy individuals with a certain health condition such as being pregnant or an asymptomatic health marker such as raised blood pressure.

Prognosis in healthcare is addressed in the context of current medical care. This care does not simply include drugs, but may range from non-pharmacological interventions, such as physiotherapy or counselling, to the ways in which healthcare is delivered and to processes of care. In this book, unless otherwise specified, we use the word 'treatment' or 'intervention' as generic terms to cover all forms of healthcare.

From taking out life insurance, to choices about what to eat, all members of the public may be interested in what their future health is likely to be. In this sense 'everyone has a prognosis', and public health, for example, is concerned with primary prevention population policies that reduce the risk of future onset of disease. However we are adopting in this textbook the arbitrary but useful definition of prognosis as restricted to the forecasting of outcomes in people who have a particular health-related condition. Here, the role of prognosis is to inform and guide healthcare professionals and policymakers, individuals, and patients and their families, in shared decision making to improve their health-related outcomes.

1.2 **Prognosis in medical practice**

A mother brings her young son, David, to the doctor (a general practitioner or 'GP'). David has a fever and is unwell, and his mother is worried. Consider three different scenarios:

1. The doctor diagnoses a throat infection likely to be caused by a common virus. She reassures mother and son, prescribing no treatment beyond fluids and rest.

2. The doctor suspects a chest infection which could be caused by a pneumonia germ (the pneumonia bacterium), and arranges urgent referral to hospital. The diagnosis is confirmed by X-ray and David is treated with an antibiotic which precisely targets the causative germ.

3. The doctor is unsure what is wrong with David but is concerned about her young patient's illness and refers him to a hospital specialist. Investigations reveal a form of cancer which affects the lymph glands of young people, called 'Hodgkin's lymphoma'. David is admitted to hospital for the most up-to-date treatment and monitoring programme.

Here we have a sick child with a common symptom but three very different diagnoses, each with their particular treatment. The three alternative scenarios are all examples of modern scientific medicine, with its emphasis on explanations based on the understanding of disease (diagnosis) and proven management or treatment strategies targeted at the underlying pathology (no specific treatment for a mild viral infection; an antibiotic known to be active in killing the bacteria which cause pneumonia; and treatments with drugs and radiation which extensive trials have shown to be capable of destroying the particular type of cancer cells in Hodgkin's disease). These examples represent the ideal logic of medical science in action. Diagnose what is wrong with the sick person and deliver appropriate management.

What is missing from these pictures of clinical practice is an account (or a prediction) of *what might happen to the patient in the future, with and without treatment*. In each of the three different scenarios, this will have been uppermost in the minds of both mother and doctor at the point when the diagnosis was made.

1. A diagnosis of viral sore throat will usually be accompanied by advice from the GP that nothing further needs to be done apart from the mother's care. The implication is that this viral infection will follow a usual pattern and run its course without causing life-threatening illness. The prognosis for David is that all will be well and he will very likely soon be better.

2. A diagnosis of chest infection caused by the pneumonia bacterium carries a more serious implication—if nothing is done, David may become sicker, and may even die. But the doctor can wrap these concerns within the reassurance that there is a treatment available which is highly likely to sort things out. If David gets the appropriate antibiotic soon, his prognosis is that he will recover because the drug can destroy the germ that causes pneumonia before it has a chance to cause serious harm.

3. Hodgkin's lymphoma also has a serious implication. This is a form of cancer which, left untreated, has a high mortality rate. However, once again, the doctor can be upbeat in explaining to David and his mother the availability of increasingly effective combinations of treatment to control and ultimately cure many patients with this disease, despite the tough experience that such treatment may entail. If he is moved to specialist care in hospital for treatment and monitoring, the prognosis for David is that he has a high chance of recovery and cure, and a successful outcome. But David and his parents will also want to know about other potential outcomes contingent on receiving treatment, such as the likelihood of side effects and their severity, or the probability of the cancer returning in the future, in order to help plan and manage expectations.

Understanding and predicting what might happen to a sick person in the future, ideally when treated and not treated, is a central element of prognosis in healthcare. Healthcare professionals have always understood that prognosis is a core part of the information that patients seek. Crucial to the mother in the examples above is understanding the likely prognosis linked to each possible situation or scenario—the risk of outcomes, including potential harm from treatment, or, more positively, the probability of recovery. In the first example she needs reassurance about the natural history of viral sore throat; in the other two scenarios, she wants the probability of recovery if appropriate treatment for the underlying diagnosis is given, and to understand the balance between potential benefits and harms from available treatments.

In the 'triad' of healthcare practice, modern diagnosis and effective treatments aim to optimize patient prognosis and improve outcomes, but the important skills of prognosis in healthcare—understanding, explaining, and forecasting future outcomes (good and bad) of sick individuals—long pre-dated the birth of scientific medicine.

1.3 A brief history of prognosis

1.3.1 Early times: prognosis dominates

The first written records of medical care in the Middle East, identified on clay tablets from the seventh century BC, already referred to the three clinical skills: 'diagnoses, prognostications, and remedies and their ingredients' (1).

From the time of Hippocrates in Greece in the fifth century BC, the medical profession in Asia and Europe focused on disease and healing as part of the natural order of things. This approach dominated medical care for the next thousand years, until a science of the human body and its ailments emerged. Porter, a medical historian, writes about this period:

> 'In the absence of decisive anatomical and physiological expertise, and without a powerful arsenal of cures and surgical skills, the ability ... to make prognoses was highly valued, and an intimate physician-patient relationship was fostered ... Success came from soothing lesser ailments and assisting people to cope with chronic conditions.' (1)

Although diagnoses were always made, they could only relate to existing prescientific knowledge about disease mechanisms and causation, and to the 'do-no-harm' approach of letting nature do its work. So the technique prized above all was prognosis or prediction, with its emphasis on observation of the sick person and on the previous experience of the physician or healthcare professional, allied to a humane and caring 'bedside manner'.

Prognosis during this pre-scientific era concerned the likely natural course of the individual with an illness, and drew on the physician's cumulative observations of previous patients with similar illness (2). Prognosis was seen as a characteristic of sick people, linked to ideas and observations about their 'constitution', and not as a characteristic of particular diseases (3). Here is Hippocrates (quoted in Porter (1)): 'It appears to me a most excellent thing for the physician to cultivate prognosis; for by foreseeing and foretelling, in the presence of the sick ... he will be the more readily believed to be acquainted with the circumstances of the sick; so that men will have confidence to entrust themselves to such a physician.'

Galen, writing in the second century AD, continued this approach, even authoring a textbook entitled 'Prognosis'. Porter (1) summarized Galen's message: 'Patient trust was essential in the healing process. It could be won by a punctilious bedside manner, by meticulous explanation, and by mastery of prognosis, an art demanding experience, observation, and logic.'

Galen's prognosis and the Hippocratic system of medicine reflected the idea of doctors providing ethical and humane care for patients, linked to a judgement of what was likely to happen in a world which did not have modern diagnostics and treatments. The effectiveness of this approach lay in its capacity to provide care which might help and promote recovery in people whose disease was self-limiting, and support patients to live with long-term but non-fatal conditions.

This idea was an important feature of medical care into the scientific era. For more than a thousand years after Galen, disease explanations and therapeutics advanced little, but prognosis remained central to medical practice and healthcare as a whole.

1.3.2 The rise of diagnosis and the decline of prognosis

As the structure and function of living organisms was unravelled from the seventeenth century on, concrete mechanisms of disease were revealed. Yet until the twentieth century, most of this understanding was not matched by effective therapies, and many doctors continued to advocate the Hippocratic ideal of letting nature do its work. In this context, prognosis obviously remained an important 'skill'. Doctors continued to predict the probable future outcomes—good or bad—of the sick patient, based on their experience taken from previous similar types of patients, and on this their prognostic ability and indeed their whole medical reputation often rested (1).

By the mid-nineteenth century, however, diagnosis of a specific pathological abnormality underlying each patient's illness was seen as the supreme skill of the physician. It was driven by new sciences, and a new knowledge and understanding of the human body, and by the availability of new diagnostic techniques, such as stethoscope auscultation, microscopy, and, by the end of the century, imaging techniques to detect underlying disease. Yet, in the continuing absence of treatments, there was little evidence that making a diagnosis had any effect on the subsequent course and outcome of the individual with the disease. Although prognosis was retreating in importance as a clinical skill, patients were yet to benefit from the diagnostic revolution. Diagnosis for diagnosis' sake ruled the roost.

Prognosis was, unfortunately, no longer perceived as a characteristic of the patient but as a characteristic of the disease (3), with less attention paid to patient-specific factors such as psychological distress, nutritional status, or educational status, which might influence the course and outcome of a person's illness. Prognosis became seen as the typical course of a disease, independent of any particular individual, and was discussed in terms of disease complications and treatment side-effects rather than the likely outcome of patients who had the disease.

By 1912, Chauffard, an eminent French physician, wrote: 'What physician, failing an accurate diagnosis, could venture a prognosis or prescribe a treatment?' (2). An American clinician, Lewis Thomas, recalled his young days on hospital wards in the 1930s when talk of treatment was restricted to surgery (4), stating:

> 'Our task for the future was to be diagnoses and explanations. Explanation was the real business of medicine. What the ill patient and his family wanted most was to know the name of the illness, and therefore if possible what had caused it.'

But still Thomas considered that, 'Most important of all was how the disease was likely to turn out.'

So prognosis was still important but was considered a characteristic of a particular disease, rather than of intrinsic value to particular individuals with the disease. This focus was intensified by the rise of the specialist clinician, the shift to hospitals, and finally the arrival of treatments to guarantee good prognoses if diagnoses were accurate. Yet prognosis itself still did not have a scientific evidence base. The modern science of diagnosis and treatment advanced, but prognosis was further relegated and disappeared from medical textbooks (3).

1.3.3 The twentieth century: prognosis continues in real-life healthcare

In the twentieth century, prognostic statements still drew heavily on the physician's experience. A UK hospital physician, Hutchison, writing in 1928 (5), and showing an early appreciation of the principles of clinical epidemiology, acknowledged that: 'GPs were better prognosticators than hospital doctors because they see lots of cases and because specialists do not have access to observe what happens to their patients in the future.'

Although Hutchison considers diagnosis the most important clinical activity, he highlights the importance of patient characteristics such as age and grip strength when judging the likelihood of surviving acute infection, and of patient habits and surroundings for successful living with chronic disease. Although he believes the major errors of prognostication arise from diagnostic error, he emphasizes they also occur when the doctor fails to notice general things about the patient (such as mood and diet) and concentrates too much on the specifics of underlying disease. Above all he spots that individual variation in outcomes challenges the assumption that diagnosis and treatment provide a standard ready-made prognosis:

> ' ... *A knowledge of the statistical rate of recovery is only of limited value in individual prognosis. If, for example, a patient is told that the mortality rate of his disease is 30 per cent, he naturally wants to know whether he is likely to be one of the unfortunate 30. It does, however, give a rough individuation of the odds against which he has to fight.*' (5)

This viewpoint sets the scene for this book and the renewed importance of prognosis in modern healthcare. High-quality prognosis research can provide the sort of objective evidence that Hutchison was looking for, about what actually happens in the future to individuals with particular diseases or health conditions, in order to inform and support prognostic estimates by healthcare professionals. These estimates should take into account not only the underlying diagnosis and available effective treatment, but also other characteristics of the individual and of their environment.

1.4 Prognosis and prognosis research in twenty-first century healthcare

In this era, all of us—including patients and public, politicians and policy-makers, healthcare and public health professionals, scientists and health researchers—want the outcomes of current healthcare to be the best achievable. Attention has turned to prognosis again to help meet this demand.

A major driver of the revived importance of prognosis has been *the new biomedical sciences*—molecular biology and the various 'omics' (e.g. genomics, proteomics, metabolomics) which study whole systems (of, for example, genes, proteins, metabolic processes) in the human body. These sciences have focused on the possibility of characterizing, in terms of structure and function at cellular level, why some individuals with particular diseases have a better prognosis than others, and who will have a different prognosis or response when given a particular treatment. This development has thrown the characterization and study of prognosis into new prominence and is a major contributor to its revival.

For example Raskin et al. pointed to genetic characteristics as a potential gap in the information to explain how melanomas (malignant tumours of melanocytes—the cells that give skin its colour) progress over time (6). They identified a genetic biomarker that was more commonly expressed in melanoma cells than in normal melanocytes and which was also associated with the outcome of decreased length of survival in patients with the tumour, that is, with patient prognosis. They concluded that this marker may be useful in practice to identify high-risk patients for targeting more aggressive treatment or as a target for new drugs specifically tailored to suppress this biomarker or its effects on the cancer cell.

Another driver of the importance of prognosis in healthcare in the twenty-first century is the *rapidly expanding amount of information* about people with diseases or health conditions—new measurements, new tests, detailed characteristics, computerized medical and personal data—all of which may be relevant to outcomes. The challenge is to determine if and how to use such information to predict future outcomes and guide treatment choices.

For example, a diagnosis is a statement about the likely pathological cause or classification of a person's current health condition. If people with the same diagnosis vary in their risk for future outcomes (i.e. they have different prognoses), such variability may lead to a revision of diagnostic labels. One case study that we use throughout this book is heart attack or, to give it the medical diagnostic pathological term, myocardial infarction (literally 'death of heart muscle cells'). When new investigations of heart muscle damage were introduced, studies revealed that the prognosis of heart attack patients, measured as twenty-eight-day mortality, varied substantially according to the results of the new tests. This led to a re-definition of the diagnostic criteria for myocardial infarction. Individuals not diagnosed before were now included because of those tests and their linked and contrasting prognoses. This is an example of how the usefulness of diagnostic classification in medical practice is driven by what it says about patient prognosis and patient management.

A contrasting example comes from a randomized trial that recruited patients presenting in primary care with low back pain. Jarvik and colleagues in the US compared patients randomized to either get X-rays or to get MRI imaging as the spinal investigation of choice (7). The people getting MRI scans had more abnormalities diagnosed and more surgical procedures performed to tackle those abnormalities. However, one year later there was no difference between the groups with respect to outcomes—back pain and disability improved to exactly the same degree in both arms of the trial. This is an example of *overdiagnosis*—'pathologies' were identified in the spine that had no impact on patient outcome. In the current medical technology era, where new tests regularly become available and are increasingly used for patients in the community as well as in primary care, estimating prognosis has become an increasingly relevant part of establishing whether the new investigations (and treatments linked to them) have any influence on the natural course of events—or whether this is overdiagnosis, leading to overtreatment that is costly, useless, or even harmful (8, 9).

The wealth of information related to health also serves to drive interest in the *wide range of characteristics that might influence prognosis* and be used to refine estimates of prognosis in the individual. This includes social, psychological, and environmental information, as well as novel biological data and, important not to forget, basic information such as age and sex. Prognosis for patients with tuberculosis (TB) is now generally good, with successful outcomes achieved by diagnosis of the disease and effective treatment, including selection of drug treatments and their mode of delivery in order to avoid or deal with antibiotic resistance. However, poorer people in socio-economically deprived areas are both more likely to get TB in the first place and more likely to have drug resistance and not to complete treatment once they have been diagnosed. Poverty identifies a group in need of targeted healthcare for achieving optimal drug delivery to deliver successful outcomes (10).

The core of healthcare is still the consultation with the individual patient and the shared decision making that takes place there. It is here that prognosis remains important to clinical, medical, and healthcare practice. Modern prognosis research aims to understand and describe the variability in patient outcomes, and what characteristics are associated with it, in order to improve patient prognosis. The ambition of prognosis research is to supply information and tools (such as *prognostic models*) to help *predict an individual's outcome* as accurately as possible given the profile of that individual; and to use that information to support the healthcare professional and patient in making shared decisions about the best strategy for lifestyle, treatment, and other care. This aspect of prognosis underpins the twenty-first century ideas of *stratified care* and *personalized* (or *precision*) *medicine*. If an individual's outcome risk or likely outcome value can be reliably predicted, in combination with their predicted response to treatment, then healthcare can be selected that is tailored to the individual, to improve outcomes.

For example, if we know that men with a particular type of prostate cancer, as characterized by biological characteristics of the tumour cell, will live as long as men without prostate cancer, and that treating them with surgery carries risks to their future health, such men can be managed differently to men with more severe types of prostate cancer. Or, if a new genetic marker is discovered that identifies people with diabetes who are at higher risk of developing diabetic eye disease, then such prognostic information can help target care and promote development and testing of new treatments for this subgroup. These are all examples of stratified care or personalized medicine, driven by prognosis research and information. We return to these topics throughout this book.

Finally politicians, public health professionals, and healthcare leaders want to understand and know *whether population-level prognosis has improved or not* in relation to changes in case finding, diagnosis, screening, treatment, or healthcare delivery and policy. This is needed in order to evaluate the impact

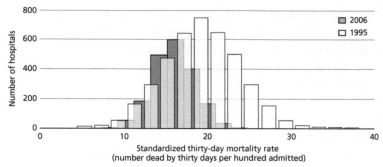

Figure 1.1 Distribution of the mortality rates across hospitals in the USA for patients admitted after heart attack, 1995 compared with 2006.

Source: reproduced with permission from Hemingway, H., et al. Prognosis research strategy (PROGRESS) 1: A framework for researching clinical outcomes. *BMJ*. 2013;346:e5595. Copyright © 2013 BMJ Publishing Group Ltd

of those changes and their cost-effectiveness as a measure of the efficiency of healthcare. For example, Figure 1.1 shows the prognosis for patients admitted to hospitals in the US in 1995 and 2006 by hospital. The average prognosis across all hospitals, measured here by the thirty-day cumulative mortality, has improved during this period, revealing the positive impact that healthcare changes during that ten-year period, such as new treatments or policies and de-livery of care, may have had on prognosis.

1.5 **Summary**

In summary, prognosis research has re-emerged at the forefront of healthcare, and this brings excitement and opportunities, but also challenges and research demands. The remainder of this book aims to inform and support people designing and undertaking prognosis research to ensure it has high standards and produces results that are fit for purpose and ultimately have a positive im-pact on health outcomes.

References

1. **Porter R** (1999) *The Greatest Benefit to Mankind: A Medical History of Humanity From Antiquity to the Present*. London: Fontana Press. pp. xxi, 833, plate 24.
2. **Chauffard A** (1913) Medical prognosis: its methods, its evolution, its limitations. *Br Med J* 2, 286–90.
3. **Christakis NA** (1997) The ellipsis of prognosis in modern medical thought. *Soc Sci Med* **44**(3), 301–15.
4. **Thomas L** (1995) *The Youngest Science: Notes of a Medicine-Watcher*. New York: Penguin Books.

5. **Hutchison R** (1928) *Some Principles of Diagnosis, Prognosis, and Treatment. A Trilogy.* Bristol, UK: John Wright and Sons Ltd.

6. **Raskin L, Fullen DR, Giordano TJ, Thomas DG, Frohm ML, Cha KB,** et al. (2013) Transcriptome profiling identifies HMGA2 as a biomarker of melanoma progression and prognosis. *J Invest Dermatol* **133**(11), 2585–92.

7. **Jarvik JG, Hollingworth W, Martin B, Emerson SS, Gray DT, Overman S,** et al. (2003) Rapid magnetic resonance imaging vs radiographs for patients with low back pain: a randomized controlled trial. *JAMA* **289**(21), 2810–8.

8. **Croft P, Altman DG, Deeks JJ, Dunn KM, Hay AD, Hemingway H,** et al. (2015) The science of clinical practice: disease diagnosis or patient prognosis? Evidence about 'what is likely to happen' should shape clinical practice. *BMC Med* **13**, 20.

9. **de Groot JA, Naaktgeboren CA, Reitsma JB,** and **Moons KG** (2017) Methodologic approaches to evaluating new highly sensitive diagnostic tests: avoiding overdiagnosis. *CMAJ* **189**, E64–8.

10. **Farmer P** (1997) Social scientists and the new tuberculosis. *Soc Sci Med* **44**(3), 347–58.

Chapter 2

A framework for prognosis research

Peter Croft, Richard D Riley,
Danielle A van der Windt, Karel GM Moons,
and Harry Hemingway

2.1 Introduction

Prognosis research aims to summarize, explain, and predict outcomes in clinically relevant populations and individuals, in order to provide prognostic information to support the treatment, counselling, and decision making used in
healthcare. The basic structure and timeline of prognosis research studies is
shown in Figure 2.1. The focus is on taking a representative sample of people
with a particular disease or health condition (the 'startpoint'), measuring characteristics of these individuals at baseline (potential 'prognostic factors'), and
then assessing the occurrence of specified outcomes or outcome values (the
'endpoints') over time.

Although thousands of studies addressing prognosis questions are published each year in the medical literature, the field has lacked a unified taxonomy or a clear distinction between different aspects or types of prognosis
research in healthcare (1). To address this, in 2013 the PROGnosis RESearch
Strategy (PROGRESS) partnership proposed a framework of four distinct but
interrelated types of prognosis research (2–5), each with a specific rationale
for studying prognosis. This overarching framework motivates the structure
and content of the subsequent parts of this book, including separate chapters for each type within Part 3. Here we provide an initial overview of the
framework.

The four types of prognosis research in the PROGRESS framework are shown
in Box 2.1. The framework begins with studies that observe and measure actual outcomes in samples of people with a particular disease or health condition of interest, providing overall summaries such as average outcome values
(e.g. 'six-month mean disability score') or outcome risks (e.g. 'percentage who

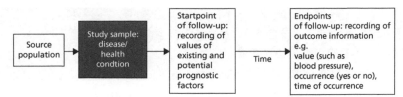

Figure 2.1 Outline structure of a typical prognosis research study.
Source: Reproduced courtesy of Danielle van der Windt.

remain off work at six months') for such people (type I). This is followed by the identification of prognostic factors that are associated with or explain the variation in outcomes across individuals (type II). Type III focuses on the combination of prognostic factors to predict outcomes in individual patients using so-called prognostic models. Type IV is concerned with finding factors that predict treatment effect in groups of similar individuals. An example of each of these types is given in Box 2.2.

Box 2.1 The PROGRESS framework for prognosis research

Among people with a given disease or health condition, four types of research investigate the following questions:

Type I: overall prognosis: what is the average outcome value, or outcome risk, in a population of interest in the context of the nature and quality of current care?

Type II: prognostic factors: which characteristics are associated with changes in the average outcome value, or outcome risk, across individuals?

Type III: prognostic models: how can we develop, validate, and evaluate the impact of models incorporating multiple prognostic factors, to predict an individual's outcome value or to estimate their outcome risk?

Type IV: predictors of treatment effect: which characteristics predict whether an individual responds to a particular treatment or not?

Source: reproduced courtesy of the authors.

Box 2.2 Example about the prognosis of patients with breast cancer for each of the four types of prognosis research

Type I: it is estimated that five out of six women diagnosed with breast cancer in the UK in 2017 will be alive in 2022.

Type II: among women diagnosed with breast cancer in the US, social isolation was associated with higher risks of future recurrence (hazard ratio (HR) 1.43, 95% confidence interval 1.15–1.77) (6), and is thus a potential prognostic factor for recurrence.

Type III: PREDICT, an online tool that clinicians can complete for an individual patient, utilizes multiple factors ('predictors') in combination (such as age, how the tumour was diagnosed, tumour pathology, and genetic receptor status) to estimate a woman's five-year survival probability after breast cancer surgery. The tool is thus a prognostic model, and predicted risks from the model show good performance when compared against observed outcomes (7).

Type IV: women with early breast cancer that was oestrogen receptor (ER) positive (i.e. they have cancer cells which attract the cancer-promoting female hormone oestrogen circulating naturally in the bloodstream) had reduced ten-year recurrence and breast cancer mortality rates if treated with an oestrogen-blocking drug (tamoxifen), whilst in women with ER-negative cancers, tamoxifen had little or no effect on recurrence or mortality. ER status is thus a predictor of tamoxifen effect (8).

Source: Reproduced courtesy of the authors.

2.2 Overall prognosis research (PROGRESS framework type I)

Type I prognosis research studies aim to provide an overall estimate of the likely course or outcome (the 'endpoints') among a group of individuals with a particular disease or health condition (the 'startpoint'), in the context of the nature and quality of healthcare available at the time and place of study. For example, in patients diagnosed with a new episode of non-specific back pain in consultation with a primary care practitioner and managed in the community, overall prognosis might be expressed in terms of the mean pain score six months after consultation; in patients diagnosed with breast cancer in a district general

---

Box 2.3 Prognosis of patients with type 1 diabetes mellitus in Wisconsin state, US

Setting: South Wisconsin.

Source population: all persons receiving primary care in South Wisconsin 1980.

Sampling frame: primary care registers.

Design: prospective cohort study 1980–2005.

Startpoint: all persons with an existing diagnosis of type 1 diabetes in 1980 (the 'baseline year').

Endpoint: severe kidney disease defined as self-reported kidney transplant or dialysis during twenty-five-year follow-up from 1980.

Overall prognosis: the proportion of patients with severe kidney disease by twenty-five years after 'baseline year' was 14.2% (95% CI, 11.9-16.5).

Source: data from Lecaire TJ, (2014) Risk for end-stage renal disease over 25 years in the population-based WESDR cohort. *Diabetes Care* 37, 381–8. Copyright © 2014 American Diabetes Association.

---

hospital it could be the proportion of patients alive at one year after the start of a particular treatment strategy.

The population recruited or identified for overall prognosis studies represents people who have the disease or health condition (i.e. the startpoint) of interest. The endpoint or endpoints of interest represent the future health outcome or outcomes of this population. See the example in Box 2.3.

Estimates of overall prognosis provide information about what is likely to happen in the future to a population of individuals with a particular disease or health condition, in order to help and support decision making by healthcare professionals, individuals, patients, insurers, and healthcare planners. This extends to assessments of new technologies in healthcare, new disease markers, new tests to diagnose disease, and new treatments, which need studies that measure overall outcomes, beneficial and hazardous, in people who are exposed to such innovations.

Overall prognosis research also provides benchmarks for healthcare funders and policymakers in evaluating the effectiveness of healthcare, for example to answer questions about whether outcomes for people with a particular startpoint have improved over time or whether outcomes are better in one population than another. Figure 2.2 shows the five-year survival for women diagnosed with breast cancer in different European countries during a particular time period

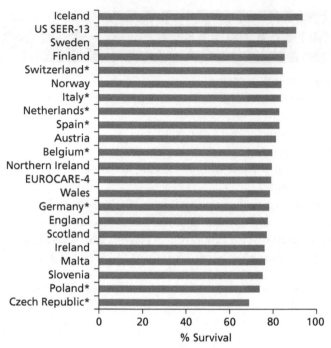

Figure 2.2 Overall prognosis research showing between-country variations in age-adjusted five-year survival among women with breast cancer.

Source: reproduced with permission from Verdecchia, A., et al. Recent cancer survival in Europe: a 2000–02 period analysis of EUROCARE-4 data. *The Lancet Oncology*. 8(9), 784-96. Copyright © 2007 Elsevier

(2000–2002) and receiving care in those countries (9). Variations might reflect differences in national policies on screening for breast cancer or in the quality or content of healthcare for women diagnosed with breast cancer.

2.3 **Prognostic factor research (PROGRESS framework type II)**

Type II prognosis research studies investigate, in groups of individuals with a specified startpoint, what characteristics are associated with changes in average outcome values or differences in outcome risk across these individuals. We call such characteristics prognostic factors. Any characteristic or measurement available at the defined startpoint is a potential prognostic factor. An example is shown in Box 2.4.

A popular approach is to screen large banks of data for evidence of associations between potential prognostic factors and outcomes. A typical example

Box 2.4 Prognosis of patients admitted to hospital with a suspected heart attack: the ECG pattern as a prognostic factor

Setting: thirteen countries in North America, Europe, Australia, and New Zealand.

Source population: all patients admitted to the participating hospitals.

Sampling frame: 373 hospitals 1993–4.

Design: prospective cohort study using data from a randomized trial.

Startpoint: 12,142 patients admitted with symptoms of a heart attack and evidence of myocardial ischaemia (restricted blood supply to the heart muscle) on the electrocardiogram.

Endpoint: death or further heart attack in first thirty days of follow-up.

Prognostic factor: pattern of waves (specifically ST segment and T wave) on the electrocardiogram measured at baseline.

Prognostic factor results: after adjusting for other factors associated with an increased risk of endpoint, the odds of thirty-day death or further heart attack were 1.62 (95% CI, 1.32–1.98) times higher for those with ST-segment depression compared with those who had T-wave inversion only. This suggests that pattern of waves is a prognostic factor, and adds prognostic value over and above other prognostic factors (a so-called independently contributing prognostic factor).

Source: data from Savonitto S, et al. (1999) Prognostic value of the admission electrocardiogram in acute coronary syndromes. *JAMA* 281, 707–13. Copyright © 1999 American Medical Association.

is provided in Figure 2.3 from a genome-wide screening study for genetic biomarkers linked with survival in women with oestrogen-receptor negative breast cancer (10).

Different values (or categories) of a prognostic factor are associated with a different expected outcome value, as measured by an absolute value (for continuous outcomes like blood pressure), or a different outcome risk or probability (for binary and time-to-event outcomes like death). Thus, prognostic factors break down a population's overall (or average) prognosis and explain variation in outcomes across individuals. This information can be used to create new subgroups of people with a particular health condition defined by the prognostic factor, to identify targets for developing new treatments based on modifying the factor, and to enhance the development of prognostic models in type III studies.

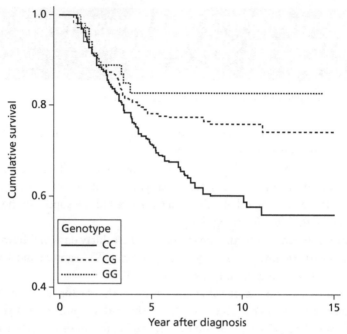

Figure 2.3 Breast cancer survival curves from a genome wide association study which was used to identify and replicate a new prognostic factor, a germline single nucleotide polymorphism in *OCA2* (C=cytosine, G=guanine).
Source: reproduced with permission from Azzato, E.M., et al. Association Between a Germline OCA2 Polymorphism at Chromosome 15q13.1 and Estrogen Receptor–Negative Breast Cancer Survival. *Journal of the National Cancer Institute*. 102(9), 650-62. Copyright © 2010 OUP

2.4 **Prognostic model research (PROGRESS framework type III)**

Type III prognosis research moves away from examining single prognostic factors to examining multiple prognostic factors ('predictors') in combination—a so-called prognostic model. These models are needed to predict future outcome values or estimate outcome risk in an individual, conditional on their own values for predictors included in the model at the startpoint of interest.

Prognostic model research incorporates studies that develop a new model (so-called model development); studies that test the predictive performance of a previously developed prognostic model in new individuals or settings (so-called external model validation), and update or tailor the model to the new setting if needed; and studies that examine the impact on health-related outcomes of using a prognostic model in daily healthcare, as compared to not using such a model. Box 2.5 is an example from the UK of one of the studies that established a prognostic model (the 'PREDICT' model) for clinicians and patients to estimate probability of future survival in women who have had surgery for early invasive breast cancer (11).

Figure 2.4 shows one of the versions of the PREDICT model now available on public websites (7) for patients and clinicians to complete, together with fictional data entered as an illustration. The model generates a risk score for five and ten-year survival.

Box 2.5 Predicting outcome in UK women after surgery for invasive breast cancer: development and validation of a prognostic model

Setting: (1) for development of model: the East Anglian region of England; (2) for external validation of model: the West Midlands region of England.

Source population: women registered with breast cancer

Sampling frame: (1) the East Anglian and (2) the West Midlands cancer registration databases.

Design: prospective cohort study using registry data linked to death certification records.

Startpoint: (1) 5694 women and (2) 5468 women, who had surgery for invasive breast cancer from 1999–2003.

Endpoint: overall survival eight years after surgery.

Multivariable analysis: a model was produced using seven prognostic factors: three general (age, whether cancer detected at screening or not, and use of chemotherapy or endocrine therapy or both), plus four ascertained at or following surgery (tumour size, tumour spread to lymph nodes, tumour severity graded from microscopic examination of tissue, and presence of oestrogen receptors (ER status) in tumour tissue).

Results: the developed prognostic model can be used to predict the probability of eight-year survival in women after surgery for invasive breast cancer. The model showed good calibration (close agreement between observed and predicted risks) and promising discrimination (separation in predicted risks between those with and without the outcome) in both development and external validation cohorts.

Source: data from Wishart GC (2010) PREDICT: a new UK prognostic model that predicts survival following surgery for invasive breast cancer. *Breast Cancer Research and Treatment* 12(1), R1. Copyright © 2010 Springer Nature.

PREDICT Tool Version 2.0: Breast Cancer Overall Survival; Input

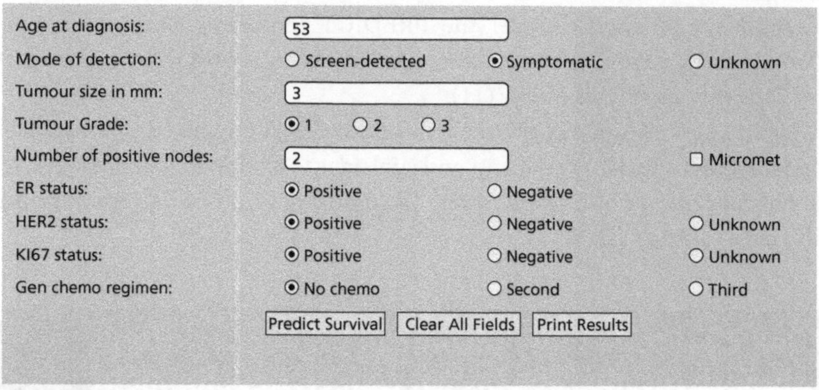

Age at diagnosis:	53		
Mode of detection:	○ Screen-detected	◉ Symptomatic	○ Unknown
Tumour size in mm:	3		
Tumour Grade:	◉ 1 ○ 2 ○ 3		
Number of positive nodes:	2		☐ Micromet
ER status:	◉ Positive	○ Negative	
HER2 status:	◉ Positive	○ Negative	○ Unknown
KI67 status:	◉ Positive	○ Negative	○ Unknown
Gen chemo regimen:	◉ No chemo	○ Second	○ Third

Predict Survival | Clear All Fields | Print Results

PREDICT Tool Version 2.0: Breast Cancer Overall Survival; Results
Five-year survival
97 out of 100 women are alive at 5 years with no adjuvant therapy after surgery
An extra 0 out of 100 women treated are alive because of hormone therapy
Ten-year survival
91 out of 100 women are alive at 10 years with no adjuvant therapy after surgery
An extra 1 out of 100 women treated are alive because of hormone therapy

Figure 2.4 Prognostic model for women with early breast cancer (Public Health England).
Source: adapted with permission from the University of Cambridge and Public Health England (www.iph.cam.ac.uk).

2.5 Predictors of treatment effect research (PROGRESS framework type IV)

The fourth type of prognosis research concerns the identification of factors, in isolation or in combination, that predict treatment effects in individuals or groups of similar individuals. The rationale is that a treatment may not work or work to the same extent for all individuals, because of specific individual characteristics of persons with a particular health condition. Therefore, type IV studies aim to identify the characteristics or factors that signal which treatments will work best for a particular individual, in terms of improved benefits and reduced harms.

Continuing the example of women with breast cancer, researchers identified that some women with breast cancer have cells in the breast tissue which contain receptors for circulating oestrogen (i.e. they are oestrogen-receptor (ER) positive) and hypothesized that oestrogen promotes cancer growth and spread, and contributes to poor prognosis. A drug (tamoxifen) was developed, designed to stop circulating oestrogen from locking to breast cancer cells. In randomized trials tamoxifen improved survival in women with early breast cancer. Box 2.6 describes an individual participant data meta-analysis of these trials designed to investigate if tamoxifen had a differential

Box 2.6 The relevance of oestrogen receptor (ER) status to the efficacy of tamoxifen therapy in improving long-term survival among women with early breast cancer

Setting: randomized controlled trials investigating the effects of tamoxifen treatment.

Source population: women with early breast cancer

Sampling frame: women randomized to receiving prevailing treatment with adjuvant tamoxifen versus prevailing treatment without adjuvant tamoxifen.

Design: individual participant data meta-analysis

Startpoint: 21457 women randomized in twenty controlled trials of five years of adjuvant tamoxifen.

Endpoints: fifteen-year mortality due to breast cancer.

Analysis: individual participant data from all included trials was obtained for the meta-analysis. The effect of adjuvant tamoxifen versus no tamoxifen (on breast cancer mortality) was separately estimated among the 10,645 women with ER-positive disease and the 10,812 women with ER-negative disease.

Results: in women with ER-positive disease, the rate of breast cancer mortality was significantly reduced by about one-third during the fifteen years in those receiving tamoxifen compared with those who were not. In women with ER-negative disease, tamoxifen had little or no effect on breast cancer mortality. There was also a statistically significant difference in treatment effects between the ER-positive and ER-negative groups (i.e. strong evidence of an interaction between treatment effect and ER status).

effect, that is, whether women with breast cancer benefited more from tamoxifen if they were ER-positive compared to ER-negative. This constitutes type IV research, and showed that ER status was indeed a predictor of the effect of tamoxifen on fifteen-year survival: those classified ER-positive had a larger relative reduction in their outcome risk after taking tamoxifen than those who were classified ER-negative. The result is summarized in Figure 2.5.

Studies of predictors of treatment effect inform rational selection and targeting of care and contribute to stratified care and personalized medicine.

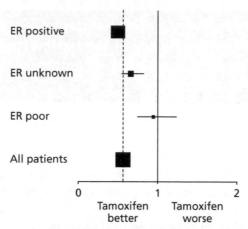

Figure 2.5 Oestrogen-receptor (ER) status and effect of tamoxifen on 15-year survival in women following surgery for breast cancer. Figures are event rate ratios.
Source: data from Early Breast Cancer Trialists' Collaborative, et al., Effect of radiotherapy after breast-conserving surgery on 10-year recurrence and 15-year breast cancer death: meta-analysis of individual patient data for 10,801 women in 17 randomised trials. *The Lancet*. 378(9804),1707–16. Copyright © 2011 Elsevier

This improves efficiency of care because fewer people receive treatments that are not going to be effective or potentially harmful, and expensive new treatments can be directed to those patients who are likely to benefit.

2.6 **Summary**

In this chapter we have provided a brief introduction to the PROGRESS research framework, and provided examples of types I to IV research and the different questions that each type seeks to address. When initiating a prognosis research study, researchers should identify which of the four types fits their objectives and the questions they want to answer. Sometimes, more than one type may be of interest. For example, researchers may want to examine prognostic factors (type II) and then develop a prognostic model (type III).

In Part 3 of the book, each of the four prognosis research types is addressed in detail, from rationale to impact, followed by a chapter on systematic reviews and meta-analysis which covers each type. However, many of the statistical methods and concepts are relevant for all four types, and therefore in the next two chapters, forming Part 2 of this book, we describe key statistical approaches that lay the foundation for the later chapters.

References

1. Hemingway H (2006) Prognosis research: why is Dr Lydgate still waiting? *J Clin Epidemiol* **59**(12), 1229–38.

2. Hemingway H, Croft P, Perel P, Hayden JA, Abrams K, Timmis A, et al. (2013) Prognosis research strategy (PROGRESS) 1: a framework for researching clinical outcomes. *BMJ* **346**, e5595.

3. Riley RD, Hayden JA, Steyerberg EW, Moons KG, Abrams K, Kyzas PA, et al. (2013) Prognosis research strategy (PROGRESS) 2: prognostic factor research. *PLoS Med* **10**(2), e1001380.

4. Steyerberg EW, Moons KG, van der Windt DA, Hayden JA, Perel P, Schroter S, et al. (2013) Prognosis research strategy (PROGRESS) 3: prognostic model research. *PLoS Med* **10**(2), e1001381.

5. Hingorani AD, Windt DA, Riley RD, Abrams K, Moons KG, Steyerberg EW, et al. (2013) Prognosis research strategy (PROGRESS) 4: stratified medicine research. *BMJ* **346**, e5793.

6. Owusu C, Margevicius S, Schluchter M, Koroukian SM, Schmitz KH, Berger NA, et al. (2016) Vulnerable elders survey and socioeconomic status predict functional decline and death among older women with newly diagnosed nonmetastatic breast cancer. *Cancer* **122**, 2579–86.

7. Public Health England. Predict v2.0: NHS England. Available from: http://www.predict.nhs.uk/predict_v2.0.html.

8. Early Breast Cancer Trialists' Collaborative, et al. (2011) Relevance of breast cancer hormone receptors and other factors to the efficacy of adjuvant tamoxifen: patient-level meta-analysis of randomised trials. *Lancet* **378**(9793), 771–84.

9. Verdecchia A, Francisci S, Brenner H, Gatta G, Micheli A, Mangone L, et al. (2007) Recent cancer survival in Europe: a 2000–02 period analysis of EUROCARE-4 data. *Lancet Oncol* **8**(9), 784–96.

10. Azzato EM, Tyrer J, Fasching PA, Beckmann MW, Ekici AB, Schulz-Wendtland R, et al. (2010) Association between a germline OCA2 polymorphism at chromosome 15q13.1 and estrogen receptor-negative breast cancer survival. *J Nat Canc Inst* **102**(9), 650–62.

11. Wishart GC, Azzato EM, Greenberg DC, Rashbass J, Kearins O, Lawrence G, et al. (2010) PREDICT: a new UK prognostic model that predicts survival following surgery for invasive breast cancer. *Breast Cancer Res* **12**(1), R1.

Part 2

Fundamental statistics for prognosis research

Chapter 3

Fundamental statistical methods for prognosis research

Richard D Riley, Kym IE Snell,
Karel GM Moons, and Thomas PA Debray

'Statistics can really save science and the world. Its mission is no less than that. It is our best tool to approach truth, describe what we know, convey with accuracy what is our residual uncertainty, and even identify what would be the best next step to decrease that uncertainty to tolerable levels. It is a valiant enterprise, fit for heroes.' (1)

3.1 Introduction

Statistical methods and principles are an essential component of medical research (2), and should form the bedrock of prognosis research (3, 4). In this chapter we outline fundamental statistical concepts and methods for prognosis research that lay the foundation for subsequent chapters.

3.2 Key statistical measures

Table 3.1 summarizes the key statistical models and measures in prognosis research of continuous, binary, and time-to-event outcomes.

3.2.1 Continuous outcomes: means, medians, and mean differences

Continuous outcomes are often of interest in medical research, such as blood pressure, weight, and pain scores. When studying a population's overall prognosis, key summary statistics for continuous outcomes are the mean and

Table 3.1 Key statistical models and measures for prognosis research studies with continuous, binary or time-to-event outcomes.

Outcome type	Examples	Key statistical models	Common measures and statistics of interest			
			Overall prognosis research	Prognostic factor research	Prognostic model research	Predictors of treatment effect
Continuous	Blood pressure of hypertension patients Pain scale score one month after hip replacement Weight gain during pregnancy	Linear regression	Mean and median outcome value Standard deviation, interquartile range, and histogram of outcome values	Mean/median outcome for different subgroups Unadjusted and adjusted mean outcome change for a one-unit increase in the factor	Predicted (expected) outcome value for individuals conditional on their predictor values Overall fit and calibration performance of developed prognostic models	Treatment effects in subgroups Differences in treatment effects across subgroups (treatment-covariate interactions), e.g. difference in mean difference
Binary	An adverse outcome during pregnancy Mortality by six months after traumatic brain injury	Logistic regression Binomial regression with log link Poisson regression with robust standard errors	Risk, cumulative incidence or incidence proportion (p) Odds (p/(1-p)) Outcome incidence per 1000 people	Outcome risk or odds for different subgroups Unadjusted and adjusted risk ratio, odds ratio, risk difference for a one-unit increase in the factor	Predicted outcome risk for individuals conditional on their predictor values Calibration and discrimination performance of developed prognostic models	Differences in treatment effects across subgroups (treatment-covariate interactions), e.g. ratio of odds ratios

Time-to-event	Time to death after breast cancer diagnosis Risk of hip revision over time after first hip replacement	Cox regression Flexible parametric survival models Competing risks models	Incidence rate (e.g. number of outcomes per 1000 person-years of follow-up) Hazard (incidence) rate over time (h(t)) Survival (Kaplan-Meier) curve (S(t)) Event curve (1-S(t)) Relative survival (e.g. survival compared to the general population)	Unadjusted and adjusted survival curves for different subgroups Unadjusted and adjusted hazard ratios for a 1-unit increase in the factor	Outcome risk predictions over time for individuals conditional on their predictor values Calibration and discrimination performance of developed prognostic models	Differences in treatment effects across subgroups (treatment-covariate interactions), e.g. ratio of hazard ratios

Source: reproduced courtesy of Richard D. Riley

median, alongside measures describing the variability of the outcome across individuals, such as the standard deviation (SD) and inter-quartile range. For example, Henschke et al. examine the prognosis of 1043 patients with non-spinal musculoskeletal pain (5), and report that after three months the mean (SD) pain intensity in the cohort had decreased from 4.8 (2.3) to 3.0 (2.6) on the eleven-point visual analogue scale (VAS), and at the twelve-month follow-up was 2.6 (2.6). An accompanying histogram of the outcome values can also be helpful, to visualize the distribution of outcome responses, especially if they do not follow a normal distribution. In the previous example, the large SD values relative to the mean values suggest that pain intensity values at three and twelve months are positively skewed. In such situations, median values are informative, along with percentile values (e.g. 25th, 75th).

In prognostic factor research, we examine how a particular factor's values correspond to changes in the mean outcome value, ideally after adjustment for other factors. For example, the difference in mean blood pressure at three months for males compared to females after adjusting for baseline blood pressure; or the change in mean pain score for every one-year increase in age after adjusting for weight. A linear regression model can be used for this purpose (see Section 3.3.1).

3.2.2 Binary outcomes: absolute risk, risk ratio, and odds ratio

Binary outcomes (events) are those that can occur within a particular time period of interest. An example is whether death occurs by six months in those with a traumatic brain injury, or whether an adverse maternal outcome occurs during pregnancy. In terms of overall prognosis, this can be summarized by the average *absolute risk* (probability, p) of the outcome occurring in a particular time period. This is also known as the cumulative incidence or incidence proportion. In a cohort study, with no loss to follow-up, it is simply the number with the outcome by the end of the time period divided by the total number in the cohort at the start of the follow-up (i.e. at the startpoint). This is often multiplied by 100%, to express risk as a percentage. For example, Krumholz et al. report that in 2006, on average across all US hospitals, the risk of death within thirty days of a heart attack was 15.8% for those patients aged > 65 years old, which is lower than the absolute risk of 18.8% recorded in 1995. The interpretation of absolute outcome risks (cumulative incidences) always requires an explicit time period being provided. For instance, in the previous example it was crucial to note the thirty-day time period, as the risk of death within thirty days is very different from the risk of death within, say, five years.

An alternative measure is the *odds* of the outcome, which is the number of individuals with the outcome divided by the number of individuals without the outcome in a certain time period; or equivalently the probability (p) that the outcome will occur in the time period divided by the probability that it will not occur in that period (i.e. odds $= p/(1-p)$). For example, in a prospective cohort study of 946 women diagnosed with early-onset pre-eclampsia, 169 had a complication by 48 hours. Therefore the estimated risk (p) of an adverse outcome by 48 hours was 0.179 ($=169/946$) or 17.9%. This corresponds to an odds of 169:777, or $0.179/(1-0.179) = 0.218$, which is approximately 3/14. Thus for every three women with an adverse pregnancy outcome by forty-eight hours there will be about fourteen without one.

In prognostic factor research, of interest is how a factor's values correspond to changes in the risk or odds of the outcome. For example, whether gestational diabetes at twenty weeks' gestation is associated with a higher risk of adverse maternal outcomes during pregnancy. Three measures that summarize the (so-called unadjusted or crude) association of a particular factor with a binary outcome are the risk difference, the risk ratio, and the odds ratio. Using diabetes as a factor of interest, these three measures can be defined as follows:

$$\text{Risk difference} = (\text{risk of outcome for diabetes group})$$
$$- (\text{risk of outcome for non-diabetes group})$$

$$\text{Risk ratio} = \frac{\text{risk of outcome for diabetes group}}{\text{risk of outcome for non-diabetes group}}$$

$$\text{Odds ratio} = \frac{\text{odds of outcome for diabetes group}}{\text{odds of outcome for non-diabetes group}}$$

Although risk differences and risk ratios are more intuitive measures, prognosis studies often report odds ratios. This is because multivariable analyses (i.e. those where multiple prognostic factors are of interest) are often more straightforward when adopting logistic regression analysis, which estimate an odds ratio for each factor after adjusting for the other included factors (see Section 3.3.2).

3.2.3 Time-to-event outcomes: survival, hazard rates, and hazard ratios

Participants in prognosis studies are usually not followed for the same length of time, and many will not experience the outcome of interest during their study follow-up. For example, an individual may choose to withdraw from the study before having the outcome of interest, may be lost to follow-up (e.g. if they move to a different county), reach the study end before an outcome has occurred, or indeed may die before the outcome of interest could have occurred (so-called competing risks, see Chapter 4). Such individuals are usually assumed to be right censored, indicating that their outcome could only occur after their

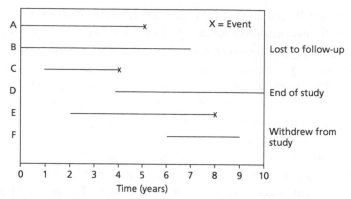

Figure 3.1 Example of survival (time-to-event) data with right censoring, for 6 individuals (A to F).
Source: reproduced courtesy of Richard D. Riley

so-called censoring time (i.e. the last follow-up time) (Figure 3.1). It is often assumed that censoring is non-informative, such that the reason for censoring is independent of the outcome occurrence. When (right) censoring occurs, it is inappropriate to simply exclude participants that are censored as they contain valuable information (i.e. that there was no outcome) up to their final follow-up time. Rather, time-to-event (survival) models are needed to include such participants in the statistical analysis up to their censoring time.

3.2.3.1 Incidence rate and hazard function

For overall prognosis of time-to-event outcomes, an important summary measure is the *incidence rate*, also known as the incidence density. This is not the same as the incidence proportion (cumulative incidence) for a binary outcome, as length of follow-up and censoring is accounted for. The incidence rate is defined as the total number of outcomes observed in the study period divided by the total number of person-years of follow-up accumulated over all individuals in the study cohort in the same period. The denominator thus accounts for the number of people in the study and the sum of their follow-up times. For example, in a registry of osteoarthritis patients that received a total hip replacement, across all patients there were 3506 hip revisions and a total follow-up duration of 858512 person-years within the study period. (6) The overall incidence rate is therefore 3506/858512, which equals 0.00408 per person-year or 4 per 1000 person-years. This suggests that in a cohort of osteoarthritis patients with hip replacement that are followed up collectively with 1000 person-years of follow-up, four individuals are expected to need a revision.

The incidence rate for the entire study period does not indicate when outcomes are more likely to occur (e.g. early or late in the follow-up period). It

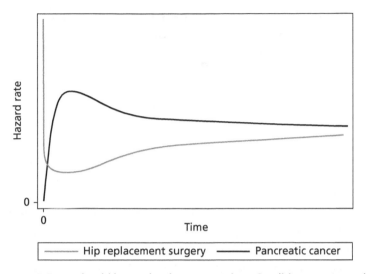

NB Focus should be on the shapes over time. Conditions are not to be compared as hazard rate (y-axis) and time (x-axis) values are not on the same scale for both conditions; in comparable periods, mortality rates are much higher for pancreatic cancer than hip replacement.

Figure 3.2 Illustration of the shape of hazard functions for mortality, over 10 years in osteoarthritis patients following a first hip replacement and over 25 months in those with advanced pancreatic cancer.

Source: adapted with permission from Snell, K.I.E. Development and application of statistical methods for prognosis research (PhD Thesis) [Ph.D.]. University of Birmingham, 2015

is unlikely that the rate is a constant over time. Two examples are shown in Figure 3.2 (7). In the ten years following hip replacement surgery, the mortality rate is higher immediately after surgery but then drops rapidly before gradually increasing again. In the twenty-five months after diagnosis of advanced pancreatic cancer, the mortality rate rapidly increases after diagnosis, before somewhat levelling out. To address this, it is preferable to model the incidence rate over time, usually denoted by the hazard function, $h(t)$. Formally, $h(t)$ is the instantaneous risk of experiencing the outcome (event) at time t conditional on the outcome having not already occurred prior to time t. The cumulative hazard function $H(t)$ is the total amount of hazard accrued up until time t (8). These functions form the foundation of survival analysis methods.

3.2.3.2 Survival function and Kaplan-Meier curve

The (cumulative) hazard function is usually the scale used for statistical modelling, but the complementary survival function, $S(t)$, is more commonly used to disseminate prognosis to health professionals and patients, as it gives the probability of being outcome free within a certain time period. That is, $S(t)$ is the probability that an individual's survival time (T, say) is longer than time t (8). It can be derived from the cumulative hazard function using $S(t) = e^{-H(t)}$.

At the population level, or for specific subgroups, $S(t)$ can be estimated using a non-parametric technique known as the Kaplan-Meier method and then plotted as Kaplan-Meier survival curves (9). This is done by estimating the survival probability at each unique outcome time (8). The estimated survival probability remains the same until the next outcome time, creating a step function. The probability of survival can only decrease over time as more patients experience the outcome. An example is shown in Figure 3.3, for survival after diagnosis of pancreatic cancer (7). Kaplan-Meier curves can be plotted for two or more groups defined by a binary or categorical factor (e.g. males and females), to give a crude (i.e. an unadjusted) estimate of the factor's prognostic effect (i.e. the difference in prognosis between two groups defined by the factor). Another important concept is relative survival (10), where the survival curve of patients with the health condition of interest is compared to the survival curve of another population, for example the general population or one with a different health condition.

The probability density function $f(t)$ represents the probability of the outcome occurring *exactly* at time t, and is an unconditional quantity with limited interpretability, also defined by $f(t) = h(t)S(t)$. The function will usually be positively skewed and, as with all probability density functions, the total area under the curve will equal one. More interpretable is the cumulative distribution of $f(t)$, referred to as $F(t)$. This provides the probability (cumulative incidence)

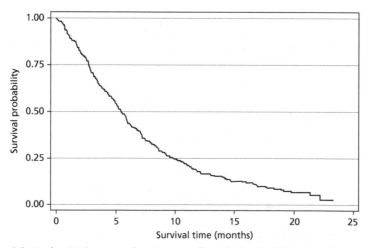

Figure 3.3 Kaplan-Meier curve showing overall survival probability after diagnosis of pancreatic cancer.

Source: adapted with permission from Snell, K.I.E. Development and application of statistical methods for prognosis research (PhD Thesis) [Ph.D.]. University of Birmingham, 2015

of the outcome occurring at any time up to and including time t, and hence $F(t) = 1 - S(t)$. When making outcome risk predictions in new individuals (e.g. based on a prognostic model), $F(t)$ is usually the main interest.

3.2.3.3 Hazard ratios and proportional hazards

It is common to assume that the hazard functions are proportional across different levels of a prognostic factor. This is convenient, as it allows prognostic effects to be summarized in terms of the hazard ratio. For example, if $h_F(t)$ and $h_M(t)$ denote the hazard functions for females and males, respectively, then the hazard ratio (HR) for males compared to females is defined as:

$$HR = \frac{h_M(t)}{h_F(t)}$$

If such an HR equals two then, assuming the two groups have proportional hazards, the hazard for males is twice that for females, at any time point t. It is important to check whether the proportional hazards assumption holds. One way to do this is graphically using 'log-log' plots in which $-\ln(-\ln(S(t))$ is plotted against $\ln(t)$. Categorical variables can be plotted by category, but continuous variables need to be categorized into groups before plotting. Lines should appear approximately parallel if the proportional hazards assumption is valid. Non-proportional (time-varying) hazard ratios can be formally examined (e.g. based on statistical significance) and quantified by including an interaction between the prognostic factor and time within a Cox regression model (see Section 3.3.3.1).

The hazard ratio compares groups over the whole follow-up period. We can also compare groups at specific time points by calculating the risk ratio by time t. For example, if $S_F(t)$ and $S_M(t)$ denote the survival functions for females and males respectively, then the risk ratio (RR) for males compared to females at one year is:

$$RR = \frac{1 - S_M(t)}{1 - S_F(t)}$$

Similarly, the odds ratio at time t could be derived by comparing the odds of the outcome by one year:

$$OR = \frac{(1 - S_M(t)) / S_M(t)}{(1 - S_F(t)) / S_F(t)}$$

3.2.4 Risk ratios, odds ratios, and hazard ratios

It is important to emphasize that risk ratios, odds ratios, and hazard ratios are different measures, and only give approximately the same value when

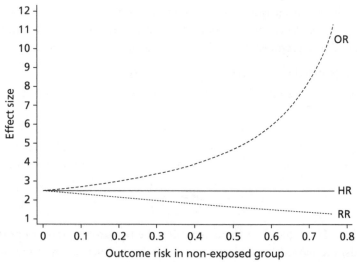

Figure 3.4 Comparison of the hazard ratio (HR), odds ratio (OR) and risk ratio (RR) for a binary prognostic factor ('exposed' versus 'non-exposed'), across different values of the outcome risk in the non-exposed group.
Source: reproduced courtesy of Richard D. Riley.

the outcome risk over the time period of interest is low (e.g. with short-term follow-up and/or when the outcome is rare). As the outcome risk increases above 5%, the three measures can rapidly diverge. This is demonstrated in Figure 3.4, where the underlying survival times are drawn from a Weibull survival distribution (11), and there is a constant hazard ratio of 2.5 for a binary prognostic factor (defined as exposed versus non-exposed) over time. The corresponding risk ratio and odds ratio are not constant: they depend on the outcome risk in the non-exposed group. As the outcome risk increases, the odds ratio, risk ratio, and hazard ratio become more disparate. For example, at a time when the outcome risk in the non-exposed group is 0.6, the odds ratio, risk ratio, and hazard ratio are 6.0, 1.5, and 2.5, respectively.

3.3 **Fundamental regression and statistical models**

'Essentially, all models are wrong, but some are useful' (12)

Most prognosis research involves statistical modelling to express and estimate prognostic relationships of interest. The most common are known as *regression models*, whereby an outcome variable is expressed (described) in terms of one or more explanatory variables (referred to here as prognostic factors or predictors).

3.3.1 Linear regression for continuous outcomes

Consider a dataset where each individual (denoted by subscript i) provides values for a set of k predictors ($X_{1i}, X_{2i},..., X_{ki}$ say) measured at a defined startpoint (e.g. at diagnosis of disease) and also a continuous outcome (Y_i, say) measured at a subsequent time point (e.g. three months after diagnosis). In this situation, a linear regression model is of the form:

$$Y_i = \alpha + \beta_1 X_{1i} + \beta_2 X_{2i} + \beta_3 X_{3i} + \cdots + \beta_k X_{ki} + e_i$$

For example, X_{1i} could be the age of the patient in years, X_{2i} could be 1 for males and 0 for females, and so on. The unknown terms ('parameters') on the right hand-side of the aforementioned equation (i.e. the βs and α) are estimated using the data at hand, usually via maximum likelihood or ordinary least squares estimation. The latter aims to yield parameter estimates that minimize the (squared) difference between the observed outcomes, Y_i, and the predicted outcomes defined by the *linear predictor* (i.e. $\alpha + \beta_1 X_{1i} + \beta_2 X_{2i} + \beta_3 X_{3i} + \cdots + \beta_k X_{ki}$). Maximum likelihood estimation aims to yield parameter estimates that maximize the probability of observing the available data, and requires distributional assumptions to be made, such as $e_i \sim N(0, \sigma^2)$. Sometimes the outcome needs to be transformed (e.g. using a natural log transformation) to more closely meet the normality assumption.

For a linear regression model without any predictors, the estimate of the intercept (referred to as 'alpha hat', $\hat{\alpha}$) is simply the mean outcome value observed in the dataset. In models involving one or more predictors, $\hat{\alpha}$ represents the mean outcome value for individuals whose predictor values are all zero. To improve interpretation, if predictors are mean-centred (i.e. we redefine X_{1i} as $(X_{1i} - \text{mean}(X_{1i}))$ and so forth), then $\hat{\alpha}$ represents the mean outcome value for an individual with mean predictor values.

For prognostic factor research, the estimates of the β terms (referred to as 'beta hat', $\hat{\beta}$) are of primary interest. Each $\hat{\beta}$ denotes the estimated change in mean outcome value (i.e. the mean difference) for a one-unit increase in the corresponding predictor, after adjusting for other predictors. For example, $\hat{\beta}_1$ may be the difference in the mean outcome for each one year increase in age, and $\hat{\beta}_2$ the difference in the mean outcome for a male compared to a female, and so on, after adjustment for other factors in the model. Therefore, each $\hat{\beta}$ reveals the added prognostic value of a particular predictor over and above others in the model. For example, Figure 3.5 shows that in patients with chronic low back pain, the predictor '*pain intensity*' (as measured by the

Final prognostic model for predicting future pain intensity, $E(Y)$, as measured by the Modified Von Korff pain scale:

$$E(Y_i) = \alpha - (0.07 \times Dose_i) + (10.7 \times (Pain\ Intensity\ after\ treatment)_i)$$
$$+ (2.95 \times (Low\ Back\ Pain{:}right\ lateral\ bending)_i)$$

where *Dose* is coded as 0, 1, 2, or 3 representing the multiple of 6 spinal manipulative therapy sessions received; *Pain Intensity* after treatment is measured by the Modified Von Korff pain scale; and *Low Back Pain: right lateral bending* is measured from 0 to 10. The intercept was not reported.

Performance of the model:

The graph below shows the poor agreement (calibration) between predicted pain intensity (x-axis) and observed pain intensity (y-axis) at follow-up, (a) in the training set used to develop the model ('apparent performance'), and (b) in the test set, which contains patients that were randomly excluded from the training set.

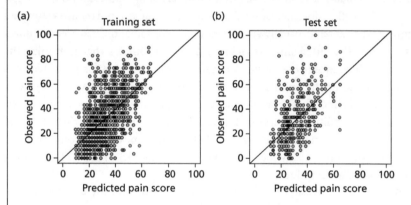

The percentage of variability explained, R^2, is 26.8% in the training set and just 6.5% in the test set. The model is therefore not useful. Additional predictors are required to improve the predictive performance. Further, as the outcome was ambiguously defined (future pain intensity between 12 and 52 weeks after treatment initiation) in this study, a more precise definition is needed with a single time point chosen for prediction.

Figure 3.5 Final model for the prediction of pain intensity (as measured by the Modified Von Korff pain scale) between 12 to 52 weeks post treatment initiation, based on predictors measured following 6 weeks treatment with spinal manipulation for the care of chronic low back pain.

Source: data from Vavrek D, Haas M, Neradilek MB, et al. Prediction of pain outcomes in a randomized controlled trial of dose-response of spinal manipulation for the care of chronic low back pain. BMC Musculoskeletal Disorders.2015; 16: 205. Copyright © 2015 Springer Nature.

Modified Von Korff pain scale after six weeks' treatment with spinal manipulation) adds prognostic value for the outcome of subsequent future pain intensity (ambiguously defined to be between twelve and fifty weeks after treatment initiation) (13). The $\hat{\beta}$ is 10.7 (95% CI: 8.84 –12.56), indicating that each one-unit increase in the pain score after treatment is associated with a 10.7 increase in the subsequent pain score, after adjusting for other predictors (dose and the right lateral bending score).

For prognostic model research, of key interest is the combination of regression coefficients (including the intercept term), in order to make predictions of the outcome in a new individual based on their predictor values. For example, one might make predictions using:

$$E(Y_i) = \hat{\alpha} + \hat{\beta}_1 X_{1i} + \hat{\beta}_2 X_{2i} + \hat{\beta}_3 X_{3i} + \cdots + \hat{\beta}_k X_{ki}$$

where $E(Y_i)$ denotes the expected value of Y_i (i.e. the actual mean outcome value) for patient i. An example of a prognostic model developed using linear regression is shown in Figure 3.5 (13). In practice, predictions of $E(Y_i)$ for new individuals are usually optimistic (too extreme) when based on regression coefficients obtained by standard estimation methods, and can be improved using penalization (shrinkage) approaches (see Chapter 4).

3.3.2 Regression for binary outcomes

For a binary outcome, the response Y_i is now defined by 0 for those without the outcome (no event) or 1 for those with the outcome (event). In this situation, Y_i follows a Bernoulli (rather than a Normal) distribution, such that linear regression is no longer appropriate. Rather, an approach such as logistic regression is needed to model the Y_i values, which can be written as:

$$Y_i \sim \text{Bernoulli}\,(p_i)$$

$$\ln\left(\frac{p_i}{1-p_i}\right) = \alpha + \beta_1 X_{1i} + \beta_2 X_{2i} + \beta_3 X_{3i} + \cdots + \beta_k X_{ki}$$

Here p_i is an individual's probability of developing the outcome Y_i, and $\ln\left(\dfrac{p_i}{1-p_i}\right)$ is the individual's log odds of the outcome. We use 'ln' and 'log' interchangeably in this book to refer to the natural logarithm transformation of a variable. This transformation is often needed during statistical modelling, to improve parameter estimation and more closely adhere to assumptions. The intercept term, α, is the baseline log-odds (where 'baseline' refers to individuals whose X values are all zero), and the $X_{1i}, X_{2i}, \ldots X_{ki}$ denote values of k included predictors. Sometimes, as described for linear regression, predictors are mean-centred to improve model estimation and the interpretation of the intercept (i.e. to represent the log-odds for an individual with mean X values). The use of a Bernoulli distribution naturally models the variation between observed outcomes Y_i and predictions of p_i, and thus there is no need to specify additional residual error terms in the model (unlike in linear regression). The model is usually estimated using maximum likelihood estimation. When there are no predictors included in the model, the estimated intercept ($\hat{\alpha}$) is simply the overall log-odds of the outcome observed in a certain time period, and can be transformed back to the odds or probability scale to summarize overall outcome risk within that time period. Extension of logistic regression to outcomes with three or more categories is possible (3). Also, if risk ratios rather than odds ratios are desired, a Poisson regression or binomial regression (with log rather than logit link) are two viable options (14, 15).

For prognostic factor research the focus is on estimating each β, to quantify the change in log odds (i.e. the log odds ratio) for each one-unit increase in the corresponding predictor. For example, $\hat{\beta}_1$ may estimate the increase in log odds for each one year increase in age, and $\hat{\beta}_2$ the log odds ratio comparing males to females, and so on. When the model includes multiple predictors, each $\hat{\beta}$ quantifies a factor's prognostic effect adjusted for (independent of) the effects of the other factors in the model. An example is shown in Table 3.2, where the added (or independent or adjusted) prognostic value of the albumin:creatinine ratio (ACR) was evaluated in regard to composite maternal and composite neonatal adverse outcomes in pregnancy (16). This shows that, after adjusting for other prognostic factors, a one-unit increase in log(ACR) is associated with a 60% increase in the odds of an adverse maternal outcome (odds ratio = 1.60, 95% CI: 1.42–1.80).

In situations of rare outcomes, a logistic regression model fitted using standard maximum likelihood estimation may give biased β estimates. That is, it may over-estimate the true odds ratio (and give very large standard errors) when numbers of outcomes are few either overall or in particular subgroups defined by the predictors. Greenland et al. note that: 'Maximum likelihood estimates of odds ratios, rate ratios, and risk ratios can have considerable upward bias when there are few or no study participants at key combinations of the outcome, exposure, and covariates, often known as *sparse data bias*' (17). This means that the odds ratio estimate is expected to be too far below or too far above 1, depending on whether the true odds ratio was below or above 1, respectively. In this situation, one strategy is to use (adaptations of) Firth's correction, which aims to remove the bias and improves upon standard logistic regression (18–20).

For prognostic model research, the focus is on using the entire linear predictor (i.e. $\alpha + \beta_1 X_{1i} + \beta_2 X_{2i} + \beta_3 X_{3i} + \cdots + \beta_k X_{ki}$) to make absolute risk predictions ($\hat{p}_i$) for new individuals conditional on their predictor values. Following

Table 3.2 Logistic regression results for the unadjusted and adjusted (independent) prognostic value of the albumin creatinine ratio (ACR) in regard to the odds of adverse maternal and neonatal outcomes, as reported by Elia et al., 2017.

Model	Variable	Composite maternal adverse outcome	
		Odds Ratio (95% CI)	p value
Unadjusted	Log ACR	1.52 (1.38–1.68)	< 0.001
Adjusted	Log ACR	1.60 (1.42–1.80)	< 0.001
	Gestational age at ACR measurement	0.88 (0.83–0.92)	< 0.001
	Maternal age	1.04 (1.08–1.08)	0.02
	Essential hypertension	0.78 (0.38–1.60)	0.52
	Pre-existing diabetes	0.68 (0.12–3.72)	0.66
	Gestational diabetes	1.02 (0.38–2.77)	0.96
	Smoking	0.85 (0.50–1.45)	0.55
	Nulliparity	0.96 (0.66–1.40)	0.83
	Social deprivation index		
	1	1	
	2	0.80 (0.46–1.41)	0.45
	3	1.10 (0.63–1.92)	0.73
	4	0.623 (0.33–1.19)	0.15
	5	0.424 (0.26–0.80)	0.01
	Body mass index		
	< 18.5	1	
	18.5–24.99	1.06 (0.32–3.50)	0.93
	25.0–29.99	1.47 (0.44–4.93)	0.54
	30.0–34.9	0.70 (0.20–2.48)	0.58
	35.0–39.9	0.50 (0.13–1.98)	0.32
	> 40.0	0.56 (0.13–2.39)	0.43
	Mean arterial blood pressure	1.02 (1.00–1.05)	0.04

Source: adapted from Elia EG, et al. Is the first urinary albumin/creatinine ratio (ACR) in women with suspected preeclampsia a prognostic factor for maternal and neonatal adverse outcome? A retrospective cohort study. *Acta Obstetricia et Gynecologica Scandinavica* 96(5), 580–88. Copyright © 2017 John Wiley & Sons, Inc. Open Access.

estimation of a logistic regression model, this is achieved by using the back-transformation of:

$$\hat{p}_i = \frac{exp(\hat{\alpha}+\hat{\beta}_1 X_{1i}+\hat{\beta}_2 X_{2i}+\hat{\beta}_3 X_{3i}+\cdots+\hat{\beta}_k X_{ki})}{1+exp(\hat{\alpha}+\hat{\beta}_1 X_{1i}+\hat{\beta}_2 X_{2i}+\hat{\beta}_3 X_{3i}+\cdots+\hat{\beta}_k X_{ki})}$$

An example is shown in Box 3.1 for women with a first trimester miscarriage and choosing expectant management (i.e. waiting for the miscarriage to happen

Box 3.1 Example of a prognostic model derived using logistic regression, and how to use it for making risk predictions for new individuals (using results shown by Casikar et al. (21))

Aim: Prediction of 'successful' outcome (e.g. no need for surgical evacuation) in women choosing expectant management (i.e. waiting for the miscarriage to happen on its own without intervention) following a first trimester miscarriage

Results: Applying to the model development dataset, the estimated logistic regression model was,

$$\log\left(\frac{\hat{p}_i}{1-\hat{p}_i}\right)=2.66+(1.48\times\text{IncompMisc}_i)-(1.63\times\text{NilBleeding}_i)-(0.07\times\text{Age}_i)$$

where $\hat{p}_i$ denotes the probability of a patient having a 'successful' outcome following expectant management. *IncompMisc* has a value of 1 if the diagnosis at primary scan is incomplete miscarriage and 0 otherwise. *NilBleeding* is 1 if there is neither bleeding nor clots and 0 otherwise. *Age* is the maternal age in years.

To calculate the predicted probability of a successful outcome for a new woman if she chose expectant management, the model was re-expressed as:

$$\hat{p}_i = \frac{exp(2.66+(1.48\times\text{IncompMisc}_i)-(1.63\times\text{NilBleeding}_i)-(0.07\times\text{Age}_i))}{1+exp(2.66+(1.48\times\text{IncompMisc}_i)-(1.63\times\text{NilBleeding}_i)-(0.07\times\text{Age}_i))}$$

Source: data from Casikar I, Lu C, Reid S, et al. (2013) Prediction of successful expectant management of first trimester miscarriage: development and validation of a new mathematical model. *Australian and New Zealand Journal of Obstetrics and Gynaecology* 53(1), 58–63. Copyright © Copyright © 2013 John Wiley & Sons.

on its own without intervention), with a logistic regression model developed for the prediction of a 'successful' outcome at fourteen days (e.g. no need for surgical evacuation) (21). As mentioned for linear regression, predictions of $\hat{p}_i$ for new individuals are usually improved after penalization (shrinkage) of the estimated regression coefficients, to reduce variability in predictions (see Chapter 4).

3.3.3 Survival models for time-to-event outcomes

The use of logistic regression is generally discouraged when predictions for longer time periods (typically longer than 3 or 6 months) are needed, and when predictions for multiple (rather than one) time points are required. It is also inappropriate when follow-up length varies across individuals (e.g. due to drop-out). To address this, we now introduce some fundamental approaches to time-to-event regression modelling, in the presence of non-informative right censored data.

3.3.3.1 Cox proportional hazards regression

The most commonly used regression approach for time-to-event outcomes is the proportional hazards model proposed by Cox (22), usually written as:

$$h_i(t) = h_0(t) \, exp\big(\beta_1 X_{1i} + \beta_2 X_{2i} + \beta_3 X_{3i} + \cdots + \beta_k X_{ki}\big)$$

where $h_i(t)$ is an individual's hazard rate of the outcome at time t. The baseline hazard term, $h_0(t)$, is similar to an intercept but is a function over time, and represents the hazard function when all predictor values are zero. Sometimes, as described for linear and logistic regression, predictors are mean-centred to improve model estimation and the interpretation of the baseline hazard (i.e. to represent the hazard rate for an individual with mean X values). Sometimes age is used as the timescale, rather than time in study, so that $h_0(t)$ summarizes the hazard rate over different ages, which Thiébaut and Bénichou suggest is preferable (23). The $X_{1i}, X_{2i}, \ldots$ terms denote values of included predictors, and each β denotes the change in log hazard rate (i.e. the log hazard ratio) for each one-unit increase in the corresponding predictor, under a proportional hazards assumption. By taking $exp(\beta)$ we obtain the hazard ratio for the corresponding predictor. For example, $\hat{\beta}_1$ may be the estimated increase in log hazard rate for each one year increase in age, and $\hat{\beta}_2$ the estimated log hazard ratio comparing males to females, and so on. As for linear and logistic regression, predictions of outcome risk in new individuals are usually more reliable after predictor effects are penalized (see Chapter 4). Also, as for logistic regression, corrections may be applied to reduce bias in estimated regression coefficients in small samples (i.e. when there is sparse data bias) (17, 24).

If there are no predictors included in the model, $h_0(t)$ becomes the overall hazard rate in the dataset, which summarizes the overall prognosis over time.

However, the commonly used partial (maximum) likelihood estimation approach proposed by Cox avoids estimating $h_0(t)$ entirely. This is appealing in prognostic factor research because it requires no assumptions to be made about the shape of the baseline hazard function. However, this also complicates the use of Cox models to make risk predictions over time (or for a certain time point) for new individuals, as now described.

3.3.3.2 Making predictions and modelling the baseline hazard

Let $\hat{S}_i(t)$ denote an individual's predicted survival probability at time t. Then, for a new individual, the predicted probability of the outcome occurring by time t can be obtained by:

$$1 - \hat{S}_i(t) = 1 - \hat{S}_0(t)^{\exp(\hat{\beta}_1 X_{1i} + \hat{\beta}_2 X_{2i} + \hat{\beta}_3 X_{3i} + \cdots + \hat{\beta}_k X_{ki})}$$

where $\hat{S}_0(t)$ is the estimated baseline survival probability at time t. However, $\hat{S}_0(t)$ is not available without $h_0(t)$. To address this, a common approach is to use the linear predictor (also known as the risk score or prognostic index, and defined by $\beta_1 X_{1i} + \beta_2 X_{2i} + \beta_3 X_{3i} + \cdots + \beta_k X_{ki}$) from the Cox model, and then produce Kaplan-Meier curves for, say, four or five groups of individuals defined by categories of this score. In this way, a new individual can be assigned to a particular category based on their score, and then the Kaplan-Meier $\hat{S}(t)$ values for a particular category can be used for making predictions over time for a new individual whose risk score falls in that category. A major drawback, however, is that all individuals within the same risk group are forced to have the same predicted survival curve, and so cannot discriminate between individuals with different actual risks in the same group.

Risk grouping can be avoided by estimating the baseline hazard (or survival) function directly. This can be achieved through a non-parametric approach after fitting the Cox model, such as the Nelson-Aalen approach (25, 26). It is often preferable to model the baseline hazard function using a fully parametric approach, such as assuming that survival times follow a Weibull distribution (11). However, parametric distributions are often not flexible enough to model complex baseline hazard shapes. A more flexible approach proposed by Royston and Parmar is to model the cumulative baseline hazard using splines (27, 28):

$$\ln(H_i(t)) = \ln(H_0(t)) + \beta_1 X_{1i} + \beta_2 X_{2i} + \beta_3 X_{3i} + \cdots + \beta_k X_{ki}$$

Here, $\ln(H_0(t))$, the baseline cumulative hazard function, is modelled using restricted cubic splines. Restricted cubic splines are used to create flexible and smooth functions that are able to fit tightly curved shapes. This is done by fitting a series of cubic functions and forcing them to join (and be smoothed) at certain points (called internal knots), whilst constraining the function to be linear in the tails (i.e. before the first internal knot and after the last internal knot). If there are zero internal knots, $\ln(H_0(t))$ becomes the baseline hazard for a Weibull model. Thus, the Royston-Parmar models are a generalization of the Weibull model (29). The degrees of freedom (df) for the baseline hazard function are calculated as df $= m +1$, where m is the number of internal knots. Royston and Lambert suggest that 2–3 df are usually adequate to model the baseline hazard function in small datasets and 4–5 df in larger datasets (29, 30).

The Royston-Parmar approach provides very similar hazard ratio estimates to those from a Cox model (28, 29), but additionally provides the baseline hazard and cumulative hazard $(H_0(t))$ functions. The baseline survival function is then obtained using $S_0(t) = exp(-H_0(t))$, and predictions for outcome risk can now be made using $\hat{F}(t) = 1 - \hat{S}_0(t)^{exp(\hat{\beta}_1 X_{1i} + \hat{\beta}_2 X_{2i} + \hat{\beta}_3 X_{3i} + \cdots + \hat{\beta}_k X_{ki})}$. This allows a potentially unique cumulative incidence to be predicted for each individual, and thus avoids the need for risk grouping. This advantage is illustrated in Figure 3.6, where predicted survival curves are shown for two individuals both from the same risk group, but whose predictions differ considerably. For example, at six months individual 1 has a predicted survival of 46% and individual 2 has a predicted survival of 29%.

3.4 Statistical measures of prognostic model performance

After a prognostic model is developed (e.g. using a regression model), it is important to quantify its predictive performance in terms of overall fit and calibration (for linear, logistic, and time-to-event models), and also discrimination (for logistic and time-to-event models). We now introduce some key measures and approaches for this purpose.

3.4.1 Overall measures of model fit

Model fit statistics measure the overall performance of the model. In particular, for continuous outcomes R^2 provides the proportion of the total variance of outcome values that is explained by the model, with values closer to one preferred. Often this is multiplied by one hundred, to give the percentage of variation explained. Generalizations of R^2 for binary and time-to-event outcomes have also been proposed, such as the Cox-Snell R^2(31), Nagelkerke's R^2(32), O'Quigley's R^2(33), Royston's R^2(34), and Royston and Sauerbrei's R^2_D(35). Other overall measures of fit are the mean-square error of predictions (the Brier score (36)), the likelihood ratio statistic, the Akaike information criterion (AIC) and the Bayesian information criterion (BIC). Chapter 7 also introduces

Context: For illustrative purposes, we developed a prognostic model (containing 10 predictors) to predict risk of mortality in patients diagnosed with advanced stage pancreatic cancer and treated with gemcitabine. We used the Royston-Parmar model framework,

$$h_i(t) = h_0(t) \exp(\beta_1 X_{1i} + \beta_2 X_{2i} + \beta_3 X_{3i} + \cdots + \beta_k X_{ki}) = h_0(t) \exp(risk\ score_i)$$

with the cumulative baseline hazard $(H_0(t) = \int_0^t h_0(u)$ where $t > 0)$ modelled using restricted cubic splines with 2 internal knots. The estimated risk score was:

$$(0.019 \times age_i) + (-0.194 \times female_i) + (0.063 \times WBC_i) + (0.522 \times (AST_i / 100)^{-0.5})$$
$$+ (0.0017 \times AP_i) + (-0.050 \times albumin_i) + (0.0012 \times LDH_i)$$
$$+ (0.080 \times ln(CA19 - 9)_i) + (-0.072 \times (Stage3or4)_i) + (0.307 \times metastasis_i)$$

where WBC = white blood cell count, AST = aspartate aminotransferase, LDH = lactate dehydrogenase. The estimated baseline hazard and cumulative hazard functions are shown below:

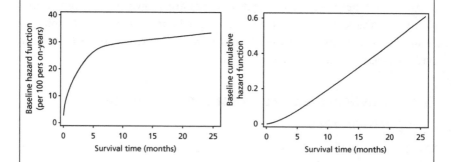

Individualised survival curve predictions: We can use the model to make individualized predictions over time for new individuals. We take the estimated baseline survival function $\hat{S}_0(t) = \exp(-\hat{H}_0(t))$ and produce a predicted survival curve using $\hat{S}_i(t) = 1 - \hat{S}_0(t)^{\exp(risk\ score_i)}$.

Survival predictions are illustrated for two individuals in the graph below. These are clearly distinct. Often researchers categorize the risk score into groups, and use the group's observed Kaplan-Meier curves (from the development dataset) to make predictions for new individuals. This only loses information. For example, in the pancreatic cancer dataset, we created four risk groups based on categories defined by the quartiles of the risk score estimated from a Cox regression model. Interestingly, the two aforementioned individuals both fall into risk group 3, and thus would have the same predicted survival curve (i.e. the Kaplan-Meier curve for risk group 3).

Figure 3.6 Comparison of individual risk predictions based on Royston-Parmar approach and predictions based on risk groups.
Source: reproduced courtesy of Richard D. Riley

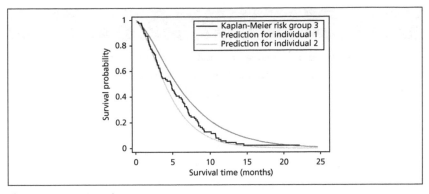

Figure 3.6 Continued

the net benefit measure, to summarize the overall clinical benefit of using the model to inform clinical decision making (37, 38).

3.4.2 Calibration statistics and plots

Calibration examines the agreement between predicted and observed outcome values (for linear regression) or between predicted and observed outcome risks (for logistic and time-to-event regression models). It should be examined across the whole spectrum of predicted values, and at each relevant time point (for time-to-event models). It can be summarized by measures such as the calibration slope (ideal value of 1), calibration-in-the-large (ideal value of 0), and the observed/expected ratio (ideal value of 1) (Box 3.2). Such measures should be derived across all individuals combined and, ideally, also in relevant subgroups.

Box 3.2 Explanation of some key measures for calibration in a prognostic model with binary or time-to-event outcomes

Observed/expected number of outcomes (O/E)

O/E summarizes the overall calibration. For binary outcomes, it provides the ratio of the total observed to have the outcome in a certain time period over the total expected to have the outcome in that same period. Thus an ideal value is 1. Values less than 1 indicate the model is over-predicting the total number of outcomes in the population, whilst values above 1 indicate the model is under-predicting the total number of outcomes in the population. For time-to-event outcomes, mean observed and expected

Box 3.2 Continued

probabilities can be used instead of total numbers of outcomes to account for censoring. Sometimes, in addition to looking at O/E across the entire dataset, O/E is reported for groups of predicted risk (e.g. by tenths of predicted risk). The O/E ratios then also give an indication of the shape of the calibration slope. Note also that sometimes the E/O ratio is presented; under-prediction then occurs for values below 1 and over-prediction for values above than 1. For continuous outcomes, an analogous measure of the O/E ratio is the mean predicted outcome value compared to the mean observed outcome value.

Calibration-in-the-large

Calibration-in-the-large is closely related to the overall O/E statistic (4), but less intuitive to interpret. For binary outcomes, it can be estimated by fitting a logistic model for the probability of the outcome (p_i) with the linear predictor (LP_i) value as a covariate (offset term),

$$\text{logit}(p_i) = \alpha + 1(LP_i)$$

where the estimate of α is the estimate of calibration-in-the-large (4). Calibration-in-the-large should be close to zero for a well calibrated model. Importantly, calibration-in-the-large may be zero and O/E may be 1 even when there is still substantial mis-calibration; that is, on average predictions may appear well calibrated, but there can be under-prediction in some predicted risk ranges (or individuals) which cancels out over-prediction (or vice versa) in other ranges (or individuals).

Calibration slope

The calibration slope is one measure of agreement between observed and predicted risk of the outcome across the whole range of predicted values (3, 4). The observed calibration slope will always be 1 in the development dataset if traditional estimation techniques (e.g. maximum likelihood estimation) are used. However, upon validation, it may often deviate from 1. A slope < 1 indicates that some predictions are too extreme (e.g. predictions close to 1 are too high, and predictions close to 0 are too low) and a slope > 1 indicates predictions are too narrow. A calibration slope < 1 is often observed in external validation studies, consistent with a lack of adjustment for over-fitting (optimism) of the model when it was developed.

Box 3.2 Continued

To estimate the calibration slope, a calibration model can be fitted in the validation dataset. For example, for a binary outcome a logistic model could be fitted as $\text{logit}(p_i) = \alpha + \hat{\beta}*LP_i$. Then, $\hat{\beta}$ is the estimated calibration slope. The calibration slope is derived using individual predicted values (for the LP), and does not require grouping. This is in contrast to the Hosmer-Lemeshow test of goodness of fit for logistic regression models, which requires arbitrary grouping of individuals and is not recommended.

Note that systematic over or under-prediction is still possible even when the calibration slope is 1, and thus it is important to consider *both* O/E (or calibration-in-the-large) and calibration slope to fully assess calibration performance, alongside calibration plots. Similarly for time-to-event outcomes, the magnitude of the baseline hazard ($h_0(t)$) may not be appropriate, even if the calibration slope is 1.

Source: reproduced courtesy of Richard D Riley.

Calibration can also be visualized graphically, using calibration plots. For example, Figure 3.5 shows poor calibration between observed pain scores and predicted pain scores from a prognostic model based on linear regression. Figure 3.7 illustrates various types of (mis)calibration for a prognostic model based on logistic regression for a binary outcome. For predictions of outcome risk (i.e. for binary or time-to-event outcomes), a calibration plot should display observed versus predicted risks, for example across tenths of predicted risk (39), or ideally by using a calibration plot with a smoothed non-linear curve generated using a LOESS smoother or splines (39, 40), or by displaying observed and predicted survival curves over time for different risk groups (41). It is helpful to add the distribution of the predicted values underneath the graph, to show the spread of risk in the dataset at hand. An example is given in Figure 3.8.

3.4.3 Discrimination statistics

Discrimination refers to how well predictions discriminate (separate) between those participants who do and do not develop the outcome of interest; therefore it is most relevant for prognostic models of binary and time-to-event outcomes (not continuous). The range of predictions on a calibration plot (e.g. separation of mean observed risk across groups defined by tenths of predicted risk) hints at the discrimination performance, as the more separated the risk groups then the better the model discriminates.

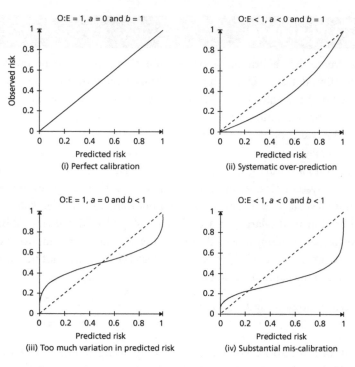

O:E = ratio of observed versus expected risk, a = calibration-in-the-large (calculated on the logit scale), b = calibration slope (calculated on the logit scale). Note that in (ii), the calibration slope is 1 (i.e. linear) on the logit scale, but becomes curved when transformed back to the probability (risk) scale shown.

Figure 3.7 Examples of the calibration performance of a prognostic model for a binary outcome.

Source: reproduced courtesy of Richard D. Riley

Discrimination is formally measured by the Concordance (C) statistic (index) (3, 42), and a value of 1 indicates the model has perfect discrimination, whilst a value of 0.5 indicates the model discriminates no better than chance. For binary outcomes, it is equivalent to the area under the receiver operating characteristic (ROC) curve. It gives the probability that for any randomly selected pair of individuals, one with and one without the outcome, the model assigns a higher probability to the individual with the outcome. Generalizations of the C statistic have been proposed for time-to-event models, most notably Harrell's C statistic (42, 43). This is the proportion (ranging also from 0.5 to 1) of all possible pairs of study participants in which the individual with the higher predicted survival probability indeed survived longer than the other individual (42). Pairs in which both individuals are

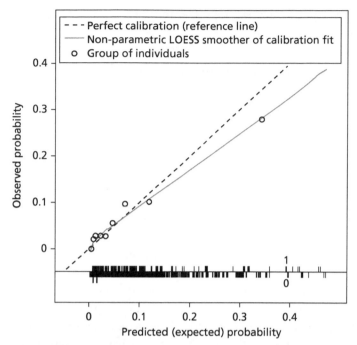

NB Distribution of predicted probability values is shown at the base of the graph for those with (1) and those without (0) the outcome

Figure 3.8 Example of a calibration plot for risk predictions from a prognostic model with a binary outcome, produced using the pmcalplot module in Stata.
Source: reproduced courtesy of Richard D. Riley

censored before the outcome occurrence, or both have the outcome at the same survival time, or where one individual is censored at an earlier time than the other individual's survival time, cannot be ordered and therefore are not included in the calculation of Harrell's C statistic. The C statistic will usually depend on the length of follow-up.

Another discrimination measure is Somer's D, which equals $(C - 0.5)/0.5$, and the discrimination slope, which is defined as the mean risk for individuals with the outcomes minus the mean risk for individuals without the outcome (44), and ranges from 0 (no discrimination) to 1 (perfect discrimination). For time-to-event outcomes Royston's D statistic is also useful (35), as it is interpreted as the log hazard ratio comparing low and high-risk groups, where these two equally sized groups are defined by dichotomizing at the median value of the linear predictor (i.e. $\hat{\beta}_1 X_{1i} + \hat{\beta}_2 X_{2i} + \hat{\beta}_3 X_{3i} + \cdots + \hat{\beta}_k X_{ki}$)

from the developed model. Higher values for the D statistic indicate greater discrimination.

3.5 Modelling non-linear prognostic effects

The association between a continuous predictor (prognostic factor) and an outcome may be non-linear. This means that the impact of a one-unit increase in the continuous predictor on the outcome changes across the spectrum of predictor values. The two most common approaches to non-linear modelling are (restricted) cubic splines and fractional polynomials. As mentioned in Section 3.3.3.2, the restricted cubic splines approach involves fitting a series of cubic functions and forcing them to join at certain locations (called internal knots), whilst constraining the function to be linear in the tails (i.e. before the first internal knot and after the last internal knot) (3, 45, 46).

Rather than describing non-linear effects through complex spline functions (involving many parameters), fractional polynomials consider a limited but flexible set of transformations to describe predictor effects (47–49). In general, for a continuous predictor X, rather than simply assuming a linear trend (i.e. including βX in the regression model), a fractional polynomial function of degree $m \geq 1$ is allowed, of the form $\sum_{j=1}^{m} \beta_j X^{p_j}$ where the fractional powers $p_1, \ldots, p_m$ are selected from a small predefined set. Royston and Sauerbrei recommend choosing powers from among $\{-2, -1, -0.5, 0, 0.5, 1, 2, 3\}$, with X^0 corresponding to $\ln(X)$(48). Powers are allowed to repeat in fractional polynomials; each time a power repeats, it is multiplied by another $\ln(X)$. For example, if power 3 is selected twice, X^3 and $X^3\ln(X)$ are used. Automated procedures in statistical software test all possible transformations of degree m to select the most appropriate transformation(s) for the data (see Section 3.6). Usually an m of 1 or 2 will suffice.

Sauerbrei et al. (50) examine the prognostic value of age for recurrence-free survival in node-positive breast cancer patients, and show that assuming a linear association for age does not reveal any prognostic effect. Similarly, categorizing age into three groups barely reveals any discrepancy in risk. However, when allowing for a non-linear relationship using fractional polynomials, there is strong and statistically significant evidence that patients have an increased risk up to an age of about forty; then, after a fairly constant risk between forty and fifty years, the risk increases again with ages over fifty-five years.

Often restricted cubic splines and fractional polynomials give similar results (51), though in some situations fractional polynomials better recover

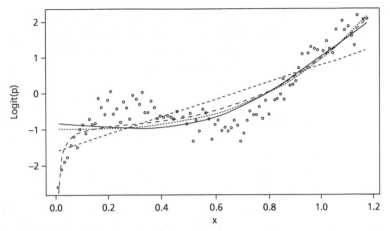

solid line: prognostic effect modelled using restricted cubic splines with three internal knots
dashed line: prognostic effect assumed; linear
dotted line: prognostic effect modelled using FPs with $m = 1$ (selected: $p_1 = 3$)
dash-dot line: prognostic effect modelled using FPs with $m = 2$ (selected: $p_1 = -1$ and $p_2 = 3$)

Figure 3.9 Comparison of fitted trends between a continuous predictor (X) and the logit transformed outcome risk (logit(p)), using restricted cubic splines and fractional polynomials (FPs).
Source: reproduced courtesy of Richard D. Riley

simpler non-linear trends, whereas splines better recover more complex trends (51). Figure 3.9 illustrates their use for a hypothetical dataset where the effect is clearly non-linear and complex. The fitted trend is very similar when either splines or fractional polynomials are used, with the only clear discrepancy in the extreme far-left of the plot when using fractional polynomial with m of 2, which may reflect overfitting. To limit the play of chance, replication of such non-linear trends is important across multiple confirmatory studies, for example in an individual participant data meta-analysis (Chapter 13) (52).

3.6 **Statistical software for prognosis research**

It is good practice for all analysis code and results to be independently validated before publication, for example by another statistician within the same department. Several statistical software packages are currently available to facilitate prognosis research. For instance, in R the default package 'stats' provides functions for standard regression modelling, and can thus be used to evaluate prognostic factors or develop multivariable prognostic models. For survival (time-to-event) models, the packages 'survival' (Cox regression) and 'flexsurv' (Royston-Parmar models) can be used. When considering penalization during model development, researchers may use 'rms' (PMLE) or 'glmnet' (LASSO and ridge regression). Alternatively, 'logistf' (logistic regression) or 'coxphf' (Cox regression) can be used to adopt Firth bias correction in small samples. Further, when considering modelling of non-linear effects, researchers may use 'mfp' or 'rms' for multivariable fractional polynomials or restricted cubic splines, respectively. The 'rms' package also incorporates functions for survival modelling, penalization, estimation of non-linear effects, calibration plots, and the assessment of (optimism-corrected) model performance. In Stata, many of the regression modelling commands are in-built, such as 'regress', 'logistic' and 'stcox' for linear, logistic and Cox regression models, respectively. The 'stpm2' command enables Royston-Parmar models to be fitted and can be installed from the SSC (Statistical Software Components) archive. To model non-linear prognostic effects, multivariable fractional polynomials can be implemented using 'mfp', and 'mkspline' used to create spline terms. For model performance, 'roctab', 'estat concordance' and 'stcstat2' estimate the C statistic for logistic, Cox and Royston-Parmar models, respectively, whilst the post-estimation module 'fitstat' computes a variety of measures of fit for many kinds of regression models. Calibration plots are possible using the 'pmcalplot' module.

3.7 **Summary**

The nuts and bolts of actually doing (and indeed, improving) prognosis research are heavily intertwined with sound statistical methods and principles. This chapter has given a detailed overview of fundamental statistical concepts and methods for prognosis research, which underpin subsequent chapters in the book. A summary of the key messages from this chapter is as follows:

◆ Statistical methods and principles form the bedrock of prognosis research.

◆ With continuous outcomes, linear regression is an important method for summarizing and predicting prognosis in terms of mean outcome values, and for deriving (adjusted) mean outcome changes to quantify prognostic factor effects.

◆ With binary outcomes, logistic regression is an important method for summarizing and predicting risk (probability) of outcome occurrence within a particular time period, and for deriving (adjusted) odds ratios to quantify prognostic factor effects.

- With time-to-event outcomes, Cox regression is a common approach for estimating (adjusted) hazard ratios to quantify prognostic factor effects, and for developing and validating prognostic models; however, as it avoids modelling the baseline hazard, it does not immediately provide absolute risks over time.

- Modelling the baseline hazard directly, for example using (flexible) parametric survival models, is advantageous for predicting absolute outcome risks over time.

- The predictive performance of a prognostic model can be measured in terms of overall fit, calibration (agreement between observed and predicted outcomes), and—for binary and time-to-event models—discrimination (separation of predicted risks between those with and without the outcome).

- Non-linear prognostic associations (trends) should be investigated between continuous predictors (factors) and outcomes, for example using fractional polynomials or (restricted) cubic splines.

References

1. **Ioannidis JP** (2014) Errors (my very own) and the fearful uncertainty of numbers. *Eur J Clin Invest* **44**(7), 617–8.
2. **Altman DG** (1991) *Practical Statistics for Medical Research*. London: Chapman and Hall.
3. **Harrell FE, Jr.** (2015) *Regression Modeling Strategies: with Applications to Linear Models, Logistic and Ordinal Regression, and Survival Analysis* (second edition). New York: Springer.
4. **Steyerberg EW** (2009) *Clinical Prediction Models: A Practical Approach to Development, Validation, and Updating*. New York: Springer.
5. **Henschke N, Ostelo RW, Terwee CB**, et al. (2012) Identifying generic predictors of outcome in patients presenting to primary care with nonspinal musculoskeletal pain. *Arthritis Care Res (Hoboken)* **64**(8), 1217–24.
6. **McMinn DJ, Snell KI, Daniel J**, et al. (2012) Mortality and implant revision rates of hip arthroplasty in patients with osteoarthritis: registry based cohort study. *BMJ* **344**, e3319.
7. **Snell KIE** (2015) Development and application of statistical methods for prognosis research (PhD Thesis). University of Birmingham.
8. **Collett D** (2014) *Modelling Survival Data in Medical Research* (third edition). London: Chapman and Hall/CRC.
9. **Kaplan EL** and **Meier P** (1958) Nonparametric estimation from incomplete observations. *J Am Stat Assoc* **53**(282), 457–81.
10. **Lambert PC, Dickman PW, Nelson CP**, et al. (2010) Estimating the crude probability of death due to cancer and other causes using relative survival models. *Stat Med* **29**, 885–95.

11. **Weibull W** (1951) A statistical distribution function of wide applicability. *J App Mech* **18**, 293–97.

12. **Box GEP** and **Draper NR** (1987) *Empirical Model-Building and Response Surfaces.* Oxford: Wiley. p. 424.

13. **Vavrek D, Haas M, Neradilek MB**, et al. (2015) Prediction of pain outcomes in a randomized controlled trial of dose-response of spinal manipulation for the care of chronic low back pain. *BMC Musculoskelet Disord* **16**, 205.

14. **Zou G** (2004) A modified poisson regression approach to prospective studies with binary data. *Am J Epidemiol* **159**(7), 702–6.

15. **Barros AJ** and **Hirakata VN** (2003) Alternatives for logistic regression in cross-sectional studies: an empirical comparison of models that directly estimate the prevalence ratio. *BMC Med Res Methodol* **3**, 21.

16. **Elia EG, Robb AO, Hemming K**, et al. (2017) Is the first urinary albumin/creatinine ratio (ACR) in women with suspected preeclampsia a prognostic factor for maternal and neonatal adverse outcome? A retrospective cohort study. *Acta Obstetricia et Gynecologica Scandinavica* **96**(5), 580–88.

17. **Greenland S, Mansournia MA**, and **Altman DG** (2016) Sparse data bias: a problem hiding in plain sight. *BMJ* **352**, i1981.

18. **Firth D** (1993) Bias reduction of maximum likelihood estimates. *Biometrika* **80**(1), 27–38.

19. **van Smeden M, de Groot JA, Moons KG**, et al. (2016) No rationale for one variable per ten events criterion for binary logistic regression analysis. *BMC Med Res Methodol* **16**(1), 163.

20. **Puhr R, Heinze G, Nold M**, et al. (2017) Firth's logistic regression with rare events: accurate effect estimates and predictions? *Statistics in Medicine* **36**(14), 2302–17.

21. **Casikar I, Lu C, Reid S**, et al. (2013) Prediction of successful expectant management of first trimester miscarriage: development and validation of a new mathematical model. *Aust NZJ Obstet Gynaecol* **53**(1), 58–63.

22. **Cox DR** (1972) Regression models and life-tables. *J Royal Stat Soc*, Series B **34**(2), 187–220.

23. **Thiébaut ACM** and **Bénichou J** (2004) Choice of time-scale in Cox's model analysis of epidemiologic cohort data: a simulation study. *Stat Med* **23**(24), 3803–20.

24. **Heinze G** and **Schemper M** (2001) A solution to the problem of monotone likelihood in Cox regression. *Biometrics* **57**(1), 114–19.

25. **Nelson W** (1969) Hazard plotting for incomplete failure data. *J Qual Tech* **1**, 27–52.

26. **Aalen OO** (1978) Nonparametric inference for a family of counting processes. *Ann Stat* **6**, 701–26.

27. **Royston P** and **Parmar MKB** (2002) Flexible parametric proportional-hazards and proportional-odds models for censored survival data, with application to prognostic modelling and estimation of treatment effects. *Stat Med* **21**, 2175–97.

28. **Lambert PC** and **Royston P** (2009) Further developments of flexible parametric models for survival analysis. *Stat Journal* **9**, 265–90.

29. **Royston P** and **Lambert PC** (2011) *Flexible Parametric Survival Analysis Using Stata: Beyond the Cox Model.* College Station, Texas: CRC Press.

30. **Rutherford MJ, Crowther MJ**, and **Lambert PC** (2015) The use of restricted cubic splines to approximate complex hazard functions in the analysis of time-to-event data: a simulation study. *J Stat Computation and Simulation* **85**(4), 777–93.

31. **Cox DR** and **Snell EJ** (1989) *The Analysis of Binary Data* (second edition). London: Chapman and Hall.

32. **Nagelkerke N** (1991) A note on a general definition of the coefficient of determination. *Biometrika* **78**, 691–92.

33. **O'Quigley J, Xu R**, and **Stare J** (2005) Explained randomness in proportional hazards models. *Stat Med* **24**(3), 479–89.

34. **Royston P** (2006) Explained variation for survival models. *Stata Journal* **6**, 83–96.

35. **Royston P** and **Sauerbrei W** (2004) A new measure of prognostic separation in survival data. *Stat Med* **23**(5), 723–48.

36. **Brier GW** (1950) Verification of forecasts expressed in terms of probability. *Monthly Weather Review* **78**(1), 1–3.

37. **Vickers AJ** and **Elkin EB** (2006) Decision curve analysis: a novel method for evaluating prediction models. *Med Decis Making* **26**(6), 565–74.

38. **Vickers AJ, Van Calster B**, and **Steyerberg EW** (2016) Net benefit approaches to the evaluation of prediction models, molecular markers, and diagnostic tests. *BMJ* **352**, i6.

39. **Altman DG, Vergouwe Y, Royston P**, et al. (2009) Prognosis and prognostic research: validating a prognostic model. *BMJ* **338**, b605.

40. **Van Calster B, Nieboer D, Vergouwe Y**, et al. (2016) A calibration hierarchy for risk models was defined: from utopia to empirical data. *J Clin Epidemiol* **74**, 167–76.

41. **Royston P** and **Altman DG** (2013) External validation of a Cox prognostic model: principles and methods. *BMC Med Res Methodol* **13**, 33.

42. **Harrell FE, Jr., Lee KL**, and **Mark DB** (1996) Multivariable prognostic models: issues in developing models, evaluating assumptions and adequacy, and measuring and reducing errors. *Stat Med* **15**(4), 361–87.

43. **Brentnall AR** and **Cuzick J** (2016) Use of the concordance index for predictors of censored survival data. *Stat Methods Med Res* 962280216680245.

44. **Yates JF** (1982) External correspondence: decompositions of the mean probability score. *Organizational Behaviour and Human Performance* **30**, 132–56.

45. **Durrleman S** and **Simon R** (1989) Flexible regression models with cubic splines. *Stat Med* **8**, 551–61.

46. **Nieboer D, Vergouwe Y, Roobol MJ**, et al. (2015) Nonlinear modeling was applied thoughtfully for risk prediction: the Prostate Biopsy Collaborative Group. *J Clin Epidemiol* **68**(4), 426–34.

47. **Sauerbrei W** and **Royston P** (1999) Building multivariable prognostic and diagnostic models: transformation of the predictors by using fractional polynomials. *J Royal Stat Soc*, Series A **162**, 71–94.

48. **Royston P** and **Sauerbrei W** (2008) *Multivariable Model-Building—a Pragmatic Approach to Regression Analysis Based on Fractional Polynomials for Modelling Continuous Variables*. Chichester: Wiley.

49. **Royston P** and **Altman DG** (1994) Regression using fractional polynomials of continuous covariates: parsimonious parametric modelling. *J Royal Stat Soc*, Series C (Applied Statistics) **43**(3), 429–67.

50. **Sauerbrei W, Royston P, Bojar H**, et al. (1999) Modelling the effects of standard prognostic factors in node-positive breast cancer. German Breast Cancer Study Group (GBSG). *Br J Cancer* 79(11–12), 1752–60.

51. **Binder H, Sauerbrei W**, and **Royston P** (2013) Comparison between splines and fractional polynomials for multivariable model building with continuous covariates: a simulation study with continuous response. *Stat Med* 32(13), 2262–77.

52. **Sauerbrei W** and **Royston P** (2011) A new strategy for meta-analysis of continuous covariates in observational studies. *Stat Med* 30(28), 3341–60.

Chapter 4

Ten principles to strengthen prognosis research

Richard D Riley, Kym IE Snell,
Karel GM Moons, and Thomas PA Debray

Evidence shows that methodology standards within prognosis research are often sub-standard (1–9). To address this, here we highlight ten principles that would strengthen the conduct, analysis, reporting, and implementation of prognosis research, building on the fundamental methods outlined in the previous chapter.

4.1 Implement protocols, analysis plans, and study registration

To improve transparency, identifiability, research standards, and reproducibility in prognosis research, all prognosis studies should have a protocol including details about the analyses to be conducted (10). A complementary analysis plan may be retained in-house, and updated over time if necessary, for example to deal with unexpected issues arising as the data is collected. Ideally studies are also registered and their protocols published.

Study registers hold an internationally agreed minimum amount of information about planned and ongoing studies, most notably of randomized studies. Given published empirical evidence about selective non-publication and reporting of prognosis studies (3, 11, 12), and unnecessary duplication of effort (13), registration of planned and ongoing prognosis studies should help to address these issues. Prognosis studies (see Chapters 5–8) can be registered in ClinicalTrials.gov; reviews of prognosis studies (see Chapter 9) can be registered in PROSPERO, and an accompanying study protocol can be published in an open-access journal such as *BMC Diagnostic and Prognostic Research* (14). Protocols describe the rationale, objectives, design (including sample size justification), methodology, statistical considerations, and organization of a study. A published or accessible protocol allows scientific peers (in principle) to replicate the study, and allows easier identification of, and access to, full study details, in order to increase opportunities for collaboration including systematic reviews and individual participant data meta-analyses. Peer review of a protocol also leads to improvements in methods, or identifies flaws, to ultimately improve study quality and analysis plans, such as the handling of continuous predictors, the approaches used for predictor selection and adjusting for model overfitting, and the estimation of treatment-covariate interactions (see subsequent items).

Importantly, study registers and protocols are not an attempt to halt exploratory prognosis research. Exploration of pre-existing and readily available data is an accepted and valuable part of current epidemiologic research practice. If a study is exploratory, this can simply be stated in the protocol, and post-hoc analyses noted in the final report.

4.2 **Do not categorize continuous predictors or outcomes**

'Categorizing continuous predictors produces models with poor predictive performance and poor clinical usefulness. Categorizing continuous predictors is unnecessary, biologically implausible, and inefficient and should not be used in prognostic model development.' (15)

It is well-documented that dichotomization of continuous predictors, such as age, blood pressure, and most biomarker values, is best avoided. Dichotomization requires choosing, often arbitrarily and via data dredging, a cut-point value to create two groups of individuals; those with values above the cut point are usually classed as high (or abnormal) and individuals below the cut point are usually classed as low (or normal). The usual argument for the approach is to aid clinical interpretation and maintain simplicity. However, it can rarely, if ever, be justified that an individual whose value is just below the cut point is completely different from an individual whose value is just above it. Furthermore, clinical decisions should be made on the absolute risk (probability) scale, not the scale of the continuous predictor itself, and as digitalization takes place in clinical practice, simplification of measured predictor values into categories is less often required.

Moreover, dichotomization reduces the power to detect genuine prognostic factors and deteriorates the predictive performance of prognostic models (4, 6, 16). In one example, dichotomizing at the median value led to a reduction in power akin to discarding a third of the data (17), whilst in another, retaining the continuous scale explained 31% more of the variability in the outcome than when dichotomizing at the median (6). Cut points of continuous predictors can also lead to data-dredging, in particular with 'optimal' cut points based on the data at hand, to minimize the associated p-value of the predictor (4). Such findings are likely to be optimistic, and are unlikely to be replicated in other data. They also hinder meta-analysis, as different studies are likely to adopt different cut points.

When continuous predictors are categorized into four or more groups, rather than dichotomizing, issues still remain regarding the number and placement of cut points, why those marginally below and marginally above cut points are considered different, and whether the range of values within the same group covers very different individuals. We recommend that continuous predictors are kept as continuous. Then, the association between predictor and outcome is either assumed to be linear (perhaps after some transformation of the data, such as a natural log transformation) or non-linear (see Chapter 3), as appropriate. A similar issue may arise for other non-binary predictors, such as ordinal (e.g. stage of cancer, pupillary reactivity) or nominal (race, ethnicity) variables. Such predictors may (arbitrarily) be entered into a model with two categories, rather than maintaining the original number of categories. Admittedly, this may be unavoidable if there are only a few participants (events) in particular categories, but otherwise is not recommended and every category should be retained instead.

Note that treatment-covariate interactions should also be examined as continuous variables where possible (e.g. when assessing whether age is a treatment effect modifier), and their relationship with the outcome may also be non-linear. Further, the dichotomization of continuous outcomes should also be avoided, as this reduces power and may lead to misleading conclusions too (18). For example, when a continuous outcome is dichotomized into normal and abnormal groups, Senn shows how within-patient variability (e.g. due to measurement error or random temporal fluctuation in the state of a patient) may lead to some individuals falling in the abnormal outcome category, even though in truth their outcome would (if measured repeatedly) have been in the normal category on average (19).

4.3 Focus on estimates and confidence intervals rather than *p*-values

'Overemphasis on hypothesis testing—and the use of p-values to dichotomize significant or non-significant results—has detracted from more useful approaches to interpreting study results, such as estimation and confidence intervals.' (20)

Current prognosis studies often focus on *p*-values to determine whether a finding is important. In particular, an emphasis is often given to those results with a corresponding *p*-value less than 0.05. In prognostic factor studies, a better approach is to focus on prognostic effect estimates (such as hazard or odds ratios, also known as predictor-outcome associations) and confidence intervals. For example, if a small study of a binary factor estimates an odds ratio of 2, with 95% confidence interval from 0.9 to 4.5, then the magnitude of the factor's prognostic effect is potentially large, even though the p-value is greater than 0.05. Conversely, in a very large cohort study, a binary factor's p-value may be highly significant, even though the corresponding odds ratio of 1.03 and 95% confidence interval of 1.01–1.05 suggest only a small prognostic effect.

Hypothesis tests are also problematic in the validation of prognostic models (e.g. the use of Hosmer-Lemeshow test of goodness of fit for logistic regression models (21)), where p-values are often used to determine whether the predictive performance of a model is acceptable. A better approach is to inspect the calibration plot, and to focus on the estimates and confidence intervals for pertinent measures such as the calibration slope, calibration-in-the-large, and O/E statistic (Chapter 3). For example, a large validation study may find the calibration slope is significantly different from 1 (i.e. p-value < 0.05), but the magnitude of miscalibration revealed by the estimate and confidence interval may only be small. Conversely, when the p-value is non-significant, the confidence interval for the calibration slope may be wide and thus calibration performance inconclusive.

Overemphasis on hypothesis testing and p-values also leads to overfitting in the development of a prognostic model (see Sections 4.4 and 4.5) (22). If predictors are selected based on their statistical significance, they are more likely to be included when their observed association with the outcome is on a random high. This leads to the apparent predictive performance of the model being exaggerated, and increases the need for penalization techniques to reduce the optimism (see next items).

Generally in this book we focus on a frequentist approach to statistical inference from prognosis research, as this leads to measures such as confidence intervals and p-values that are familiar to most readers. However, often a Bayesian approach is more helpful (23); in particular, it leads to probabilistic statements about the magnitude of a factor's prognostic effect (e.g. there is a probability of 0.85 that the factor's hazard ratio is > 1.2), and the magnitude of a model's predictive performance (e.g. there is a probability of 0.25 that the model's calibration slope is between 0.9 and 1.1) (24).

4.4 **Do not select predictors based on univariable analysis**

When developing a prognostic model, many researchers prefer to keep the included set of predictors to a minimum in order to reduce the complexity of the model when used in practice. This motivates their use of predictor selection methods based on observed predictor-outcome associations in the model development dataset. A common—but misleading—approach is univariable screening (25), where decisions for predictor inclusion in the model are based on p-values for observed unadjusted predictor-outcome associations (26). This is not a sensible strategy, as what matters is the association of a predictor with the outcome after adjustment for other predictors, since in practice the relevant predictors are used (by healthcare professionals and patients) in combination. For example, when developing a prognostic model for risk of recurrent venous thromboembolism, Ensor et al. found that the unadjusted prognostic effect of age was non-significant from univariable analysis, but that the adjusted effect was significant and even in the opposite direction in multivariable analysis (27).

Hence, when applying selection methods to remove predictors based on their observed association with the outcome in the development dataset, it is better to start from a full model that includes all potentially relevant predictors. Then, a backwards selection approach can be applied to remove seemingly unnecessary (non-contributing) predictors (28), based on adjusted estimates in the full multivariable model. This can still lead to overfitting and optimism, especially in small datasets. Appealing alternative approaches are elastic net and the LASSO, which also starts with a full model but simultaneously performs predictor selection and, if needed, penalization of each predictor-outcome association to address overfitting (see next item) (29).

Generally our preferred approach is to entirely avoid predictor selection based on observed predictor-outcome associations in the development dataset. Rather, the researcher then pre-defines a set of predictors (e.g. based on previous evidence and clinical acceptability) and includes them all in the model regardless of the statistical significance of their associations with the outcome (30). If the pre-defined set is still considered too large then, before estimating predictor-outcome associations, reduction could be based on collapsing correlated predictors into a single predictor or by removing predictors highly correlated with other predictors (31). Techniques such as principal components are useful for this purpose (32).

In prognostic factor research, automated selection methods can also be avoided, as the aim is not to develop a parsimonious model, but rather to examine how a new factor (or factors) add(s) prognostic value over and above other (established) prognostic factors. Therefore, a full model forcing in all the existing factors is needed to obtain the fully adjusted associations of the new factors of interest with the outcome.

4.5 Improve prognostic models through shrinkage and penalization

Traditional estimation techniques, such as ordinary least squares or maximum likelihood estimation, are usually adequate when the focus is on the prognostic effects of particular predictors, and the sample size is not small (33, 34). Surprisingly, however, such methods are usually not optimal when the focus is on developing a model for making outcome predictions in new individuals. That is, predictions of outcome risk (from logistic or time-to-event regression models) or outcome values (from linear regression) are usually optimistic (i.e. too extreme) for new individuals when based on regression coefficients obtained by traditional methods. This phenomenon is known as overfitting, and can be addressed by using penalization (shrinkage) approaches. Penalization techniques shrink (in fact, introduce bias in) the estimated predictor-outcome associations towards the null to reduce the variability of predictions in new datasets, thereby improving the mean-square error of the predictions. This apparent contradiction of improving model performance by introducing bias is also known as Stein's paradox (35). A related concept is regression to the mean. For example, in a logistic regression model the predictor-outcome associations (odds ratios) are shrunk toward 1, so that predicted risks in new individuals show less variability (i.e. pulled away from 0 and 1 toward the mean risk), and subsequently have lower mean-square error. The concept of shrinkage to minimize mean-square error corresponds to finding an optimal trade-off between bias and variance of estimates.

Figure 4.1 illustrates the need for shrinkage of a simple linear regression model. The expected shrinkage will usually increase as the sample size and/or number of outcomes decreases, as the number of considered predictors increases, and with the use of automated predictor selection procedures (see previous item). Unfortunately, many prognostic model development studies do not consider penalization techniques or shrinkage. Important approaches, including uniform shrinkage via bootstrapping, the LASSO, elastic net, and ridge regression, will be discussed in Chapter 7.

4.6 Quantify difference in treatment effects between subgroups

In prognosis research aimed to identify predictors of treatment effect, the intention is to identify genuine differences in treatment effect for individuals across different values of a particular predictor. A common error when doing so is to examine the significance of treatment effects in each predictor subgroup separately, rather than examining the *difference* in treatment effect between subgroups, that is, estimating a treatment-covariate interaction.

Altman and Bland consider this eloquently (36), showing a meta-analysis of fourteen trials of women aged on average < 60 years that gave a summary risk ratio of 0.67 (95% CI: 0.46–0.98; P = 0.03), which was statistically

Consider a prognostic model written as a linear regression model, which is of the form:

$$Y_i = \mu_i + e_i = \alpha + \beta_1 X_1 + \beta_2 X_2 + \beta_3 X_3 + \ldots + e_i$$

Two important points are:

(i) the model has the *observed* (continuous) outcome Y_i as the dependent response variable, but the mean (μ_i) is our desired response when making predictions for new individuals conditional on a particular set of predictor values; and

(ii) due to the residual error (e_i), the Y_i values are more spread out than the underlying mean values.

When estimating the unknown parameters on the right hand side of the equation, traditional methods (e.g. maximum likelihood estimation) are based on minimising the error between the predicted values and the observed Y_i values, and not on the error between the predicted values and the mean values.

To show this, consider that the mean (μ_i, for blood pressure say) for a patient is drawn randomly from a $N(110,100)$ distribution, and their observed blood pressure (Y_i value) is then drawn from a $N(\mu_i,5)$ distribution. Given a random sample of 100 such patients, and using maximum likelihood estimation to fit a linear regression of Y_i against μ_i (i.e. $Y_i=\alpha+\beta\mu_i+e_i$) then the estimated regression slope ($\hat{\beta}$) is approximately 1.

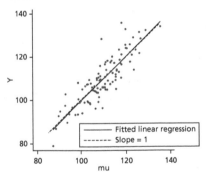

However, using the same dataset, if we rather fit a linear regression of μ_i against Y_i (i.e. we fit $\mu_i=\alpha+\beta Y_i+e_i$) then the estimated slope ($\hat{\beta}$) is much less than 1:

Figure 4.1 Graphical illustration of the need for shrinkage (penalisation) of regression coefficients to improve predictions from developed prognostic models.
Source: reproduced courtesy of Richard D. Riley

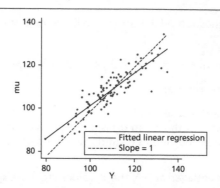

In a real dataset we do not know the true mean values, and can only fit a linear regression with Y_i values as the response. So we must anticipate that our estimated slope coefficients (i.e. $\hat{\beta}_1$, $\hat{\beta}_2$ etc) from a traditional estimation of a regression model need to be shrunk (and the intercept updated accordingly) to improve subsequent predictions of the mean outcome (μ) in new individuals. The expected shrinkage will usually increase as the sample size (and number of events for binary and time-to-event outcomes) decreases, as the number of candidate predictors increases, and with the use of automated predictor selection procedures based on p-values.

Figure 4.1 Continued

significant, and a meta-analysis of eight trials of women aged ≥ 60 that gave a summary risk ratio of 0.88 (0.71–1.08; P = 0.22), which was not statistically significant. These results might wrongly be used to infer that younger women experience a larger treatment effect. However, the treatment-age interaction estimate (i.e. the difference in log risk ratios) was -0.273, leading to a ratio of risk ratios of 0.76 (= $exp(-0.273)$) with a corresponding 95% confidence interval of 0.49–1.17, and a p-value of 0.2, indicating only weak evidence to support a differential treatment effect in younger and older women. A related mistake is to assume that the interaction would be non-significant if the two subgroups have effect estimates with 95% confidence intervals that overlap (37).

Another pertinent issue is that a treatment-covariate interaction may appear important when comparing odds ratios between groups, but is not when comparing risk ratios. This is because the treatment effect as measured by the odds ratio is dependent on the magnitude of the baseline risk (e.g. in the control group), and becomes less similar to the risk ratio as the baseline risk increases (see Chapter 3). When subgroups are defined by values or categories of a prognostic factor, they have different baseline risks. Therefore, when comparing treatment effects for two subgroups, their ratio of odds ratios may not be 1, even when their ratio of risk ratios is 1. This is well-illustrated by Shrier and Pang (38), and often referred to as the non-collapsibility of the odds ratio (39). The risk ratio scale may also be problematic as, unlike the odds ratio, its value is bounded. For example,a risk ratio cannot be greater than 2 when baseline risk is 0.5 or higher. Changes in baseline risk across subgroups may therefore lead to differences in risk ratios but not odds ratios, or vice versa; similarly a hazard ratio may be constant across covariate values, even when the risk ratio and odds ratio are not. In other words, treatment-covariate interactions may depend on the scale of analysis.

4.7 Use multiple imputation to deal with missing data

Missing values, for either predictors or outcomes, occur in all types of medical research (40). Arguably, prognosis research studies may suffer more from missing data than other types of medical studies as they are often based on data that were collected for other purposes. It is common for researchers to discard participants with missing data, and perform a so-called available case or complete-case analysis, such that statistical analyses delete any participants' data that contain a missing value on one of the analysed variables (predictors or outcomes). However, a small number of missing values in each of several predictors can result in a large number of participants being excluded from a multivariable analysis. Simply excluding participants with any missing data will always reduce sample size; but this lowers statistical power and precision to detect and estimate prognostic effects, and often leads to biased estimates as well (41). Available or complete-case analysis does not affect the validity of the results if the deleted participant records are a completely random subset of the original study sample. However, it leads to biased results when the excluded participants differ in (un) observed case-mix characteristics (i.e. in predictor or outcome distribution) as compared to the participants without missing values. Then, the sample with completely observed records has become a selective sample from the original study sample. Such selection bias will (likely) yield biased estimates of predictor-outcome associations and thus inappropriate prognostic models compared to what would be obtained if the whole dataset (without any missing values) had been obtained and analysed. Use of a separate category of a (categorical) predictor to indicate the presence of a missing value (i.e. the so-called missing indicator method) also leads to biased results in prognosis studies (42).

Regardless of the amount of missingness, it is thus mandatory to have a sense of whether participants with any missing data are a completely random subset of those with completely observed data. Authors should show the distributions (%, mean, or medians with dispersion measures) of the predictors and outcomes between the group of study participants with completely observed data and the group with at least one missing value for any of the study variables. If the two groups are similar for all study variables, a complete or available case analysis will not lead to bias, although will still be inefficient. Theoretically, the reasons for missing values may still depend on non-observed variables that may influence the prognostic factor or model performance estimates, but this is unlikely if the number of study variables, on which the two groups are found to be similar, is large. If the two groups are different, there is a strong indication that the completely observed participants are a selective subset of the original study sample. Instead of simply omitting individuals with any missing value or using the missing indicator method, authors should consider multiple imputation of the missing values based on the observed values of the other study variables.

Multiple imputation is advocated as the most appropriate method to handle missing data, as it leads not only to the least biased and thus most valid results, but also to the most appropriate standard errors and p-values (41). With multiple imputation one creates multiple copies of the dataset, with the missing values replaced by imputed values of that variable (predictor or outcome) drawn from their predicted distribution using the other observed data (i.e. other predictors and, crucially, also the outcome (43)). This assumes missing data are *missing at random*, that is, they occur according to a certain probability that depends on the observed data. As a result, missing values can be predicted based on the values of other observed predictors and outcomes. At least twenty copies are recommended (41), although a rule of thumb is for the number of copies (K) to be greater than or equal to the percentage of participants with one or more missing values in the dataset (44). In very large datasets (e.g. containing many thousands of individuals), this may be computationally challenging. Because variation in imputed values reflects uncertainty of estimating the predicted distribution, the analysis of multiple imputed datasets helps to acknowledge that imputed values are, in fact, unknown. Then, standard statistical analyses can be applied on each imputed dataset which in turn are combined using Rubin's rules to produce an overall estimate (and standard error) for each regression coefficient or measure of interest (e.g. C statistic or calibration slope when validating a prognostic model) that accounts for the uncertainty in the imputed values (45).

Multiple imputation can typically only use the variables that are included and thus observed in the study to impute missing values in that study. If data are likely to be missing only due to *unobserved* variables—which cannot be inferred from the study data itself—then multiple imputation cannot solve the problem of missing data. Such missing data are referred to as 'missing not at random'. In that situation, sensitivity analyses may be useful, to ascertain whether conclusions are robust when making different assumptions about the missing data mechanism.

It is also important for the statistical model used for multiple imputation to be consistent ('congenial') with the statistical model used for data analysis, as otherwise substantial bias may appear in the subsequent analysis (46). This implies that researchers should carefully consider which variables should inform the imputation model, and how their functional form should be specified. Problems may, for instance, appear when investigating non-linear relationships or between-study heterogeneity, without accommodating for this complex nature of the (missing) data during imputation (e.g. by assuming linearity and homogeneity).

4.8 Consider the potential for competing risks

In the analysis of time-to-event outcomes, competing risks refer to events which, if they occur first, prevent a primary outcome of interest from occurring. This issue is especially relevant when competing events are common, for instance in frail populations or studies with a very long follow-up. For example, consider the risk over time of a second hip replacement (revision) after receiving a first hip replacement. During follow-up if a patient dies then a second hip replacement cannot subsequently occur, and thus death is a competing risk. If patients with the competing event are simply censored at the competing event time, then the analyst creates an artificial world where only the outcome of interest can occur. This leads to inflated estimates and predictions of outcome risk, especially when the competing event is common.

This is illustrated by Wolbers et al. (47) for ten-year risk predictions of coronary heart disease in patients aged over fifty-five years based on three survival models: a standard Cox regression model (which wrongly censors individuals at their competing event time), the Fine and Gray model, and the cause-specific hazards model. The latter two models account for competing risks (48), and their predicted risks calibrate closely to the observed risks, but the predicted risks from the Cox model are systematically too large. For example, when defining 'high-risk' patients as those with a predicted risk > 20%, then the Cox model suggests 18% of the population are 'high risk' but the Fine and Gray model suggests only 8% are.

Thus, for deriving absolute risk predictions it is important to account for prevalent competing events, which Berry et al. define as: 'when the proportion of subjects experiencing a competing risk is equal or greater to the proportion of subjects experiencing the primary outcome, or when follow-up exceeds five years' (49). This rule-of-thumb is only approximate, and unpublished work (Teece et al., personal communication) suggests competing risks may be influential in other situations. An extended concept is multi-state modelling (48), and further explanation and illustration is given in Chapter 15.

4.9 **Use reporting guidelines when publishing prognosis research**

Transparent and complete reporting is important because meta-analysis, decision modelling, and clinical decision making rely on the available information being complete and not a biased subset. However, deficiencies in reporting in published prognosis studies are common (1, 7, 11, 12, 50–53), with omission of rudimentary results and methods such as the number of patients and events, the time points(s) for outcome prediction, the number of considered prognostic factors (predictors), and the estimated predictor-outcome associations with their confidence intervals.

Selective reporting is also a concern (4, 11). To address this, reporting guidelines should be adhered to. Reporting Recommendations for Tumor Marker Prognostic Studies (REMARK) provides guidelines for prognostic factor studies, with most items also relevant for overall prognosis studies (54, 55); TRIPOD provides guidelines for studies developing, validating and/or updating (extending) prognostic (prediction) models (56, 57); and Consolidated Standards of Reporting Trials (CONSORT) is pertinent for studies of predictors or subgroups of differential treatment effect (58, 59).

4.10 **Encourage reproducibility in prognosis research**

'Attempts to corroborate statistically significant subgroup differences are rare; when done, the initially observed subgroup differences are not reproduced.' (60)

Unfortunately, there is currently an overemphasis on identifying new prognosis research findings (e.g. by seeking new prognostic factors or by developing new prognostic models), rather than aiming to reproduce previous findings (e.g. about the prognostic effect of a particular factor, or the predictive performance of an existing prognostic model). Many seemingly 'novel' prognosis research findings will not replicate in new studies, due to the exploratory nature of the original primary study, and because analysis strategies often lead to chance findings and overfitting, as discussed above. Therefore reproducibility studies aiming to confirm or replicate the original findings, or to see if they generalize to different populations and settings, should be given more prominence and priority in prognosis research (3, 61–63). Notable examples are confirmatory prognostic factor studies (Chapter 6) and external validation studies of prognostic model performance (Chapter 7), or of predictors of treatment effect (Chapter 8). A growing opportunity for examining replication and reproducibility across multiple populations is an individual participant data (IPD) meta-analysis (see Chapter 13) (62, 64).

4.11 **Summary**

Adherence to the ten principles outlined would strengthen the robustness and translation of prognosis research findings in the medical literature. The items echo recommendations of previous methodology studies, systematic reviews, and empirical evaluations (1–3, 10, 11, 16, 50, 51, 53, 65–70), including those of the STRATOS (STRengthening Analytical Thinking for Observational Studies) initiative (70). We encourage researchers, reviewers and journal editors to embrace such practice.

References

1. **Mallett S, Royston P, Waters R,** et al. (2010) Reporting performance of prognostic models in cancer: a review. *BMC Medicine* **8**, 21.

2. **Steyerberg EW, Moons KG, van der Windt DA,** et al. (2013) Prognosis Research Strategy (PROGRESS) 3: prognostic model research. *PLoS Med* **10**(2), e1001381.

3. **Hemingway H, Riley RD,** and **Altman DG** (2009) Ten steps towards improving prognosis research. *BMJ* **339**, b4184.

4. **Altman DG, Lausen B, Sauerbrei W,** et al. (1994) Dangers of using 'optimal' cutpoints in the evaluation of prognostic factors. *J Natl Cancer Inst* **86**(11), 829–35.

5. **Holländer N** and **Sauerbrei W** (2007) On statistical approaches for the multivariable analysis of prognostic marker studies. In: **Auget J-L, Balakrishnan N, Mesbah M,** et al., eds. *Advances in Statistical Methods for the Health Sciences*. Boston: Birkhäuser. pp. 19–38.

6. **Royston P, Altman DG,** and **Sauerbrei W** (2006) Dichotomizing continuous predictors in multiple regression: a bad idea. *Stat Med* **25**(1), 127–41.

7. **Sauerbrei W** (2005) Prognostic factors—confusion caused by bad quality of design, analysis and reporting of many studies. In: **Bier H,** ed. *Current Research in Head and Neck CancerAdvances in Oto-Rhino-Laryngology*. Basel: Karger. pp. 184–200.

8. **Sauerbrei W, Holländer N, Riley RD,** et al. (2006) Evidence-based assessment and application of prognostic markers: the long way from single studies to meta-analysis. *Communications in Statistics* **35**, 1333–42.

9. **Schumacher M, Holländer N, Schwarzer G,** et al. (2012) Prognostic factor studies. In: **Crowley J, Hoering A,** eds. *Handbook of Statistics in Clinical Oncology* (third edition), Boca Raton, Florida, US: Chapman and Hall/CRC. pp. 415–70.

10. **Peat G, Riley RD, Croft P,** et al. (2014) Improving the transparency of prognosis research: the role of reporting, data sharing, registration, and protocols. *PLoS Med* **11**(7), e1001671.

11. **Kyzas PA, Loizou KT,** and **Ioannidis JP** (2005) Selective reporting biases in cancer prognostic factor studies. *J Natl Cancer Inst* **97**(14), 1043–55.

12. **Riley RD, Abrams KR, Sutton AJ,** et al. (2003) Reporting of prognostic markers: current problems and development of guidelines for evidence-based practice in the future. *Br J Cancer* **88**(8), 1191–8.

13. **Perel P, Edwards P, Wentz R,** et al. (2006) Systematic review of prognostic models in traumatic brain injury. *BMC Med Inform Decis Mak* **6**, 38.

14. **Moons KGM, Cook N,** and **Collins G** (2007) A new community for those involved and interested in diagnosis and prognosis. *Diagnostic and Prognostic Research* 1(1), 5.

15. **Collins GS, Ogundimu EO, Cook JA,** et al. (2016) Quantifying the impact of different approaches for handling continuous predictors on the performance of a prognostic model. *Stat Med* 35(23), 4124–35.

16. **Altman DG** and **Royston P** (2006) Statistics notes: the cost of dichotomising continuous variables. *BMJ* 332,1080.

17. **MacCallum RC, Zhang S, Preacher KJ,** et al. (2002) On the practice of dichotomization of quantitative variables. *Psychol Meth* 7, 19–40.

18. **Senn S** and **Julious S** (2009) Measurement in clinical trials: a neglected issue for statisticians? *Stat Med* 28(26), 3189–209.

19. **Senn S** (2004) Individual response to treatment: is it a valid assumption? *BMJ* 329(7472), 966–8.

20. **Gardner MJ** and **Altman DG** (1986) Confidence intervals rather than P values: estimation rather than hypothesis testing. *BMJ* 292(6522), 746–50.

21. **Hosmer DW** and **Lemeshow S** (1980) A goodness-of-fit test for the multiple logistic regression model. *Communications in Statistics* A10, 1043–69.

22. **Derksen S** and **Keselman HJ** (1992) Backward, forward and stepwise automated subset selection algorithms: Frequency of obtaining authentic and noise variables. *British Journal of Mathematical and Statistical Psychology* 45(2), 265–82.

23. **Bayes T** (1764) An essay toward solving a problem in the doctrine of chances. *Philosophical Transactions of the Royal Society* 53, 418.

24. **Snell KI, Hua H, Debray TP,** et al. (2016) Multivariate meta-analysis of individual participant data helped externally validate the performance and implementation of a prediction model. *J Clin Epidemiol* 69, 40–50.

25. **Mallett S, Royston P, Dutton S,** et al. (2010) Reporting methods in studies developing prognostic models in cancer: a review. *BMC Medicine* 8, 20.

26. **Sun GW, Shook TL,** and **Kay GL** (1996) Inappropriate use of bivariable analysis to screen risk factors for use in multivariable analysis. *J Clin Epidemiol* 49(8), 907–16.

27. **Ensor J, Riley RD, Jowett S,** et al. (2016) Prediction of risk of recurrence of venous thromboembolism following treatment for a first unprovoked venous thromboembolism: systematic review, prognostic model and clinical decision rule, and economic evaluation. *Health Technol Assess* 20(12), i–xxxiii, 1–190.

28. **Mantel N** (1970) Why stepdown procedures in variable selection. *Technometrics* 12, 621–25.

29. **Tibshirani R** (1996) Regression shrinkage and selection via the lasso. *J Royal Statist Soc B* 58, 267–88.

30. **Harrell FE, Jr.** 2015 *Regression Modeling Strategies: with Applications to Linear Models, Logistic and Ordinal Regression, and Survival Analysis* (second edition). New York: Springer.

31. **Steyerberg EW, Balmaña J, Stockwell DH,** et al. (2007) Data reduction for prediction: A case study on robust coding of age and family history for the risk of having a genetic mutation. *Statistics in Medicine* 26(30), 5545–56.

32. **Harrell FE, Jr.** (2015) Chapter 8: Case Study in Data Reduction. *Regression Modeling Strategies: With Applications to Linear Models, Logistic and Ordinal Regression, and Survival Analysis.* New York: Springer. pp. 161–80.

33. **Nemes S, Jonasson JM, Genell A**, et al. (2009) Bias in odds ratios by logistic regression modelling and sample size. *BMC Medical Research Methodology* **9**(1), 56.
34. **Firth D** (1993) Bias reduction of maximum likelihood estimates. *Biometrika* **80**(1), 27–38.
35. **Stein C** (1956) Inadmissibility of the usual estimator of the mean of a multivariate normal distribution. *Proceedings of the Third Berkeley Symposium on Mathematical Statistics and Probability* **1**, 197–206.
36. **Altman DG** and **Bland JM** (2003) Interaction revisited: the difference between two estimates. *BMJ* **326**(7382), 219.
37. **Austin PC** and **Hux JE** (2002) A brief note on overlapping confidence intervals. *J Vasc Surg* **36**(1), 194–5.
38. **Shrier I** and **Pang M** (2015) Confounding, effect modification, and the odds ratio: common misinterpretations. *Journal of Clinical Epidemiology* **68**(4), 470–74.
39. **Greenland S, Robins MR**, and **Pearl J** (1999) Confounding and collapsibility in causal inference. *Statistical Science* **14**, 29–46.
40. **Little JA** and **Rubin DB** (2002) *Statistical Analysis with Missing Data*. New York: John Wiley and Sons.
41. **Sterne JA, White IR, Carlin JB**, et al. (2009) Multiple imputation for missing data in epidemiological and clinical research: potential and pitfalls. *BMJ* **338**, b2393.
42. **Groenwold RH, White IR, Donders AR**, et al. (2012) Missing covariate data in clinical research: when and when not to use the missing-indicator method for analysis. *CMAJ* **184**(11), 1265–9.
43. **Moons KG, Donders RA, Stijnen T**, et al. (2006) Using the outcome for imputation of missing predictor values was preferred. *J Clin Epidemiol* **59**(10), 1092–101.
44. **White IR, Royston P**, and **Wood AM** (2011) Multiple imputation using chained equations: issues and guidance for practice. *Stat Med* **30**(4), 377–99.
45. **Rubin DB** (1976) Inference and missing data. *Biometrika* **63**, 581–92.
46. **Meng X-L** (1994) Multiple-imputation inferences with uncongenial sources of input. *Statistical Science* **9**(4), 538–58.
47. **Wolbers M, Koller MT, Witteman JCM**, et al. (2009) Prognostic models with competing risks methods and application to coronary risk prediction. *Epidemiology* **20**, 555–61.
48. **Putter H, Fiocco M**, and **Geskus RB** (2007) Tutorial in biostatistics: competing risks and multi-state models. *Stat Med* **26**(11), 2389–430.
49. **Berry SD, Ngo L, Samelson EJ**, et al. (2010) Competing risk of death: an important consideration in studies of older adults. *Journal of the American Geriatrics Society* **58**(4), 783–87.
50. **Kyzas PA, Denaxa-Kyza D**, and **Ioannidis JP** (2007) Quality of reporting of cancer prognostic marker studies: association with reported prognostic effect. *J Natl Cancer Inst* **99**(3), 236–43.
51. **Bouwmeester W, Zuithoff NP, Mallett S**, et al. (2012) Reporting and methods in clinical prediction research: a systematic review. *PLoS Med* **9**(5), 1–12.
52. **Rifai N, Altman DG**, and **Bossuyt PM** (2008) Reporting bias in diagnostic and prognostic studies: time for action. *Clin Chem* **54**(7), 1101–3.
53. **Mallett S, Timmer A, Sauerbrei W**, et al. (2009) Reporting of prognostic studies of tumour markers: a review of published articles in relation to REMARK guidelines. *Br J Cancer* **102**(1), 173–80.

54. **McShane LM, Altman DG, Sauerbrei W**, et al. (2005) Reporting recommendations for tumor marker prognostic studies (REMARK). *J Natl Cancer Inst* **97**(16), 1180–4.

55. **Altman DG, McShane LM, Sauerbrei W**, et al. (2012) Reporting recommendations for tumor marker prognostic studies (REMARK): explanation and elaboration. *PLoS Med* **9**(5), e1001216.

56. **Collins GS, Reitsma JB, Altman DG**, et al. (2015) Transparent Reporting of a multivariable prediction model for Individual Prognosis Or Diagnosis (TRIPOD): The TRIPOD Statement. *Ann Intern Med* **162**, 55–63.

57. **Moons KG, Altman DG, Reitsma JB**, et al. (2015) Transparent Reporting of a multivariable prediction model for Individual Prognosis Or Diagnosis (TRIPOD): explanation and elaboration. *Ann Intern Med* **162**(1), W1–73.

58. **Campbell MK, Elbourne DR**, and **Altman DG** (2004) CONSORT statement: extension to cluster randomised trials. *BMJ* **328**(7441), 702–8.

59. **Schulz KF, Altman DG, Moher D** (2010) CONSORT 2010 Statement: updated guidelines for reporting parallel group randomised trials. *BMJ* **340**, c332.

60. **Wallach JD, Sullivan PG, Trepanowski JF**, et al. (2017) evaluation of evidence of statistical support and corroboration of subgroup claims in randomized clinical trials. *JAMA Internal Medicine* **177**(4), 554–60.

61. **Debray TP, Vergouwe Y, Koffijberg H**, et al. (2015) A new framework to enhance the interpretation of external validation studies of clinical prediction models. *J Clin Epidemiol* **68**(3), 279–89.

62. **Riley RD, Ensor J, Snell KI**, et al. (2016) External validation of clinical prediction models using big datasets from e-health records or IPD meta-analysis: opportunities and challenges. *BMJ* **353**, i3140.

63. **Justice AC, Covinsky KE**, and **Berlin JA** (1999) Assessing the generalizability of prognostic information. *Annals of Internal Medicine* **130**(6), 515–24.

64. **Debray TPA, Riley RD, Rovers MM**, et al. (2015) Individual participant data (IPD) meta-analyses of diagnostic and prognostic modeling studies: guidance on their use. *PLoS Med* **12**(10), e1001886.

65. **Hemingway H, Croft P, Perel P**, et al. (2013) Prognosis research strategy (PROGRESS) 1: a framework for researching clinical outcomes. *BMJ* **346**, e5595.

66. **Hingorani AD, Windt DA, Riley RD**, et al. (2013) Prognosis research strategy (PROGRESS) 4: stratified medicine research. *BMJ* **346**, e5793.

67. **Riley RD, Hayden JA, Steyerberg EW**, et al. (2013) Prognosis research strategy (PROGRESS) 2: prognostic factor research. *PLoS Med* **10**(2), e1001380.

68. **Kyzas PA, Denaxa-Kyza D**, and **Ioannidis JP** (2007) Almost all articles on cancer prognostic markers report statistically significant results. *European Journal of Cancer* **43**(17), 2559–79.

69. **Sauerbrei W, Royston P**, and **Binder H** (2007) *Variable Selection for Multivariable Model Building, with an Emphasis on Functional Form for Continuous Covariates.* FDM-Preprint 98: University of Freiburg.

70. **Sauerbrei W, Abrahamowicz M, Altman DG**, et al. (2014) STRengthening analytical thinking for observational studies: the STRATOS initiative. *Stat Med* **33**(30), 5413–32.

Part 3

Undertaking prognosis research

Chapter 5

Overall prognosis research

Danielle A van der Windt, Harry Hemingway, and Peter Croft

5.1 Introduction

Chapter 2 summarized the PROGRESS framework, which classifies prognosis research based on four different types of prognosis questions, each of which requires a different approach to study design and analysis. This chapter will provide a definition and describe the basic design of *overall prognosis research*, described as type I fundamental prognosis research in the PROGRESS framework (1). Overall prognosis research provides crucial information for a wide range of stakeholders, including patients, healthcare professionals, policymakers, and researchers, and contributes to the understanding and definition of diseases and their expected consequences or course (i.e. outcomes). This chapter will explain the main aspects of study design of an overall prognosis research study, including the definition of startpoints and endpoints, and discuss the most relevant sources of potential bias that should be guarded against. We will also address the importance of evidence regarding overall prognosis for the design and interpretation of other types of prognosis research, and for the rationale, design, and consequences of research into diagnosis and treatment.

5.2 Overall prognosis

5.2.1 What is overall prognosis?

Overall prognosis refers to the most likely average outcome of a group of individuals with a certain disease or health condition in the context of available care. In the era of modern medicine it is unlikely for overall prognosis to reflect the natural history of a condition in isolation from any care or treatment at all. Overall prognosis may be influenced by self-management and lifestyle decisions, diagnostic investigations, referrals and treatment. It is therefore essential to interpret overall prognosis estimates within the context of the time and place of their observation. It is also important to realize that overall prognosis summarizes the overall outcome (or outcome risk) within the target population, averaged across all individuals with the startpoint of interest. However, outcomes (and outcome risk) are likely to vary across groups of individuals, due to, for example, variability in the distribution of age, gender, and spectrum or severity of the health condition across populations.

This means that overall prognosis research will draw on the same classic triad of time, place, and person that provides a structure for epidemiological descriptions of the incidence of disease in a specific population. For example, in a population-based cohort of children from Leicestershire with type I diabetes newly diagnosed before the age of seventeen years between 1940 and 1989, the overall prognosis was 30.6 deaths per 10,000 person-years of follow-up (2). This example highlights the importance of the definition of a startpoint or health state in the target population, as well as of time and place. Early identification of diabetes type I and healthcare provision for patients with this diagnosis may vary over time and between geographical areas.

Although overall prognosis is often expressed as an absolute probability (risk) or rate of an outcome (e.g. survival, complication of a health condition, or time to recovery), overall prognosis may also be presented as mean values on a continuous measure of the outcome. Figure 5.1 describes the course of pain intensity in people presenting with musculoskeletal pain in Dutch general practice,

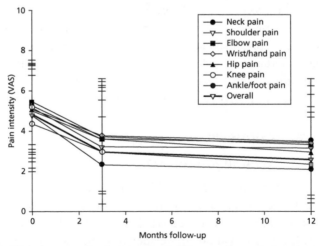

Figure 5.1 Clinical course of pain intensity (0–10) over 12 months in cohort participants (n=1,123) presenting with non-spinal musculoskeletal pain in general practice (The Netherlands, 2001–2002).

Source: reproduced with permission from Henschke, N. et al. Identifying generic predictors of outcome in patients presenting to primary care with nonspinal musculoskeletal pain. Arthritis Care & Research. 64(8), 1217-24. Copyright © 2012 by the American College of Rheumatology

who completed questionnaires at baseline, three months and twelve months follow-up (3). Overall prognosis in this study shows a very similar mean pattern of pain improvement, regardless of the location of pain at presentation.

5.2.2 **The importance of context**

As explained above, overall prognosis reflects the observed average outcome of a certain disease or health condition for a specific group of individuals (i.e. the startpoint in PROGRESS terminology) in a particular context (1). Overall prognosis research should provide sufficiently well-characterized estimates of prognosis in the target population group to allow investigation of variation in prognosis between relevant subgroups of individuals, in order to describe and understand differences between geographical areas, healthcare settings, and subgroups with different characteristics. Furthermore, in order to allow interpretation of estimates of overall prognosis in groups with a specific health condition, especially where the outcome concerns a measure of general health (including death or survival), estimates are often compared to or standardized against the occurrence of the outcome in a general population sample (e.g. relative survival, see Section 5.3.3).

Researchers also need to take into account that overall prognosis in a particular population may change over time, due to changes in:

- The nature and spectrum of the disease or health condition
- The content, quality, and effectiveness of care
- The populations being studied (change in case mix, e.g. distribution of age, co-morbidities, sociodemographic variables)
- The definition and recording of outcomes

For example, in 2009 Cancer Research UK published survival data for women with breast cancer diagnosed between 2002 and 2007 in thirty European countries (4). The results showed that five-year, age-adjusted relative survival was below the European average of 82% for the Central European countries, England, Wales, and Scotland (78–79%), whereas women diagnosed with breast cancer in other European countries appeared to have better overall prognosis (relative survival up to 87%). A subsequent analysis (5), investigating temporal changes in breast cancer mortality, showed wide variability in changes over time in breast cancer mortality, UK nations having larger relative reductions compared with other countries (see Figure 5.2). Large reductions in mortality were achieved in countries that combined high mortality in the late 1980s, high participation in newly developed nationwide screening programmes, rapid adoption and easy access to new treatments, and restructuring of healthcare services towards specialized breast clinics and multidisciplinary management.

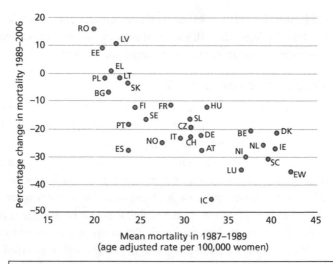

Figure 5.2 Percentage changes in breast cancer mortality in European countries during 1989-2006 according to the mean breast cancer mortality in 1987–9.
Source: reproduced with permission from Autier, P., et al. Disparities in breast cancer mortality trends between 30 European countries: retrospective trend analysis of WHO mortality database. BMJ (Clinical research ed). 2010;341:c3620. Copyright © 2010 BMJ

This example highlights the importance of providing context to the interpretation of estimates of overall prognosis, in terms of time, place, and healthcare provision, and shows how high-quality prognosis research can contribute to a better understanding of variations in overall prognosis and to the planning of healthcare service provision.

5.3 **Conducting overall prognosis research**

5.3.1 **Study design**

The basic design of an overall prognosis study is that of a cohort study, identifying relevant individuals with the disease or health condition of interest from a source population and following them up over time to collect data regarding the outcome of interest. Prognosis studies are ideally designed prospectively by developing a new bespoke cohort to investigate the prognosis of the health condition of interest. An example of such a bespoke prospective cohort study is an investigation of the prognosis of people with polymyalgia rheumatica (PMR) in primary care. The protocol for this study, including a detailed description of study setting, case definition, and recruitment processes (startpoint), and data collection regarding baseline characteristics, healthcare received (primary care consultations, diagnostic tests, medications, referrals), and outcomes over two-year follow-up, was published separately ahead of analysis and reporting (6).

The design of a prospective cohort study, including identification of potential participants, informed consent procedures, data collection, and long-term follow-up is expensive and time consuming. Access to electronic healthcare records and the availability of national registries, which are common in cancer, cardiovascular disease, and surgical interventions, have made it possible to design prognosis cohort studies using existing data. For example, a study using data from a UK cardiovascular disease registry (MINAP) linked to primary care data and national mortality data, investigated the risk of myocardial infarction and other cardiovascular outcomes in patients presenting with chest pain between 2002 and 2009 in UK primary care (7).

Prognosis studies based on data routinely collected in healthcare are much less expensive than prospectively designed cohort studies, make optimal use of existing data, and enable data analysis and reporting of results within a short timescale. However, researchers have to depend fully on the quality and completeness of available data to identify cohort participants, define startpoints, describe management over the course of follow-up, and extract data regarding outcomes. Important data may be lacking, for example regarding patient-reported outcomes, and the risk of selection bias and information bias is likely to be higher, as explained in Section 5.4. Use of electronic healthcare data in prognosis research is considered in more detail in Chapter 14.

5.3.2 **Startpoint**

The startpoint of a prognosis cohort is defined as: 'people with a certain baseline health state or condition'. Given the importance of context, a clear definition of the startpoint is crucial. This includes: (1) a clear case definition describing the baseline health state of interest, and (2) description of study setting, including time and place. The need for a clearly defined startpoint is just as important in a historical cohort study design when using existing data from routinely collected health records. In a study investigating the prognosis of heart failure in UK primary care (8), the startpoint was defined as: all patients recorded with newly diagnosed heart failure in a national primary care database (Clinical Practice Research Datalink, CPRD) from 1 January 1997 to 26 March 2010, with the definition of heart failure based on a pre-specified algorithm using a set of disease and symptom codes. People under thirty years of age (heart failure unlikely), or whose CPRD practices did not submit data for at least one year before the diagnosis of heart failure (prior data required to define new heart failure) were excluded from the study.

When investigating overall prognosis of a certain disease or health condition, researchers will aim, ideally, to identify a cohort of individuals in a severity stage or at a time point when estimating prognosis matters to individuals and their healthcare professionals in order to inform decisions regarding self-management, treatment, or referral. Individuals will not always present early in the course of their condition, or may not be diagnosed until the disease or health problem has already progressed. Therefore, prognosis cohorts are often defined from the moment individuals first consult in healthcare. In such patient cohorts, the duration of symptoms may vary widely. This is likely to impact on estimates of overall prognosis. When measured, such variability can be taken into account, and subgroups defined, for which separate estimates of overall prognosis can be provided. Nevertheless, defining a patient cohort based on first presentation or new diagnosis of a health problem can make it easier to specify the startpoint, and resulting estimates of prognosis may be more relevant to both patients and healthcare professionals.

5.3.3 Endpoint

Any health outcome considered important by patients, healthcare professionals, and researchers, can be examined as a potential endpoint in overall prognosis research. As mentioned in Chapter 3, binary and time-to-event outcomes are often summarized by a cumulative incidence (e.g. proportion of pregnant women developing pre-eclampsia during pregnancy) or as an incidence rate (e.g. number of outcomes per 1000 years of follow-up in women newly diagnosed with breast cancer), respectively, or for a continuous outcome a mean (or median) value is often reported (e.g. mean change on a patient-reported measure of physical function twelve months after first presenting in general practice with low back pain). When summarizing an outcome, researchers should clarify the associated time frame, and provide an accompanying measure of precision for the overall estimate (e.g. 95% confidence interval for an incidence rate, standard deviation for a continuous outcome).

Relative or standardized estimates of an outcome allow calculation of the expected impact of a condition on health outcomes in the population. In cancer, relative survival methods are commonly applied, which estimate the survival probability of people with a condition relative to the expected survival without the condition, obtained from national population life tables stratified by age, sex, calendar year, and other covariates (9). For example, by comparing the observed survival to expected survival in a comparable general population

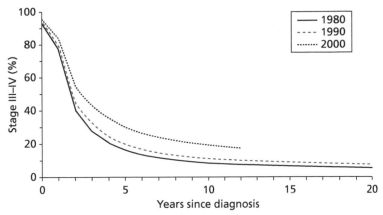

Figure 5.3 Cumulative relative survival among white women aged 50–59 years diagnosed with advanced stage ovarian cancer in 1980, 1990, and 2000 based on models adjusted for age, race, year of diagnosis, and time since diagnosis.
Source: reproduced with permission from Wright, J.D., et al. Trends in relative survival for ovarian cancer from 1975 to 2011. Obstetrics & Gynecologyl. 125(6), 1345–52. Copyright © 2015 Wolters Kluwer

sample, it is possible to estimate the excess risk of mortality due to a specific condition, and calculate potential gain from intervention.

Relative survival was used to investigate population trends over time in women with ovarian cancer in the US from 1975 to 2011 (10). Reductions in excess mortality were noted over time, illustrated by Figure 5.3, which shows notable improvement in cumulative relative survival for women with stage III or IV ovarian cancer diagnosed between 1980, 1990, and 2000, adjusted for age, race, year of diagnosis, and time since diagnosis. The excess hazard of mortality was lower for women diagnosed in 2006, ranging from 0.49 (95% CI 0.44–0.55) when compared with women diagnosed in 1975 to 0.93 (95% CI 0.87–0.99) when compared with women diagnosed in 2000.

5.4 **Potential sources of bias in overall prognosis research**

As in all research, when designing a cohort study to investigate prognosis, risk of bias needs to be taken into account. When investigating overall prognosis the main sources of bias are related to selection bias and information bias, and these will be discussed in more detail below. Several tools and checklists have been developed to assess methodological quality or risk of bias of cohort studies, or more specifically prognosis studies (e.g. Newcastle Ottawa Scale, CASP, NICE checklist, QUIPS, PROBAST). The Quality In Prognosis Studies (QUIPS) tool (11) or Prediction model Risk Of Bias ASsessment Tool (PROBAST) (12, 13) which were designed to assess the risk of bias of prognostic factor studies and prognostic model studies respectively, can also be used to assess risk of bias in overall prognosis studies, as different bias domains are scored separately. This makes it possible to only score those domains that are relevant for overall prognosis research (study participation, study attrition, outcome measurement).

5.4.1 Selection bias

To assess the risk of selection bias, one needs to judge to what extent the study sample is representative of the source population from which the study sample was drawn and which was specified to address the study question. In prognosis research, a clear definition of the startpoint (people with a given baseline health state, in the context of setting, time, and place) is important to make this judgement. In a prospective cohort study, bias can arise at baseline when potential participants are incorrectly identified, invited to or excluded from the cohort (*participation bias*), and during follow-up when cohort participants may withdraw or data on outcomes may be missing (*attrition bias* or *selective loss to follow-up*). It is not always easy to assess this risk of bias. It requires a judgement as to whether the study sample, either at baseline or by the end of follow-up, still adequately reflects the population of interest. The QUIPS tool or PROBAST offer guidance, and propose 'signalling questions' that can help to assess the risk of *participation bias*, for example:

- Is the source population clearly described?
- Is the recruitment period (time) and place of recruitment described?
- Are in- and exclusion criteria clearly described and appropriate, including diagnostic criteria or case definition?
- Is response rate among those eligible sufficiently high?
- Is there an informative description of the baseline study sample?

An overall prognosis study would be considered to have a low risk of participation bias if there is a high participation of eligible and consecutively recruited individuals with characteristics similar to those in the source population. This ensures that the probability or distribution of the outcome observed in the study sample is likely to be close to the overall prognosis in the source population. Conversely, a study would be considered as having high risk of participation bias if the participation rate is low, the study sample has a different case mix (e.g. different age and gender distribution) to the source population, a selective rather than consecutive sample of eligible individuals has been included in the study, and it is likely that participation is associated with the outcome of interest (11). For example, if people with less healthy lifestyle behaviours (smoking, more frequent alcohol use, less physical activity) are less likely to take part in a study investigating cardiovascular outcomes among patients diagnosed with type II diabetes, the study might underestimate the risk of cardiovascular complications due to the study sample being somewhat healthier than the target population of patients with type II diabetes.

Attrition concerns the loss of information during follow-up, due to cohort participants dropping out from the study or not providing data on the outcome by the time point of interest. The QUIPS tool and PROBAST propose signalling questions to assess the risk of bias related to *attrition*, including:

◆ Is response rate to follow-up assessment adequate?

◆ Are reasons for loss to follow-up provided and unlikely to be related to study outcomes?

◆ Are baseline characteristics described for those lost to follow-up?

◆ Are key baseline characteristics of those lost to follow-up similar to those remaining in the study?

A study has a low risk of attrition bias if the study sample at the end of follow-up (or at the time of measuring the outcome) is still representative of the original study sample. This will require high follow-up rates, or information that reassures the investigator that any loss to follow-up is unlikely to influence estimates of overall prognosis, with reasons for study withdrawal unlikely to be related to study outcomes, and the baseline characteristics of those lost to follow-up similar to participants remaining in the study.

The risk of selection bias, and this holds for both participation and attrition bias, is likely to be higher in historical cohort studies, where cohort membership is defined using existing data from available data sources. Investigators will have to depend on available data to define their sample, apply appropriate selection criteria and identify outcomes, which may not be ideal for their specific study question. Furthermore, awareness of outcome data in historical cohorts may potentially influence how individuals are selected into the study, increasing the risk of selection bias. For example, in a study investigating the prognosis of inflammatory back pain (spondyloarthritis), using data from patients included in a French multicentre (DESIR) cohort (14), participants with missing data on the outcome (poor function at two-year follow-up) were excluded from the analysis. Analysis of baseline characteristics indicated that those lost to follow-up were more often smokers and had a lower educational level. Further analysis showed that both smoking and educational level were strongly associated with poor function at two years in those remaining in the study. Even though the association between these prognostic factors and the outcome is still likely to be valid, overall prognosis (absolute risk of poor functional outcome) is likely to be underestimated in this sample, which included a smaller proportion of people with high risk of poor functional outcome compared to the full DESIR cohort.

5.4.2. Information bias

In overall prognosis research, the risk of information bias is relevant for measuring the outcome. In order to limit the risk of information bias when designing an overall prognosis study, investigators need to: (1) provide a clear definition of the outcome; (2) use methods to measure the outcome that are sufficiently reliable and valid; and (3) use the same outcome for all study participants. Poor methods for measuring outcomes may result in misclassification, leading to underestimation or overestimation of overall prognosis. The risk of information bias may be particularly high when outcome assessment is influenced by awareness or knowledge of baseline characteristics of cohort participants. Participants who are older and have more severe symptoms or more advanced disease at baseline are more likely to be classified as having a poor outcome than those who are younger or have milder disease characteristics.

An independent outcome assessment is more difficult to achieve when endpoints are based on subjective, patient-reported outcome measures, such as quality of life or activity limitations. However, this should not distract from the need to provide evidence on patient-reported outcome measures in overall prognosis research, given the importance to patients of information regarding the likely future course of symptoms and disease, and their impact on everyday life.

5.5 Importance of evidence from overall prognosis research

Estimates of overall prognosis from high-quality cohort studies provide simple, descriptive information regarding the likely course of a disease or health condition for a particular group of individuals. This type of evidence may at first glance have less appeal than evidence regarding prognostic factors (Chapter 6), prognostic models (Chapter 7), or predictors of treatment effect (Chapter 8), which may more directly inform clinical decision making and impact on health and disease outcomes for individuals. However, the importance of estimates of overall prognosis to patients, clinicians, and policymakers should not be underestimated, nor for the design and interpretation of other types of research.

5.5.1 **Informing patients, clinicians, and policymakers**

When individuals consult a healthcare professional or are diagnosed with a certain health condition, they commonly have questions regarding their prognosis: what is the risk of complications, how long will it take for symptoms to resolve, what are the long-term consequences, how can treatment improve my prognosis? Information on overall prognosis is important for individuals to understand the average outcomes in people similar to them, and for healthcare professionals to assess how best to inform and care for groups of patients with a particular disease or health condition. Despite this, patients and healthcare professionals have reported that prognosis is only discussed in a minority of healthcare encounters, suggesting that there are barriers to effective communication of overall prognosis, and that patients' information needs regarding prognosis are unknown (15, 16). Healthcare professionals will ideally have access to estimates of prognosis that take account of their geographical location, healthcare context, and characteristics of their patient population (case mix).

Information on overall prognosis (or outcomes of care) offers the opportunity to audit and compare services. This then sets benchmarks for quality of care in order to identify outliers, including high-performing services as well as services where interventions to support quality improvement may be needed. Figure 5.4 provides an example of overall prognosis research investigating variations in mortality in patients admitted with acute myocardial infarction. The results demonstrate that in the UK, compared to Sweden, there is substantially higher standardized (case-mix adjusted) thirty-day mortality rates for patients admitted with acute myocardial infarction, as well as greater variability in mortality between hospitals. Although there may be multiple explanations for these differences, the authors conclude that the results are likely to reflect the differing ability of nationwide health systems to improve the quality of care across all hospitals (17). This example shows how overall prognosis research can provide public health policymakers with data to model the population burden of diseases, and estimate the health gain to be achieved through healthcare delivery (1).

5.5.2 **Defining disease or health conditions**

A disease or health condition is often defined based on underlying pathology or cause of the condition (diagnosis), but this is not always possible or helpful in terms of clinical decision making. For example, for subjectively reported illnesses such as mental health problems or pain syndromes, a diagnosis may not always be possible, whereas an estimate of prognosis, based on symptoms,

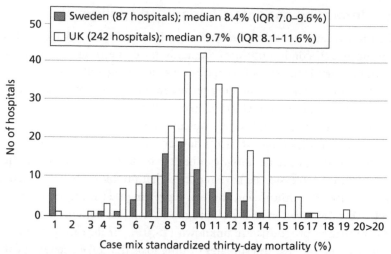

Figure 5.4 Example of overall prognosis research, investigating international differences in mortality rate within 30 days of admission in patients with acute myocardial infarction in the UK and Sweden.

Source: reproduced with permission from Chung, S.C., et al. Comparison of hospital variation in acute myocardial infarction care and outcome between Sweden and United Kingdom: population based cohort study using nationwide clinical registries. BMJ (Clinical research ed). 2015;351:h3913. Copyright © 2015 BMJ

signs, and other patient characteristics may be feasible and inform decisions regarding treatment or referral. In low back pain, diagnostic imaging (radiography, magnetic resonance imaging, computed tomography) has contributed little to understanding the prognosis of most back pain (18, 19), and randomized clinical trials have indicated that referral for lumbar spine radiography in primary care is associated with increased health costs, but does not lead to reductions in pain or improvement in function (20, 21). Investigation of long-term back pain trajectories, on the other hand, has identified patient groups with variable overall prognosis (recovering, mild, fluctuating, severe-chronic) and increasing complexity of their pain problem (22). Identification of clinically important groups of individuals based on overall prognosis supports a prognostic definition of back pain rather than classification based on imaging findings or current episode duration (acute versus low back pain) (23). The low back pain example is discussed further in Chapter 10.

5.5.3 Importance of prognosis for diagnosis and screening

Diagnostic classification of a disease or health condition is important when it can inform clinical decision making and prognosis in individuals with that diagnosis (24, 25). Using the example of back pain, diagnostic classification, or the use of a diagnostic test, may not always lead to a better estimation of future patient outcomes. Therefore, when investigating the clinical utility of diagnostic classification, the added value of new diagnostic tests or procedures, or the clinical and cost-effectiveness of a diagnostic screening programme, evidence of impact on the overall prognosis of a disease or health condition is essential (26). However, the 'downstream consequences' of using diagnostic tests or procedures are not always investigated, with most diagnostic research focusing on the assessment of diagnostic test accuracy (sensitivity and specificity), rather than impact on patient outcomes (27).

A thorough understanding of disease course and overall prognosis is fundamental to the design and evaluation of a diagnostic screening programme, as illustrated by the controversy regarding the utility of prostate-specific antigen (PSA) screening for prostate cancer, which can have a mild, non-life threatening course in many men, and where screening might lead to overdiagnosis and overtreatment (28, 29). In order to decide on the opportunity and feasibility of screening, information is needed regarding the accuracy of the diagnostic test, but also regarding overall prognosis in individuals with the condition. This applies particularly to the time period (the detectable pre-clinical phase) from first measurable manifestations of the disease (here: changes in PSA) to the onset of symptoms and signs that may lead to individuals presenting and being diagnosed in healthcare without the need for screening. Conditions that develop and deteriorate quickly (poor prognosis) may be missed through screening, or require more frequent screening compared to slowly developing conditions, which may have a better prognosis. This also means that screening programmes are more likely to detect non-progressive or slowly progressing disease with no or weak life-threatening potential (length-time bias).

Once conditions are identified through screening, evidence on overall prognosis is essential to assess whether early identification and subsequent treatment actually leads to improved prognosis in the screened population. In the case of prostate cancer, prognosis should be measured in terms of relative (age-adjusted) survival (see Section 5.3.3), as early identification of disease may result in patients living longer from the time of diagnosis, without necessarily affecting mortality (lead-time bias). A simulation study investigating the potential cost-effectiveness of plausible PSA screening strategies for prostate cancer showed that screening may lead to a modest increase in life years, but that a gain in quality-adjusted life years and benefit in terms of cost-effectiveness was only achieved with conservative screening strategies (infrequent screening and additional tests and procedures only for those with high PSA levels) and in combination with a conservative management approach for those with low-risk disease

(30). This example illustrates the importance of evidence on overall prognosis for estimating the risk of lead-time and length-time bias, and assessing the feasibility and utility of diagnostic screening programmes.

5.5.4 Importance for interpreting value of prognostic factors and models

Without clear information on overall prognosis it is not easy to interpret the information arising from prognostic factor or prognostic model studies. If prognosis shows little variability at the patient level, and is either highly favourable or highly unfavourable in the vast majority of patients, results from prognostic tests or models may add little information. This is similar to the clinical utility of diagnostic tests, where the predictive value (posterior probability) of tests is unlikely to deviate strongly from the overall prevalence (prior probability) of the condition, if prevalence is either very high (e.g. > 90%) or very low (e.g. < 10%). Prognostic factors and models may offer more information and help to better discriminate between those with poor or good outcome, if prognosis varies across individuals.

For example, in 298 patients presenting with low back pain in primary care, a lack of improvement of back pain at multiple time points during the one-year follow-up occurred in 112 (37%) of participants, indicating variability in prognosis across individuals in this population (31). A history of previous episodes of back pain was strongly associated with poor outcome (odds ratio 3.92, 95% CI 2.39–6.44), discriminating reasonably well between patients with a low versus increased risk of poor outcome, as illustrated in Figure 5.5a, adding relevant information regarding the likely future course of back pain. Deriving an

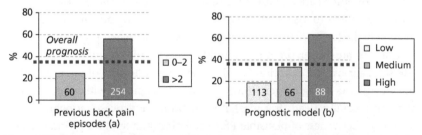

Figure 5.5 Example illustrating the ability to better predict the future likely course of low back pain using a single prognostic factor (a) or prognostic model (b), relative to the estimate of overall prognosis in the population.

Source: data from Jellema, P., et al. Prediction of an unfavourable course of low back pain in general practice: comparison of four instruments. Br J Gen Pract. 57(534):15-22. Copyright © 2007 Royal College of General Practitioners.

optimal prognostic model based on five clinical or psychological characteristics enabled stratification of the risk into three categories (C statistic for discrimination 0.72, 95% CI 0.66–0.79). Although considerable uncertainty regarding the likely future course of symptoms remains, the majority of participants could be classified as being at either low (n = 113, 19%) or high risk (n = 88, 64%) of poor outcome. The added value of the model is reflected by the difference between these predicted probabilities tailored to the individual and the average risk estimate that summarizes overall prognosis in the population (37%, see Figure 5.5b). Chapter 3 explained how to estimate and interpret measures of the predictive performance (discrimination and calibration) of prognostic models, and further discussion is given in Chapter 7.

5.5.5 Importance for designing and interpreting trials

When designing a randomized trial to investigate the effectiveness of one or more treatments, estimates of overall prognosis are important to argue the relevance of the trial question, as investigators will need to demonstrate the need to improve patient outcomes above and beyond their likely future course in the context of current care. If the overall prognosis in the trial population is good, or comparable to that for the general population, then the trial may be considered low priority for funding. Information on overall prognosis will subsequently inform the sample size calculation for the proposed trial: what is the expected (minimally important) difference in outcome between participants receiving the treatment of interest compared to the control arm? The control arm may receive a placebo intervention, but in many pragmatic trials the control arm will be offered treatment according to current clinical practice or guidance, allowing wider generalizability and more easy translation of trial results into routine healthcare. Accurate estimates of overall prognosis are therefore essential for a realistic and appropriate sample size calculation, as is demonstrated in Figure 5.6.

For a binary (or time-to-event) outcome and given a specific expected treatment effect size (here a risk ratio of 0.5), the required sample size per trial arm will strongly depend on the expected outcome risk (or rate) in the control arm. Overestimation of the outcome risk (rate) at the design stage may result in an underpowered trial that is unlikely to demonstrate the expected treatment effect with sufficient precision.

Once the results of a trial have become available, policymakers and healthcare professionals will need to understand the impact of the treatment effect in the population of interest, as this will vary considerably depending on overall prognosis. Table 5.1 illustrates how the absolute reduction in risk (risk difference) and number needed to treat for a specific treatment effect (stable risk ratio of

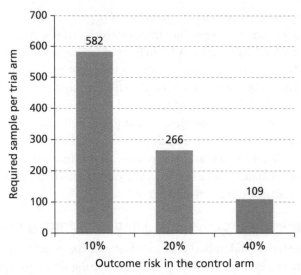

Figure 5.6 Required sample size per trial arm, given an expected risk ratio (RR) of 0.5 and increasing outcome risk (overall prognosis) in the control arm (significance level (α) = 0.05 and power (1-β) =0.90).
Source: reproduced courtesy of Danielle van der Windt

0.5) varies with the probability of the outcome in the population. Together with costs, potential harm, and acceptability of the treatment, this will influence decisions regarding the implementation or reimbursement of the treatment. Investigators may be inclined to conduct trials in populations with relatively high event rates (e.g. in secondary care rather than primary care settings), as smaller sample sizes may be required, and/or larger absolute effects may be achieved. However, when translating results of trials to a different context and to populations with potentially different overall prognosis, it is important to consider implications in terms of wider applicability and benefit of the treatment.

Table 5.1 Illustration of how the impact (risk difference, NNT) of a specific treatment effect (risk ratio 0.5) can vary depending on overall prognosis in the population of interest.

Target population	Outcome risk (overall prognosis)	Risk ratio (RR)	Risk difference (RD)	Number needed to treat (NNT)
Low risk	0.05	0.5	0.025	40
Medium risk	0.20	0.5	0.10	10
High risk	0.40	0.5	0.20	5

Source: reproduced courtesy of Danielle van der Windt.

5.6 **Summary**

In this chapter we have defined overall prognosis as the average future outcome in people with a certain disease or health condition (startpoint), emphasizing the importance of estimating prognosis in the context of current diagnostic and treatment practices. The essential components of the design of an overall prognosis study have been described and the main potential sources of bias (selection bias and information bias) have been discussed. Although overall prognosis research is descriptive in nature, we have argued that information regarding overall prognosis is central to healthcare: from a basic understanding of the categories we choose to call disease, through to understanding how variations in healthcare may influence individual health outcomes. We have illustrated the importance of obtaining estimates of overall prognosis to inform individuals, healthcare professionals, and policymakers, and for understanding the utility of prognostic factors and prognostic models. We have demonstrated why accurate estimates of overall prognosis are essential to arguing the case for designing a trial, to calculating the required sample size of a trial, and to understanding the results of a trial in terms of generalizability and population impact.

5.6.1 **Summary points**

- Overall prognosis research investigates the average outcomes of people with a certain disease or health condition in the context, time and setting of current healthcare.

- Estimates of overall prognosis can be expressed in several ways, depending on the definition of the outcome (endpoint), and may include absolute measures (e.g. average outcome risk or mean outcome value at a specific future time point) or relative measures (e.g. mortality rate relative to that expected in a general population).

- The basic design of an overall prognosis study is a prospective or historical cohort, with a clearly defined startpoint (i.e. a disease or health condition in the context of time, place, and available healthcare). Cohorts may be established as part of a newly designed prospective study, but are increasingly identified from routinely collected electronic healthcare data or disease registries, as long as sufficient data are available to define appropriate start and endpoints.

- Information regarding overall prognosis is important: for people to understand the average outcomes of their condition and to be able to plan their life activities; for healthcare professionals to consider need for treatment or referral to subsequent care; for policymakers to plan resources and monitor quality of care; and for funders to prioritize conditions and people whose overall prognosis requires most improvement.

♦ Estimates of overall prognosis inform the design of other types of prognosis research, such as prognostic factor research, prognostic model research, and research to identify predictors of treatment effect.

♦ Estimates of overall prognosis are crucial to understand the relevance of diagnostic or disease classifications, and the consequences of introducing new diagnostic tests and procedures.

♦ Overall prognosis may identify unanticipated benefits or harms of treatment, clarify where new interventions are required to improve prognosis, and inform the design of clinical trials.

References

1. Hemingway H, Croft P, Perel P, Hayden JA, Abrams K, Timmis A, et al. (2013) Prognosis research strategy (PROGRESS) 1: a framework for researching clinical outcomes. *BMJ* 346, e5595.

2. McNally PG, Raymond NT, Burden ML, Burton PR, Botha JL, Swift PG, et al. (1995) Trends in mortality of childhood-onset insulin-dependent diabetes mellitus in Leicestershire: 1940–1991. *Diabet Med* 12(11), 961–6.

3. Henschke N, Ostelo RW, Terwee CB, and van der Windt DA (2012) Identifying generic predictors of outcome in patients presenting to primary care with nonspinal musculoskeletal pain. *Arthritis Care Res* (Hoboken) 64(8), 1217–24.

4. Cancer Research UK (2017) Breast Cancer Survival in the UK compared to Europe 2017 (available from: http://www.cancerresearchuk.org/health-professional/cancer-statistics/statistics-by-cancer-type/breast-cancer/survival#heading-Four).

5. Autier P, Boniol M, La Vecchia C, Vatten L, Gavin A, Hery C, et al. (2010) Disparities in breast cancer mortality trends between thirty European countries: retrospective trend analysis of WHO mortality database. *BMJ* 341, c3620.

6. Muller S, Hider S, Helliwell T, Bailey J, Barraclough K, Cope L, et al. (2010) The epidemiology of polymyalgia rheumatica in primary care: a research protocol. *BMC Musculoskelet Disord* 13, 102.

7. Jordan KP, Timmis A, Croft P, van der Windt DA, Denaxas S, Gonzalez-Izquierdo A, et al. (2107) Prognosis of undiagnosed chest pain: linked electronic health record cohort study. *BMJ* 357, j1194.

8. Koudstaal S, Pujades-Rodriguez M, Denaxas S, Gho J, Shah AD, Yu N, et al. (2017) Prognostic burden of heart failure recorded in primary care, acute hospital admissions, or both: a population-based linked electronic health record cohort study in 2.1 million people. *Eur J Heart Fail* 19(9), 1119–27.

9. Rutherford MJ, Dickman PW, and Lambert PC (2012) Comparison of methods for calculating relative survival in population-based studies. *Cancer Epidemiol* 36(1), 16–21.

10. Wright JD, Chen L, Tergas AI, Patankar S, Burke WM, Hou JY, et al. (2015) Trends in relative survival for ovarian cancer from 1975 to 2011. *Obstet Gynecol* 125(6), 1345–52.

11. **Hayden JA, van der Windt DA, Cartwright JL, Cote P,** and **Bombardier C** (2013) Assessing bias in studies of prognostic factors. *Ann Intern Med* **158**(4), 280–6.

12. **Wolff RF, Riley RD, Whiting PF, Westwood M, Collins GS, Reitsma JB,** et al., **on behalf of the PROBAST group** (2019) PROBAST: a tool to assess the risk of bias and applicability of prediction model studies. *Ann Int Med* (in press).

13. **Moons KGM, Wolff RF, Riley RD, Whiting PF, Westwood M, Collins GS,** et al., **on behalf of the PROBAST group** (2019) PROBAST: a tool to assess the risk of bias and applicability of prediction model studies—explanation and elaboration. *Ann Int Med* (in press).

14. **Lukas C, Dougados M,** and **Combe B** (2016) Factors associated with a bad functional prognosis in early inflammatory back pain: results from the DESIR cohort. *RMD Open* **2**(1), e000204.

15. **Mallen CD, Peat G, Porcheret M,** and **Croft P** (2007) The prognosis of joint pain in the older patient: general practitioners' views on discussing and estimating prognosis. *Eur J Gen Pract* **13**(3), 166–8.

16. **Mallen CD** and **Peat G** (2009) Discussing prognosis with older people with musculoskeletal pain: a cross-sectional study in general practice. *BMC Fam Pract* **10**, 50.

17. **Chung SC, Sundstrom J, Gale CP, James S, Deanfield J, Wallentin L,** et al. (2015) Comparison of hospital variation in acute myocardial infarction care and outcome between Sweden and United Kingdom: population based cohort study using nationwide clinical registries. *BMJ* **351**, h3913.

18. **de Schepper EI, Koes BW, Oei EH, Bierma-Zeinstra SM,** and **Luijsterburg PA** (2016) The added prognostic value of MRI findings for recovery in patients with low back pain in primary care: a one-year follow-up cohort study. *Eur Spine J* **25**(4), 1234–41.

19. **Chou R** and **Shekelle P** (2010) Will this patient develop persistent disabling low back pain? *JAMA* **303**(13), 1295–302.

20. **Kerry S, Hilton S, Dundas D, Rink E,** and **Oakeshott P** (2002) Radiography for low back pain: a randomised controlled trial and observational study in primary care. *Br J Gen Pract* **52**(479), 469–74.

21. **Kendrick D, Fielding K, Bentley E, Miller P, Kerslake R,** and **Pringle M** (2001) The role of radiography in primary care patients with low back pain of at least six weeks duration: a randomised (unblinded) controlled trial. *Health Technol Assess* **5**(30), 1–69.

22. **Dunn KM, Campbell P,** and **Jordan KP** (2013) Long-term trajectories of back pain: cohort study with seven-year follow-up. *BMJ Open* **3**(12), e003838.

23. **Kongsted A, Kent P, Axen I, Downie AS,** and **Dunn KM** (2016) What have we learned from ten years of trajectory research in low back pain? *BMC Musculoskelet Disord* **17**, 220.

24. **Dinant GJ, Buntinx FF,** and **Butler CC** (2007) The necessary shift from diagnostic to prognostic research. *BMC Fam Pract* **8**, 53.

25. **Croft P, Altman DG, Deeks JJ, Dunn KM, Hay AD, Hemingway H,** et al. (2015) The science of clinical practice: disease diagnosis or patient prognosis? Evidence about 'what is likely to happen' should shape clinical practice. *BMC Med* **13**, 20.

26. **Lord SJ, Irwig L,** and **Bossuyt PMM** (2009) Using the principles of randomized controlled trial design to guide test evaluation. *Medical Decision Making* **29**(5), E1–E12.

27. **Staub LP, Dyer S, Lord SJ,** and **Simes RJ** (2012) Linking the evidence: intermediate outcomes in medical test assessments. *Int J Technol Assess Health Care* **28**(1), 52–8.

27. **Kim EH** and **Andriole GL** (2015) Prostate-specific antigen-based screening: controversy and guidelines. *BMC Med* 13, 61.

29. **Guessous I, Cullati S, Fedewa SA, Burton-Jeangros C, Courvoisier DS, Manor O**, et al. (2016) Prostate cancer screening in Switzerland: 20-year trends and socioeconomic disparities. *Prev Med* 82, 83–91.

30. **Roth JA, Gulati R, Gore JL, Cooperberg MR**, and **Etzioni R** (2106). Economic analysis of prostate-specific antigen screening and selective treatment strategies. *JAMA Oncol* 2(7), 890–8.

31. **Jellema P, van der Windt DA, van der Horst HE, Stalman WA**, and **Bouter LM** (2007) Prediction of an unfavourable course of low back pain in general practice: comparison of four instruments. *Br J Gen Pract* 57(534), 15–22.

Chapter 6

Prognostic factor research

Richard D Riley, Karel GM Moons,
Jill A Hayden, Willi Sauerbrei, and
Douglas G Altman[†]

6.1 Introduction

The previous chapter outlined the importance of examining the overall prognosis in clinically relevant populations defined by, for example, diagnosis of a particular disease or health condition in the context of current care. However, an individual's prognosis may be very different from the overall (average) prognosis, and this motivates research to identify factors that are associated with differences in prognosis across individuals. We call this *prognostic factor research*.

A prognostic factor is any variable that, among people with a given health condition (i.e. a startpoint), is associated with (the risk of) a subsequent clinical outcome (i.e. an endpoint). Different values (or categories) of a prognostic factor are associated with a better or worse prognosis. For example, in many cancers tumour grade at the time of histological diagnosis is a prognostic factor because it is associated with time to subsequent disease recurrence or death. This is illustrated in Figure 6.1, where the clearly distinct survival curves, the unadjusted hazard ratio estimates greater than one, and the finding of a significant log-rank test result (p = 0.01) suggest tumour grade is a prognostic factor for recurrence or mortality in breast cancer patients treated with tamoxifen (1, 2). Each grade represents a group of patients with a different average prognosis. In this way, the overall prognosis for the whole clinical population (here defined by having breast cancer and receiving tamoxifen treatment) is broken down into relevant strata, thereby enhancing the prognostic information available for clinicians and their patients.

Other names for prognostic factors include *prognostic variables, prognostic indicators, prognostic determinants*, or *predictors*. Indeed, the labels used are often inconsistent both within and across disease fields. In cancer, prognostic factors are usually referred to as prognostic markers to address factors that are associated with outcomes (prognosis) of untreated individuals, whereas the

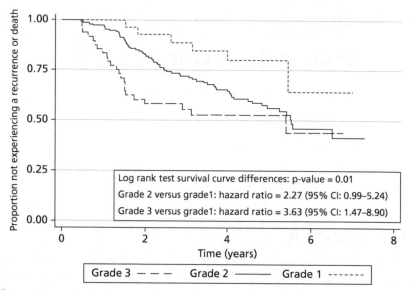

Figure 6.1 Unadjusted, Kaplan-Meier disease-free survival curves for three groups of breast cancer patients defined by tumour grade status (1, 2 or 3), (Schumacher et al., 1994) derived from a study involving 246 breast cancer patients treated with tamoxifen (with a total of 94 cancer recurrences or deaths over a possible 7 years of follow up).

Source: reproduced from Riley, R.D., et al. Prognosis Research Strategy (PROGRESS) 2: prognostic factor research. PLoS Med.10(2):e1001380. Copyright © 2013 Riley et al. Open Access.

term *predictive* markers is typically used for factors that are associated with differential treatment effects (see Chapter 7). However, this distinction (prognostic versus predictive) is not explicitly used in other clinical areas. We here prefer the term prognostic factors, as this is more inclusive and reinforces the idea that many prognostic factors are not biomarkers, may predict the outcome of untreated and treated individuals, and are not necessarily causally related to an outcome. Two related terms are *risk factors* and *confounders*. Risk factors usually refer to exposures that are causally associated with the onset of a disease, although the term is also sometimes used when considering whether a specific factor is causally related to subsequent outcomes after disease onset. Confounders, for example within observational studies that aim to examine intervention effects, are essentially prognostic factors that distort the true relationship between a particular intervention and outcome when that factor's values are not balanced between those receiving the intervention or not.

Prognostic factor research aims to identify factors that are associated with differences in prognosis, and how such factors can be used to improve patient or treatment outcomes. Thousands of prognostic factor studies are published each year, and it is undoubtedly the most common form of prognosis research. A crude search of the PubMed database for articles with the terms 'prognostic factor' or 'prognostic marker' in the title or abstract shows an exponential growth observed over time, with over four thousand articles per year from 2015 onwards (Figure 6.2). Given the inconsistent nomenclature in prognostic factor research (2), these numbers are likely to be a substantial underestimate.

Unfortunately, alongside this dramatic growth in publications, an increasing body of evidence has highlighted severe limitations in the conduct of prognostic factor studies (3–6): they are often poorly designed (7, 8), badly analysed (9, 10), and poorly reported (11–13). For these reasons, many published prognostic associations are at high risk of bias. Furthermore, few prognostic factor studies provide a clear message about the implications of their findings for clinical practice, randomized trials, or further research (2). Such problems are making prognostic factor research notorious in some disease areas. It has even been labelled as a 'playground' for researchers looking for significant *p*-values and quick publications to further academic careers (4, 14, 15). In cancer prognostic factor studies, Kyzas and colleagues suggest 'investigators may tend to conduct opportunistic studies on the basis of specimen availability rather than on thoughtful design' (16). Hemingway et al. refer to this as a 'what's in the

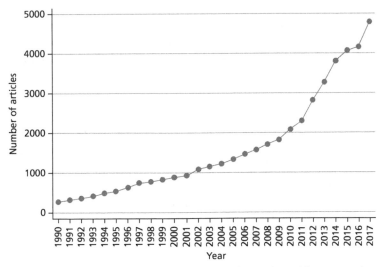

Figure 6.2 Number of citations identified in PubMed over time with 'prognostic factor' or 'prognostic marker' in the title or abstract (search conducted on 24th January 2018).
Source: reproduced courtesy of Richard D. Riley

freezer?' approach (15), in which the investigator apparently argues: 'given the data we already have, what abstract can be produced to allow a junior colleague to present at a conference?'

Though this state of play is worrying, in the remainder of this chapter we paint a more optimistic future for the prognostic factor field, by focusing on novel examples, clinical impact, and good research practice. We begin by focusing on the broad scope of potential prognostic factors to be researched, and outline why and how they may help improve clinical outcomes. We then propose different phases of prognostic factor research, that move from initial exploratory studies to larger confirmatory studies, to encourage a move toward higher quality and replicability of research evidence. Key guidance for conduct, analysis, and reporting is provided, and numerous examples are used throughout.

6.2 Types of prognostic factors

There are many different types of prognostic factors. Though often ignored amidst the drive for more complex or genetic measures, many simple and routinely collected patient characteristics may be prognostic, such as age, BMI, smoking, and blood pressure. For example, Ensor et al. identified that age and sex are prognostic factors for the risk of recurrence of venous thromboembolism following treatment for a first unprovoked venous thromboembolism (17).

In many diseases, the most researched prognostic factors are so-called biomarkers (3). Biomarkers include a diverse range of biological (including genomic (18), transcriptomic (19), proteomic, metabolomic), pathological, imaging, clinical, and physiological variables. For example, in children with neuroblastoma, elevated levels of MYCN oncogene expression are associated with a shorter time to recurrence and death (20). Symptoms, and behavioural and psychosocial characteristics, may also be prognostic. For example, in the field of low back pain, psychosocial factors, including maladaptive pain coping and co-morbid depression, and higher levels of functional limitation at clinical presentation are associated with worse outcomes (21). Co-morbidities are also well-known prognostic factors. For example, in patients with chronic kidney disease, co-morbidities are common and associated with a poorer survival rate, independent of other established prognostic factors (22).

Prognostic factors may also be measured outside the individual, at an ecological level (in which the exposure of individuals is inferred), such as area-level social deprivation, healthcare access and quality, and physical environment. For example, mortality and morbidity rates in patients with coronary heart disease vary by socioeconomic group (rates are higher in lower socioeconomic groups), and by geographical area (rates are highest in Wales, north-west

England, and northern England and the Yorkshire regions, and lowest in south-east England) (23).

Some prognostic factors are defined as amalgamations of two or more variables (potentially even hundreds of variables in high-dimensional settings such as omics research). For example, the stage of disease in cancer is associated with a worse time to death or recurrence, and is thus a prognostic factor. However, it is itself defined by other prognostic factors including Tumour size, Nodal status, and Metastasis ('TNM staging'). In chronic kidney disease, the urinary albumin/creatinine ratio is a prognostic factor for progression and thus the risk of adverse outcomes (24). Changes in variables over a period of time before the startpoint may also be prognostic. For example, in patients undergoing a thyroidectomy the percentage change in parathyroid hormone level (pre-surgery to six hours post-surgery) is suggested as a prognostic factor for subsequent onset of hypocalcaemia by forty-eight hours post-surgery (25). In hypertensive patients, the nocturnal fall in systolic blood pressure is suggested as a prognostic factor for cardiovascular event risk (26). More generally, an individual's pattern over time in a particular variable may be prognostic. For example, in patients with acute heart failure, a persistently high (defined by > 60 ng/m) soluble growth stimulation expressed gene 2 (sST2) level was found to be a prognostic factor for increased mortality risk (27).

The amount of variability in a characteristic over time may also be a prognostic factor. For example, in patients with previous transient ischaemic attack or hypertension, Rothwell et al. suggest that visit-to-visit variability in systolic blood pressure is a prognostic factor for stroke (28); specifically, the larger the variability in blood pressure over the previous few years, the larger the increased risk of stroke, even after adjusting for the mean blood pressure over time.

6.3 **Importance and potential use of prognostic factors**

Prognostic factors have a broad array of potential uses in healthcare and clinical research, as follows.

6.3.1 **Refining definitions of diseases and health conditions**

A fundamental role of prognostic factors is to aid or refine the definition of a disease or health condition (29), to provide average prognosis summaries for specific groups of similar individuals (30). Diagnosis of cancer is usually accompanied by the stage of disease, and specifically in breast cancer patients is usually classed as either HER2 positive or negative breast cancer. HER2 (human epidermal growth factor) is a protein that affects the growth of breast cancer cells, and thus high HER2 levels are prognostic for a worse outcome risk. Subsequently, patients are typically classed as either 'positive' or 'negative' HER2 breast cancer patients, with the former referring to those with a very high number of HER2 receptors which are likely to stimulate the cancer cells to divide and grow quickly. This dichotomization of continuous variables such as HER2 is sub-optimal, however (see Chapter 4).

Another example of a prognostic factor used to further classify disease is CD4 count. This was not initially included in the definition of AIDS, but with evidence that it was a strong prognostic factor (associated with a range of measures of disease progression) and biologically important, it became included in the diagnostic criteria for AIDS. We anticipate further classifications and subdivision of disease based on (multiple) prognostic factors in the coming years, especially with the use of genomics and evaluation of gene expression signatures (31).

6.3.2 Informing treatment recommendations and individual patient management

A single prognostic factor can be used to inform treatment choices. For example, considering HER2 and breast cancer again, treatments such as trastuzumab (Herceptin) have been developed to target HER2, and are thus used to reduce the risk of poor outcomes in HER2 positive patients (32, 33). In 2008, the use of drug-eluting stents in the treatment of coronary artery disease was restricted, by the National Institute for Health and Clinical Excellence (NICE), to patients with a specific vessel anatomy, as this was a key prognostic factor for the probability of restenosis (23). Patients with this anatomy had a worse prognosis and thus were considered to have a greater potential to gain from receiving drug-eluting stents than patients without it. Conversely, the identification of new prognostic factors may also widen the set of patients considered suitable for treatment, if they expand the group of patients considered at high risk.

6.3.3 Building blocks for prognostic models

To improve the accuracy of outcome prediction for individuals, multiple prognostic factors can be combined to form a prognostic model (34). For example, based on a logistic or Cox regression model, a prediction equation is obtained that is a weighted linear combination of multiple prognostic factors (a multivariable model; see Chapter 3). For example, a prognostic model developed to help identify patients with traumatic brain injury who are likely to have an unfavourable six-month outcome (35) includes the prognostic factors of age, motor score, pupillary reactivity, CT characteristics, and laboratory variables. Prognostic models for predicting individual outcome risk are being used in clinical practice, such as the GRACE score in acute myocardial infarction or the Adjuvant! score in breast and other cancers. They enable improved patient counselling, inform treatment decisions, and enable risk classifications which further subdivide patients into different strata based on their predicted risk. Prognostic models are considered in detail in Chapter 7.

6.3.4 Potential predictors of treatment effect

The current drive toward stratified medicine requires the identification of factors associated with more benefit or less harm from a specific intervention ('predictors of treatment effect', Chapter 8) (36). Prognostic factors (or prognostic models based on multiple prognostic factors) are natural to consider for this role. First, they identify patients at higher risk. Thus, if a treatment works equally well for all individuals, then those at a higher risk will benefit the most, as their absolute risk reduction due to the treatment will be largest. An example of a prognostic factor that also predicts treatment response is HER2 in breast cancer. Trastuzumab is given to those who are HER2 positive, due to the specific targeting of this drug at over-expression of HER2 (37). HER2 is also associated with unfavourable outcome regardless of treatment. Thus it is both a prognostic factor and a predictor of treatment effect (38).

Relatively few prognostic factors are also predictors of treatment effect (39), and controversy often exists about whether a factor is both. For example, NICE recommend use of gefitinib for the first-line treatment of non-small cell lung cancer only in those patients who tested positive for Epidermal Growth Factor Receptor Tyrosine Kinase (EGFR-TK) status (40). However, contrary to initial findings (41), there is now increasing evidence that EGFR-TK is not an independent prognostic factor (42, 43). We return to predictors of treatment effect in Chapter 8 (44), and confusion across multiple prognosis studies is considered in detail within Chapter 9 on systematic reviews.

6.3.5 Use for monitoring disease progression

Clinicians also use prognostic factors to monitor changes in disease status and treatment response over time (45). For example, measurement of haemoglobin A1c (HbA1c) levels in people with diabetes allows clinicians, with one blood test, to assess the average serum glucose values over the previous 120 days, and make inferences about how well interventions have controlled glucose levels (46). Evidence that HbA1c is a prognostic factor (strongly associated with the risk of subsequent vascular events) influenced guideline recommendations that it should be routinely assessed (47). Other examples of prognostic factors being used for monitoring include CD4-count in HIV infection, blood pressure or temperature in critical care medicine, and carcinoembryonic antigen (CEA) levels in colorectal cancer (48).

6.3.6 **Development of new interventions**

Prognostic factors may influence the development of new interventions, or new applications of existing interventions, under the assumption of a causal relationship between the factor and subsequent outcome. Every causal factor is prognostic because it directly or indirectly causes future outcomes, and so effectively modifying a causal prognostic factor has the potential to change the disease course in the patients of interest. An example of a prognostic factor in low back pain with evidence of causality is the psychological behavioural factor 'fear avoidance beliefs' (FAB), which has subsequently informed intervention strategies. This factor describes exaggerated pain perceptions and fear of experiencing pain, leading to avoidance of activities that are perceived to cause pain. Evidence supporting an association between FAB during an acute episode of low back pain and subsequent chronic disability and return-to-work outcomes includes several prospective cohort studies, synthesized in systematic reviews (49, 50). Clinicians and researchers hypothesized that FAB may be a modifiable prognostic factor and have recommended patient management to decrease fear avoidance and promote normal activities (e.g. through graded activity exposure) (51, 52). A randomized trial in primary care settings evaluated an intervention that used fear-reducing and activating techniques and found a decrease in low back pain-related disability compared to usual care (53).

Another prognostic factor with strong evidence of causality is HER2 in breast cancer. An excess of HER2 receptors is considered causal as it propagates the development and spread of cancer cells, and thus prognostic as it increases the risk of poor outcomes. Indeed, it was only by understanding the causal mechanism that treatments such as trastuzumab were specifically developed to block the HER2 receptors, and thus reduce tumour growth, whilst even alerting the body's immune system to destroy cancer cells. Many other prognostic factors are potentially modifiable, which could stimulate new interventions aimed at modifying the factor. For example, mild anaemia is prognostic in stable coronary artery disease (54), and glucose measured at admission is prognostic in traumatic brain injury (55, 56).

The benefit of modifying a (potentially) causal prognostic factor on subsequent patient outcomes is best evaluated through a randomized trial. Most prognostic factors will not be causal, and are merely associated with the true (often unknown) causal factors; thus their modification will often not improve outcomes, unfortunately. As in aetiological research, it is very difficult to establish whether a particular factor is truly causal, and one must consider multiple sources of evidence from high-quality studies (57). For example, is there repeated confirmation (from multiple studies) that the factor is prognostic? Does the factor retain prognostic value even after adjustment for other factors? Is there evidence of how the factor fits on the causal pathway from disease to outcome, and an understanding of the (biological) mechanism involved? If so, the final evidence for the benefit of modification will then be studies (usually randomized trials) that demonstrate causality in the sense that changing the factor improves the outcome.

The example of homocysteine in coronary artery disease illustrates some of the key issues for examining causality of a prognostic factor, as summarized by Wald et al. (58). A meta-analysis of sixteen cohort studies suggested that, after adjusting for other prognostic factors (confounders), lower homocysteine levels are associated with a better prognosis in terms of coronary death and non-fatal myocardial infarction. This supports evidence from a meta-analysis of eighty genetic studies that used a Mendelian randomization design to adjust for confounders. Thus homocysteine appears a prognostic factor. However, a meta-analysis of seven randomized trials of folate supplementation, which is known to lower homocysteine, did not show any benefit in terms of improved patient outcome. This may imply that homocysteine is not causal, as modifying it did not improve outcome; however, conversely it may be that homocysteine is causal but that folate supplementation does not lower it sufficiently to improve outcome, or that the causal pathway is more complex (i.e. one would need to modify more than just homocysteine). Thus, causal prognostic factor inferences are problematic, notably when only non-randomized data are used, and should be made with due caution. We do not consider causality again in this chapter.

6.3.7 **Aiding design and analysis of clinical research**

Prognostic factors can be important in the design and analysis of clinical research, including randomized trials where stratified randomization (or minimization) may be used to ensure treatment groups are balanced across levels of a prognostic factor (59). For example, a cluster randomized trial of different approaches for targeted case-finding of individuals with chronic obstructive pulmonary disease (COPD) used block randomization with variable block size, but also balanced by key practice characteristics deemed prognostic, including deprivation index, ethnic origin (percentage of white patients), and age (60).

If prognostic factor values are not balanced across treatment groups being compared then they may mask the true effect of an intervention on disease outcome, and potentially lead to a spurious 'finding'. Thus, as mentioned earlier, prognostic factors are potential confounding factors in the evaluation of interventions using either observational studies or randomized trials with baseline differences between treatment groups, and thus should be adjusted for in the statistical analysis to limit or reduce potential confounding. Royston et al. (61) demonstrate how in a randomized trial of azathioprine versus placebo in patients with primary biliary cirrhosis, a Cox regression ignoring imbalance in the strong prognostic factor of serum bilirubin concentration, produces an unadjusted treatment effect estimate that is not statistically significant (HR = 0.83, 95% CI: 0.57–1.22, p = 0.348); however, after adjusting for imbalance in bilirubin (suitably modelled on its continuous scale) within the Cox model, the treatment effect is substantially larger and statistically significant (HR = 0.61, 95% CI: 0.41–0.91, p = 0.015), suggesting azathioprine is beneficial. This is perhaps an extreme case, and in most sufficiently powered randomized trials large sample sizes are unlikely to give important baseline imbalances in prognostic factors. However, in small or moderately sized trials, and especially in non-randomized studies, baseline differences in a prognostic factor are more likely.

Even in randomized trials with no baseline imbalance, adjusting for prognostic factors may gain power to detect a genuine treatment effect (as prognostic factors explain variation in outcomes across individuals) (62–65). Further, in some statistical models (most notably logistic regression), omission of important prognostic factors may lead to biased effect estimates (66–68). For such reasons, researchers may pre-specify that statistical analyses will be adjusted for key prognostic factors, regardless of baseline imbalances. In the aforementioned COPD trial, for example, adjustment was pre-specified for deprivation index, ethnic origin (percentage of white patients), and age (60).

6.4 Conducting prognostic factor research studies

We now describe the key components to consider when initiating, designing, analysing, and reporting a prognostic factor study.

6.4.1 Phases of prognostic factor research

Different phases of prognostic factor research have been proposed (7, 57). Broadly, prognostic factor evidence should evolve from initial *exploratory* studies that aim to explore the prognostic value of many (perhaps hundreds or even thousands) of factors, to *confirmatory* studies that seek to evaluate the added prognostic value (i.e. after adjustment for established prognostic factors) of one or a few factors previously identified as promising. Researchers should pre-specify whether their planned study is exploratory or confirmatory, and outline their objectives in the context of previous findings.

6.4.1.1 Exploratory studies

Exploratory (hypothesis-generating) prognostic factor studies are important to generate new candidates for, and initial evidence to support, novel prognostic factors, and can be considered as phase I (7, 57). In particular, there is a growing role for hypothesis free, 'biology agnostic', exploratory studies to discover previously unsuspected prognostic factors. These studies are often driven by the availability of biological data or material and new analytical technologies to support the use of 'omic' approaches to discover potential prognostic factors, for example using DNA (genomics), RNA (expression products, transcriptomics), proteins (proteomics), or metabolites (metabolomics) (31, 69, 70). Such studies usually do not focus on one (or even a few) specific prognostic factors, but rather investigate many factors (e.g. thousands of genetic variants) and their association with the outcome. Using statistical methods and bioinformatics, those factors with the most promising prognostic associations are identified for further research. Such exploratory prognostic factor approaches also benefit from sound biological reasoning and an understanding of the causal pathway from the onset of disease or condition to subsequent outcome, to 'home in' more quickly on the important factors. Though such biomarker research is always a hot topic, researchers should also not overlook exploration of whether much more easily accessible clinical information and individual characteristics (e.g. blood pressure, age) are equally or even more prognostic than these more cumbersome to measure factors (71).

6.4.1.2 Confirmatory studies

'The number of cancer prognostic markers that have been validated as clinically useful is pitifully small, despite decades of effort and money invested in marker research.' (72)

Exploratory prognostic factor studies are prone to chance findings, especially when a large number of factors are explored. Therefore, it is imperative that promising findings from exploratory studies are evaluated again in new confirmatory prognostic factor studies, which can be considered as phase II (57). Confirmatory studies should be characterized by pre-specified (hypothesis driven) objectives to establish the prognostic value of one or a few factors discovered in the exploratory studies. They should be well-designed and adhere to high methodological standards (see Section 6.4.2), and include assessment of each factor's prognostic value over and above (independent from) other, perhaps established and more easy to measure, prognostic factors. Confirmatory studies will often show that results from the exploratory phase do not hold. An excellent confirmatory study is by Wolbers et al. (73), who evaluate whether the rate of CD4 cell decline prior to therapy has prognostic value over and above current CD4 cell count in 2820 HIV-infected patients. After adjusting for established prognostic factors (including CD4 cell count, viral load, and age), the hazard ratio for AIDS or death was 1.01 (95% CI: 0.97–1.04) for each 10 cells/µl per year reduction in CD4 cell decline. Thus, the authors conclude that CD4 cell slope does not add additional prognostic value.

Ideally, replication of prognostic factor evidence should emerge over multiple, independent confirmatory studies. These might be identified and synthesized in a systematic review and meta-analysis (Chapter 9). Unfortunately, confirmatory studies are rare relative to exploratory prognostic factor studies, perhaps driven by a desire to discover something 'new', rather than replicating existing findings. This is illustrated by a systematic review of prognostic factors in neuroblastoma, which found that the median number of the 260 articles per factor was only one (Figure 6.3). With growing awareness from journals and researchers that replication is important, it is hoped that the situation will improve in the coming years.

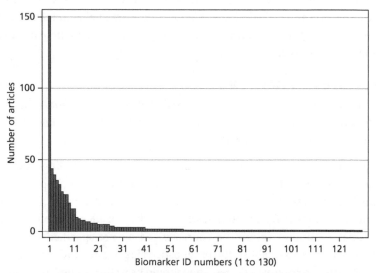

Figure 6.3 Number of articles examining the prognostic value of each of 130 biomarkers in neuroblastoma, as identified by the review of Riley et al.
Source: data from Riley, R.D. et al. A systematic review of molecular and biological tumor markers in neuroblastoma. Clinical Cancer Research. 10(1 Pt 1), 4-12. Copyright © 2004 AACR Publications; and Riley R.D., et al. Reporting of prognostic markers: current problems and development of guidelines for evidence-based practice in the future. Br J Cancer. 88(8), 1191-8. Copyright © 2003 Macmillan Publishers Limited

6.4.1.3 Research combining both exploratory and confirmatory phases

With growing access to individual participant data (IPD) from multiple sources, such as registries and previous studies (75), exploratory and confirmatory phases may occur within the same research project. For example, Dalerba et al. (76) search for novel prognostic factors in patients with stage II colon cancer. In an exploratory phase, the authors obtained 2329 gene-expression arrays from primary human colon epithelial tissues from a repository (containing 214 from normal colon samples and 2115 from colon-cancer samples), and used bioinformatics methods to search for markers of colon epithelial differentiation. This identified sixteen candidate markers, but only one of these encoded a protein that could be studied using immunohistochemical analysis: the CDX2 gene. In 466 of the 2115 colon cancer patients with follow-up information, Cox regression identified a large unadjusted and adjusted prognostic effect of CDX2 in regard to disease-free survival. To immediately validate their work, a dataset of 314 human tissues with colon cancer from the Cancer Diagnosis Programme of the National Cancer Institute (NCI-CDP) was obtained with follow-up information. After five years, the observed proportion of disease-free individuals was 48% and 71% in the CDX2-negative and CDX2-positive groups, and the adjusted HR for CDX2 (negative versus positive groups) was 2.42 (95% CI: 1.36–4.29) (Table 6.1). Further validation in a prospectively collected cohort with consecutively recruited patients, and CDX2 analysed on its continuous scale (compared to dichotomization), is still warranted.

In another example, Azzato et al. (18) performed a genome-wide association study with no prior hypotheses about which of thousands of candidate genes would be prognostic, and identified an association between a variant in the gene called OCA2 and survival among women with oestrogen receptor negative breast cancer. The authors then immediately used individual participant data from fifteen additional studies to confirm that OCA2 had prognostic value.

6.4.2 **Design of confirmatory prognostic factor studies**

We now concentrate on how to conduct a confirmatory prognostic factor study, though many aspects are also relevant for exploratory studies (e.g. ideally using a prospective design). Guidance for those planning and undertaking confirmatory studies has been suggested before (3, 7, 8), and we draw on the main recommendations here. Researchers should strive to ensure high standards of study quality, design, and analysis, and try to emulate the standards set by randomized trials (77). This includes the need for study registration and a published

Table 6.1 Multivariable Cox regression results for the exploratory and confirmatory ('validation') analyses of CDX2 as a prognostic factor in colon cancer.

Factor	Hazard ratio	95% CI	*p*-value
Exploratory data (n = 216)			
CDX2-negative versus CDX2-positive	3.44	1.60–7.38	0.002
Adjustment factors:			
Tumour stage, according to increase in stage	3.28	2.15–4.99	< 0.001
Tumour grade, according to increase in grade	0.99	0.56–1.74	0.96
Age (continuous)	0.99	0.97–1.01	0.46
Male versus female	1.20	0.89–1.61	0.24
Validation data (n = 314)			
CDX2-negative versus CDX2-positive	2.42	1.36–4.29	0.003
Adjustment factors:			
Tumour stage, according to increase in stage	2.71	1.92–3.84	< 0.001
Tumour grade, according to increase in grade	0.79	0.61–1.03	0.08
Age (continuous)	1.00	0.99–1.02	0.68
Male versus female	0.91	0.61–1.35	0.63

Source: reproduced courtesy of Richard D. Riley, using data from Dalerba P, et al. (2007) Prognostic biomarker in stage ii and stage III colon cancer. New Engl J Med 374, 211–22. Copyright © 2007 NEJM Group.

protocol (see Chapter 4), ideally a prospective approach, and suitable statistical analysis. Box 6.1 summarizes our key recommendations.

6.4.2.1 Prospective or retrospective cohort design

A prospective rather than retrospective design is preferable for prognostic factor studies as it enables the definition of clear inclusion criteria, the collection of more complete baseline and follow-up data, and the standardization of data and its recording (including measurement methods for prognostic factors and outcomes, timings and definitions of startpoints and endpoints, recording of therapeutic procedures, and reasons for drop-out). For example, Adab et al. set up a new prospective cohort study in patients with COPD because 'there are no primary care COPD cohorts with case-found patients and few with patients representing the full range of disease severity, particularly those with mild to moderate disease and diverse socioeconomic mix' (78). A prospective approach also allows prognostic factors and outcomes to be clearly defined in advance, with measurements of factors and outcomes blinded (when needed) to prevent information bias. It also facilitates the production of protocols and analysis plans, to reduce the potential for data dredging and thus chance findings (type I errors). For reasons of time or costs, sampling of patients from an existing cohort rather than using the full cohort may be applied. Examples are case-cohort and nested case-control designs. Such sampling strategies must be chosen with care, as selectively choosing or omitting participants may bias the sample relative to the population of interest and affect the generalizability of the prognostic effect estimates (79–81).

Prospective cohort studies are typically expensive and time consuming, with much dedication required from study investigators over many years, from initiation to end of follow-up. Therefore analyses of existing cohort studies or datasets dominate the prognosis literature. In particular, there is increasing availability of datasets including routinely collected or real life participant data, for example obtained from electronic health records, both in primary (47) and secondary care. The advantages of such datasets are that they include the entire case mix of participants encountered in daily practice, and all data commonly documented and used in daily practice of these individuals, and there is increasing possibility to link these datasets to other registries and data sources (mortality and morbidity registries) (48) to enable examination of the complete 'patient journey'. Existing cohorts and datasets are also useful for setting up nested case-control and case-cohort studies for prognosis research purposes.

However, there are key limitations of the usefulness of routine care, real-life (even when linked) datasets. In particular, concerted efforts are required to harmonize the type and quality of data collected across healthcare practices and settings, and how (which measurement methods and blinded observers) and when it is recorded (measured), to mimic the higher standards possible within a prospective predesigned cohort study. For example, standardization of definitions and timings of routinely collected startpoints, factors, and endpoints across different practices, regions, and countries, is required as otherwise they are difficult to synthesize. Further, a major limitation of the use of existing, notably routine care, data is that new and emerging prognostic factors are unlikely to have been collected historically. However, the increased existence of biobanks and their linkage to routine care datasets, allows re-analysis of stored human material or data for new prognostic factors (biomarkers), with immediate linkage to follow-up data (82–84).

For many diseases and health conditions, there is a lack of high-quality data to evaluate prognostic factors. Researchers, and research funders, should help establish new large-scale and prospective cohorts to address this gap. The COPD cohort study of Adab et al. was initiated for this reason, funded by the National Institute for Health Research in the UK (78). Also, an often underutilized resource for prognostic factor research is existing data from previously conducted randomized trials. Trials often record many prognostic factors, if only to determine comparison of baseline prognostic differences of the randomized groups; they have both a treated and an untreated group (sometimes even a care-as-usual group in case of pragmatic randomized trials); have excellent baseline and follow-up information; and the randomization of treatment may be considered an advantage. For example, in traumatic brain injury, the IMPACT collaborators have synthesized individual participant data from many randomized trials in order to identify prognostic factors (59). Nonetheless, a key limitation of trial data is whether the findings generalize beyond the potentially selective, homogeneous participants recruited.

6.4.2.2 Startpoints, prognostic factors, and endpoints

High-quality, predesigned prognostic factor (cohort, case-cohort, or nested case-control) studies have high standards throughout the whole process (85), from deciding the inclusion criteria and recruitment strategy, to defining the startpoint and prognostic factor measurements, to accurate follow-up and outcome recording (Box 6.1). In particular, researchers must identify the targeted

Box 6.1 Key guidance for conducting a confirmatory prognostic factor study

- ◆ Plan the study carefully, write a protocol, and register the study.
- ◆ Specify primary objectives in relation to prognostic factor(s) and outcome(s) under study. Identify any secondary objectives.
- ◆ Adopt a prospective cohort study design or, if not feasible, another study design using reliable and well-defined existing cohort data (e-health records, biobanks, trials).
- ◆ Define a clear startpoint that is clinically meaningful and of interest for prognosis, including context (with or without treatments received), and specify time and place of recruitment.
- ◆ Specify inclusion and exclusion criteria so that included participants reflect the population(s), setting(s), and treatments of interest.
- ◆ For prospective studies, recruit individuals consecutively, or at random, to avoid selection bias.
- ◆ Measure the factors of interest, as well as other prognostic factors to be adjusted for, at the startpoint from which prognosis inferences are desired.

Box 6.1 Continued

- Ensure, if applicable, that outcome assessments are blinded to prognostic factor information (and vice versa in case of retrospective studies).

- Use clear definitions and methods of measurement that are validated and available in practice, for all factors and outcomes.

- Monitor patients regularly, so that key outcomes and their timings are known, to minimise patient drop-out, and understand the reasons for drop-out when it occurs.

- Perform a sample size calculation to ensure the study is powered to answer the questions of interest.

- Use a statistical model suitable for the outcome data of interest (e.g. logistic regression for a binary outcome, Cox regression for a time-to-event outcome), and deal with loss to follow-up (e.g. censor individuals at their drop-out time).

- Consider continuous factors on their continuous scale (and not by dichotomization), and ideally examine non-linear trends using fractional polynomials or splines.

- Avoid complete-case only analyses and rather account for the missing data, for example using multiple imputation.

- Evaluate the added value of each prognostic factor of interest, by adjusting for existing (established) prognostic factors and, if necessary, treatment. Selection procedures are often unnecessary.

- For time-to-event outcomes, consider the potential for prognostic factor effects (hazard ratios) to vary over time (non-proportional hazards).

- Perform sensitivity analyses to assess impact of assumptions made (e.g. regarding data inclusion or modelling techniques).

- Report the study methods and findings according to the REMARK guidelines, and include key recommendations for further research.

Source: reproduced courtesy of Richard D Riley.

health startpoints, settings, and treatment policies for which they want to evaluate prognosis. Clear inclusion and exclusion criteria are then needed to ensure a participant sample from this target population and setting. Ideally a consecutive (or, if not possible, random sample from a consecutive sample) should be taken to avoid selection bias. Startpoints, outcomes, and prognostic factors should be measured using valid methods that would also be used in practice. If an existing dataset is used, requiring assessment of outcomes and factors (e.g. using stored data or material from a biobank), these assessments must be made blind for each other, notably when measurements require subjective interpretation. Also, the prognostic factors should be measured at their intended moment of use, that is, at the moment of intended outcome prediction, as otherwise quantified effects of the prognostic factors may be biased (86). Follow-up should also be as complete as possible, with reasons for any drop-out ideally known.

6.4.2.3 Sample size

An adequate sample size is important for confirmatory prognostic factor studies. However, whereas small effects (e.g. a hazard ratio less than 1.20) are often relevant in RCTs comparing two treatments, typically larger effects are of interest in prognostic factor studies (such as greater than a hazard ratio of 1.5 for a binary factor). The sample should be large enough to detect such an effect when it exists. This is fundamental when setting up a new prospective cohort study. Even for retrospective cohort studies, which use an existing (convenience) cohort typically with a fixed sample size, it is important to establish the potential power of the available sample size. In particular, identifying low power and precision should signal that the dataset is too small to reliably answer the objectives, and so additional data are required.

Sample size calculations are relatively straightforward for prognostic factor effects measured by unadjusted (univariable) mean differences (for continuous outcomes), odds ratios (for binary outcomes), or hazard ratios (for time-to-event outcomes), and available in most software packages. In particular, the sample size calculations for unadjusted results are the same as those for parallel-group randomized trials (87–89), and thus require specification of the size of true prognostic effect one wishes to be able to detect (θ), the type I error (α), the desired statistical power, and the standard deviation of the factor (σ). For a binary or time-to-event outcome, the total number of events required is approximately (8, 90),

$$D = \left(Z_{1-\frac{\alpha}{2}} + Z_{power} \right)^2 / (\sigma \times \theta)^2$$

where θ is the ln odds ratio or ln hazard ratio, and Z values are as defined in Box 6.2. For a binary factor, σ is approximately equal to $\sqrt{\pi(1-\pi)}$, where π is the proportion of patients in the positive group. Where loss to follow-up is expected, the sample size will need to be inflated to account for this (Box 6.2).

Box 6.2 Example of sample size calculations for a prognostic factor study

Hsieh and Lavori consider whether the natural log of the amount of blood urea nitrogen is a prognostic factor for overall mortality rate in a cohort study of sixty-five patients with multiple myeloma (90). The authors aim to detect (based on statistical significance) a ln hazard ratio (θ, say) of 1 and they assume a standard deviation (σ) of 0.3126 for ln blood urea nitrogen.

Their proposed sample size equation is:

$$D = (Z_{1-\frac{\alpha}{2}} + Z_{power})^2 / (\sigma \times \theta)^2$$

Here, D is the total number of deaths, α is the type I error (e.g. 0.05 for 5% error), *power* is the chosen power (e.g. 0.80 for 80% power), and $Z_{1-\frac{\alpha}{2}}$ and Z_{power} are the values of a standard normal distribution corresponding to probabilities of being below the value of $\left(1-\frac{\alpha}{2}\right)$ and *power*, respectively.

Applying this equation for the research question at hand, with a power of 80% and a type I error of 5%, the number of deaths required is derived by $D = (1.96 + 0.84)^2 / (0.3126 \times 1)^2 = 80.23$.

For an adjusted hazard ratio, the sample size needs to be inflated to account for correlation of log blood urea nitrogen and adjustment factors. The authors consider eight adjustment factors, and estimate that 0.1837 is the proportion of variation explained (ρ^2) by a linear regression of ln blood urea nitrogen against the eight factors. Thus, the VIF = $1/(1 - \rho^2)$ = $1/(1 - 0.1837)$ = 1.225, and the required D is 80.23 × VIF = 80.23 × 1.225 = 99 (rounded up). Assuming that by end of follow-up 73.8% of patients will die, a total sample size of 99/0.738 = 135 patients is required (again rounding up).

Source: data from Hsieh FY, et al. (2000) Sample-size calculations for the Cox proportional hazards regression model with nonbinary covariates. *Controlled Clinical Trials*. 21(6), 552–60. Copyright © Elsevier.

The major complication for confirmatory studies is that adjusted rather than unadjusted prognostic factor effect estimates should be the focus. Adjusted effects are typically smaller than unadjusted ones. They are typically obtained from regression analyses that adjust for other prognostic factors that are potentially correlated with the factors of interest. The sample size ideally needs to account for such correlations, which will usually inflate the sample size compared to that for unadjusted prognostic effects, as standard errors of effects usually increase when adjusting for correlated factors due to their collinearity. For binary factors, Hsieh et al. provide a formula for sample size needed for adjusted effects from a logistic regression model (91, 92), and this was extended for time-to-event data by Schmoor et al. (93) They showed that one should multiply the number of events needed for an unadjusted analysis by a variance inflation factor (VIF) of $1/(1-\rho^2)$, where ρ is the correlation between the values of the factor of interest and the values of an adjustment factor. If there are multiple adjustment factors, then ρ relates to the multiple correlation coefficient between the factor of interest and the combination of all other factors (such that ρ^2 is the proportion of variance explained by a regression of the factor of interest against all the adjustment factors, referred to as R^2 in chapter 3) (91, 92). Hsieh and Lavori extend this work to consider sample size for a continuous factor (90, 94), and again show that this VIF is appropriate. An example is given in Box 6.2.

6.4.3 Analysis of prognostic factor studies

Guidance to improve the statistical methods of prognostic factor studies is given in Box 6.1. In particular: to write statistical analysis plans; to analyse continuous factors on their continuous scale, thereby avoiding the use of arbitrary cut points to categorize them (10, 61, 95, 96); to examine non-linear relationships, for example using fractional polynomials or a spline approach (9, 97, 98); to focus on effect estimates and confidence intervals, rather than just p-values (11); to examine a factor's prognostic value over (adjusted for) existing prognostic factors; and to examine time-dependent prognostic effects. These and further issues are discussed in detail in Chapters 3 and 4, and elsewhere (98, 99). Also, the STRATOS (Strengthening Analytic Thinking for Observational Studies) initiative works on guidance for relevant topic areas (http://www.stratos-initiative.org).

Unfortunately, most researchers consider unadjusted (univariable) prognostic effects, but far fewer examine adjusted effects (11), even though a main objective of confirmatory studies should always be to establish if a factor adds prognostic value over established factors. When researchers do perform multivariable analyses, they typically incorporate a selection procedure (such as based on p-values from univariable analyses) to identify a final set of adjustment factors to include in the multivariable analysis. This is often not sensible as the aim is to identify factors that add prognostic value, and not to develop a parsimonious model. Therefore, as advocated in aetiological research to identify independent risk factors, adjustment for established prognostic factors should be routine (i.e. not based on their statistical significance) and pre-specified. In this way, the study will build explicitly on existing knowledge. Hence item 17 in the REMARK reporting guidelines (100, 101): 'Among reported results, provide estimated effects with confidence intervals from an analysis in which the marker and standard prognostic variables are included, regardless of their statistical significance.' Treatment should also be included as an adjustment factor in cohorts where treatments varied across participants (102).

Finally, many prognostic factors (such as some biomarkers, blood pressure) are measured with error. As the variation due to this error is typically unknown, measurement error is rarely accounted for. As a consequence, and especially when the variation is large, prognostic factor effect estimates will tend to be downwardly biased (e.g. hazard ratios and odds ratios closer to 1) and/or too precise (103). If repeated measurements of the factor are taken in a small time period, then the variability can be measured and measurement error accounted for. For example, Crowther et al. (104) investigate the prognostic value of systolic blood pressure (as a continuous variable) for stroke in patients with diabetes. The hazard ratio comparing two individuals with SBP 1 mmHg apart was smaller and more precise when ignoring measurement error (HR = 1.11; 95% CI: 1.05–1.17) than when accounting for it (HR = 1.20; 95% CI: 1.11–1.30). A related issue is when considering repeated measurements over a longer time period, and whether a longitudinal profile of factor values is prognostic. In such situations, a joint longitudinal and survival model will often be helpful, to account for measurement error and censoring over time simultaneously (105, 106). Chapter 15 considers this scenario further.

6.4.4 Reporting prognostic factor studies

Full and transparent reporting of the conduct, analysis, and results of prognostic factor studies is essential to help establish new prognostic factors; resolve ongoing debate over the prognostic value of existing factors; identify good-quality from low-quality research; facilitate systematic reviews and meta-analyses in the field (15, 107), and ultimately help decision makers use prognostic factor evidence. The REMARK reporting guidelines provide recommendations for prognostic factor studies in the field of oncology (100, 101), and the checklist is given in Box 6.3 (101). Almost all the items are applicable also to other, non-cancer disease areas. In addition to the items mentioned, we also emphasize

Box 6.3 Checklist of reporting recommendations for tumour marker prognostic studies (REMARK) (as sourced from McShane et al. (101))

Item to be reported

Introduction

1. State the marker examined, the study objectives, and any pre-specified hypotheses.

Materials and methods

Patients

2. Describe the characteristics (e.g. disease stage or co-morbidities) of the study patients, including their source and inclusion and exclusion criteria.

3. Describe treatments received and how chosen (e.g. randomized or rule-based).

Specimen characteristics

4. Describe type of biological material used (including control samples) and methods of preservation and storage.

Assay methods

5. Specify the assay method used and provide (or reference) a detailed protocol, including specific reagents or kits used, quality control procedures, reproducibility assessments, quantitation methods, and scoring and reporting protocols. Specify whether and how assays were performed blinded to the study endpoint.

Study design

6. State the method of case selection, including whether prospective or retrospective and whether stratification or matching (e.g. by stage of disease or age) was used. Specify the time period from which cases were taken, the end of the follow-up period, and the median follow-up time.

7. Precisely define all clinical endpoints examined.

8. List all candidate variables initially examined or considered for inclusion in models.

Box 6.3 Continued

9. Give rationale for sample size; if the study was designed to detect a specified effect size, give the target power and effect size.

Statistical analysis methods

10. Specify all statistical methods, including details of any variable selection procedures and other model-building issues, how model assumptions were verified, and how missing data were handled.

11. Clarify how marker values were handled in the analyses; if relevant, describe methods used for cut point determination.

Results

Data

12. Describe the flow of patients through the study, including the number of patients included in each stage of the analysis (a diagram may be helpful) and reasons for drop-out. Specifically, both overall and for each subgroup extensively examined report the numbers of patients and the number of events.

13. Report distributions of basic demographic characteristics (at least age and sex), standard (disease-specific) prognostic variables, and tumour marker, including numbers of missing values.

Analysis and presentation

14. Show the relation of the marker to standard prognostic variables.

15. Present univariable analyses showing the relation between the marker and outcome, with the estimated effect (e.g. hazard ratio and survival probability). Preferably provide similar analyses for all other variables being analysed. For the effect of a tumour marker on a time-to-event outcome, a Kaplan-Meier plot is recommended.

16. For key multivariable analyses, report estimated effects (e.g. hazard ratio) with confidence intervals for the marker and, at least for the final model, all other variables in the model.

17. Among reported results, provide estimated effects with confidence intervals from an analysis in which the marker and standard prognostic variables are included, regardless of their statistical significance.

Box 6.3 Continued

18. If done, report results of further investigations, such as checking assumptions, sensitivity analyses, and internal validation.

Discussion

19. Interpret the results in the context of the pre-specified hypotheses and other relevant studies; include a discussion of limitations of the study.
20. Discuss implications for future research and clinical value.

Source: reproduced with permission from McShane LM, et al. (2005) Reporting recommendations for tumor marker prognostic studies (REMARK). *Journal of the National Cancer Institute* 97(16), 1180– 4. Copyright © 2005 OUP.

the usefulness of graphical displays, such as Kaplan-Meier survival curves for unadjusted prognostic factor effects (Figure 6.1), adjusted survival curves that account for the adjustment for other prognostic factors (108), and plots of non-linear trends across the range of a continuous factor (109).

We also emphasize that full reporting is needed for all prognostic factor studies that are conducted, and not just those which show the most promise. For example, incomplete and selective reporting are two key reasons why the prognostic value of p53 remains a source of confusion in bladder cancer (14, 110). Sekula et al. reviewed German studies evaluating p53 in bladder cancer and identified sixteen, of which five were unpublished mainly due to 'a loss of interest of the investigators' (111). Such poor reporting severely limits meta-analysis (Chapter 9) (11, 111).

6.5 Summary

In this chapter, we have described how prognostic factors play an important role toward improving health outcomes, including within clinical practice, healthcare research and the development, evaluation, and targeting of interventions. Historically, prognostic factor research has been sub-standard, but the quality of future studies can be raised by a concerted effort from funding bodies, journal editors, reviewers, and the prognosis research community. We outlined good practice criteria for the design, conduct, analysis, and reporting. In particular, more focus on confirmatory studies is required, with improved analysis methods, and clear and unbiased reporting of all results.

Many of the uses of prognostic factors—such as informing diagnosis, tailoring treatment decisions, and monitoring patients—constitute a health technology for clinical practice. Therefore, subsequent research must examine the impact of using prognostic factors to inform clinical decisions. This requires decision modelling techniques (24, 46) and randomized trials (112) to examine the actual impact of implementing prognostic factors—in terms of costs and healthcare outcomes. Currently such studies are rare, and indeed the nature and extent of evidence required must be clarified. Further consideration of this issue in relation to prognostic models and predictors of treatment effect is given in Chapters 7 and 8. A summary of the key messages from this chapter is now provided.

6.5.1 **Summary points**

- A prognostic factor is any variable that, among people with a given startpoint (e.g. diagnosis of disease), is associated with (the risk of) a subsequent outcome (e.g. death).

- Prognostic factors include simple and established measures, such as demographics, symptoms, signs, and stage of disease, but increasingly studied are novel biomarkers and genetic information.

- Different values of a prognostic factor are associated with a different prognosis; thus, prognostic factors break down (stratify) and enhance the overall prognosis summaries described in Chapter 5.

- Prognostic factors have many potential uses; for example they may help define disease at diagnosis, inform clinical and therapeutic decisions, provide the building blocks for prognostic models, enhance the design and analysis of research studies (including randomized trials), and help identify targets for new interventions.

- Prognostic factor research usually involves a prospective cohort study to identify factors that have prognostic value, over and above (independent of) other (e.g. established) prognostic factors.

- Exploratory prognostic factor studies are important to identify new or the most promising prognostic factors from a large number of possible factors; however, they must be labelled as exploratory due to their potential for chance findings.

- Initial exploratory evidence about a prognostic factor must be replicated in new confirmatory prognostic factor studies that, ideally, are suitably powered, registered, and protocol-driven, with a pre-specified statistical analysis plan.

- Prospectively planned cohort studies are the ideal for both exploratory and confirmatory research, but may not be practical. Existing data from electronic healthcare databases and disease registries may provide large and immediate cohorts, but factors and outcomes of interest may be (selectively) missing or not recorded at the requisite time points.

♦ Confirmatory studies should examine the added (independent) prognostic value of a factor; that is, its prognostic effect after adjusting for (independent of) other, for example established, prognostic factors.

♦ Statistical analysis is enhanced by handling missing data using multiple imputation (rather than complete-case analysis), by analysing continuous factors on their continuous scale with examination of potential non-linear prognostic trends, and by considering time-dependent prognostic effects.

♦ The REMARK guidelines should be adhered to for transparent reporting of a prognostic factor study, including all factors and outcomes considered.

♦ Greater translation is needed regarding how particular prognostic factors can be used to improve clinical outcomes or the design and analysis of future research studies.

References

1. **Schumacher M, Bastert G, Bojar H,** et al. (1994) Randomized 2×2 trial evaluating hormonal treatment and the duration of chemotherapy in node-positive breast cancer patients. German Breast Cancer Study Group. *J Clin Oncol* **12**(10), 2086–93.

2. **Riley RD, Hayden JA, Steyerberg EW,** et al. (2013) Prognosis Research Strategy (PROGRESS) 2: prognostic factor research. *PLoS Med* **10**(2), e1001380.

3. **Riley RD, Sauerbrei W,** and **Altman DG** (2009) Prognostic markers in cancer: the evolution of evidence from single studies to meta-analysis, and beyond. *Br J Cancer* **100**(8), 1219–29.

4. **Rifai N, Altman DG,** and **Bossuyt PM** (2008) Reporting bias in diagnostic and prognostic studies: time for action. *Clin Chem* **54**(7),1101–3.

5. **Simon R** (2001) Evaluating prognostic factor studies. In: **Gospodarowicz MKea,** ed. *Prognostic Factors in Cancer*. New York: Wiley-Liss. pp. 49–56.

6. **Sauerbrei W** (2005) Prognostic factors—confusion caused by bad quality of design, analysis and reporting of many studies. In: **Bier H,** ed. *Current Research in Head and Neck Cancer, Advances in Oto-Rhino-Laryngology*. Basel: Karger. pp.184–200.

7. **Altman DG** and **Lyman GH** (1998) Methodological challenges in the evaluation of prognostic factors in breast cancer. *Breast Cancer Res Treat* **52**(1–3), 289–303.

8. **Simon R** and **Altman DG** (1994) Statistical aspects of prognostic factor studies in oncology. *Br J Cancer* **69**(6), 979–85.

9. **Holländer N** and **Sauerbrei W** (2006) On statistical approaches for the multivariable analysis of prognostic marker studies. In: **Auget J-L, Balakrishnan N, Mesbah M,** et al., eds. *Advances in Statistical Methods for the Health Sciences*. Boston: Birkhäuser. pp. 19–38.

10. **Altman DG, Lausen B, Sauerbrei W**, et al. (1994) Dangers of using 'optimal' cutpoints in the evaluation of prognostic factors. *J Natl Cancer Inst* **86**(11), 829–35.

11. **Riley RD, Abrams KR, Sutton AJ**, et al. (2003) Reporting of prognostic markers: current problems and development of guidelines for evidence-based practice in the future. *Br J Cancer* **88**(8), 1191–8.

12. **Kyzas PA, Loizou KT**, and **Ioannidis JP** (2005) Selective reporting biases in cancer prognostic factor studies. *J Natl Cancer Inst* **97**(14), 1043–55.

13. **Sekula P, Mallett S, Altman DG**, et al. (2017) Did the reporting of prognostic studies of tumour markers improve since the introduction of REMARK guideline? A comparison of reporting in published articles. *PLoS One* **12**(6), e0178531.

14. **Schmitz-Dräger BJ, Goebell PJ, Ebert T**, et al. (2000) p53 immunohistochemistry as a prognostic marker in bladder cancer. Playground for urology scientists?. *Eur Urol* **38**, 691–99.

15. **Hemingway H, Riley RD**, and **Altman DG** (2009) Ten steps towards improving prognosis research. *BMJ* **339**, b4184.

16. **Kyzas PA, Denaxa-Kyza D**, and **Ioannidis JP** (2007) Quality of reporting of cancer prognostic marker studies: association with reported prognostic effect. *J Natl Cancer Inst* **99**(3), 236–43.

17. **Ensor J, Riley RD, Jowett S**, et al. (2016) Prediction of risk of recurrence of venous thromboembolism following treatment for a first unprovoked venous thromboembolism: systematic review, prognostic model and clinical decision rule, and economic evaluation. *Health Technol Assess* **20**(12), i-xxxiii, 1–190.

18. **Azzato EM, Tyrer J, Fasching PA**, et al. (2010) Association between a germline OCA2 polymorphism at chromosome 15q13.1 and estrogen receptor-negative breast cancer survival. *J Natl Cancer Inst* **102**(9), 650–62.

19. **Mostertz W, Stevenson M, Acharya C**, et al. (2010) Age and sex-specific genomic profiles in non-small cell lung cancer. *JAMA* **303**, 535–43.

20. **Riley RD, Heney D, Jones DR**, et al. (2004) A systematic review of molecular and biological tumor markers in neuroblastoma. *Clin Cancer Res* **10**(1 Pt 1), 4–12.

21. **Chou R** and **Shekelle P** (2010) Will this patient develop persistent disabling low back pain? *JAMA* **303**, 1295–302.

22. **Fraser SD, Roderick PJ, May CR**, et al. (2015) The burden of comorbidity in people with chronic kidney disease stage 3: a cohort study. *BMC Nephrol* **16**, 193.

23. **National Institute for Health and Clinical Excellence** (2008) *NICE Technology Appraisal Guidance 152: Drug-Eluting Stents for the Treatment of Coronary Artery Disease* (part review of NICE technology appraisal guidance 71). London: NICE.

24. **Levey AS, Eckardt KU, Tsukamoto Y**, et al. (2005) Definition and classification of chronic kidney disease: a position statement from Kidney Disease: Improving Global Outcomes (KDIGO). *Kidney Int* **67**(6), 2089–100.

25. **Noordzij JP, Lee SL, Bernet VJ**, et al. (2007) Early prediction of hypocalcemia after thyroidectomy using parathyroid hormone: an analysis of pooled individual patient data from nine observational studies. *J Am Coll Surg* **205**(6), 748–54.

26. **Salles GF, Reboldi G, Fagard RH**, et al. (2016) Prognostic effect of the nocturnal blood pressure fall in hypertensive patients: the ambulatory blood pressure collaboration in patients with hypertension (ABC-H) meta-analysis. *Hypertension* **67**(4), 693–700.

27. **Tang WH, Wu Y, Grodin JL,** et al. (2016) Prognostic value of baseline and changes in circulating soluble ST2 levels and the effects of nesiritide in acute decompensated heart failure. *JACC Heart Failure* **4**(1), 68–77.

28. **Rothwell PM, Howard SC, Dolan E,** et al. (2010) Prognostic significance of visit-to-visit variability, maximum systolic blood pressure, and episodic hypertension. *Lancet* **375**(9718), 895–905.

29. **Von Korff M** and **Miglioretti DL** (2005) A prognostic approach to defining chronic pain. *Pain* **117**(3), 304–13.

30. **Hemingway H, Croft P, Perel P,** et al. (2013) Prognosis research strategy (PROGRESS) 1: a framework for researching clinical outcomes. *BMJ* **346**, e5595.

31. **Micheel CM, Nass SJ,** and **Omenn GS** (2012) *Evolution of Translational Omics: Lessons Learned and the Path Forward.* Washington, DC: The National Academies Press.

32. **Balduzzi S, Mantarro S, Guarneri V,** et al. (2014) Trastuzumab-containing regimens for metastatic breast cancer. *Cochrane Database Syst Rev* (6), CD006242.

33. **Moja L, Tagliabue L, Balduzzi S,** et al. (2012) Trastuzumab-containing regimens for early breast cancer. *Cochrane Database Syst Rev* (4), CD006243.

34. **Steyerberg EW, Moons KG, van der Windt DA,** et al. (2013) Prognosis Research Strategy (PROGRESS) 3: prognostic model research. *PLoS Med* **10**(2), e1001381.

35. **Steyerberg EW, Mushkudiani N, Perel P,** et al. (2008) Predicting outcome after traumatic brain injury: Development and international validation of prognostic scores based on admission characteristics. *PLoS Medicine* **5**(8), 1251–61.

36. **Trusheim MR, Berndt ER,** and **Douglas FL** (2007) Stratified medicine: strategic and economic implications of combining drugs and clinical biomarkers. *Nat Rev Drug Discov* 287–93.

37. **Cooke T, Reeves J, Lanigan A,** et al. (2001) HER2 as a prognostic and predictive marker for breast cancer. *Ann Oncol* **12**(1), S23–8.

38. **Ballman KV** (2015) Biomarker: predictive or prognostic? *J Clin Oncol* **33**(33), 3968–71.

39. **Clark GM** (2008) Prognostic factors versus predictive factors: Examples from a clinical trial of erlotinib. *Mol Oncol* **1**(4), 406–12.

40. **National Institute for Clinical Excellence** (2010) *NICE Technology Appraisal Guidance 192: Gefitinib for the First-line Treatment of Locally Advanced or Metastatic Non-small-cell Lung Cancer.* London: NICE.

41. **Volm M, Efferth T,** and **Mattern J** (1992) Oncoprotein (c-myc, c-erbB1, c-erbB2, c-fos) and suppressor gene product (p53) expression in squamous cell carcinomas of the lung. Clinical and biological correlations. *Anticancer Res* **12**(1), 11–20.

42. **Kim YT, Seong YW, Jung YJ,** et al. (2013) The presence of mutations in epidermal growth factor receptor gene is not a prognostic factor for long-term outcome after surgical resection of non-small-cell lung cancer. *J Thorac Oncol* **8**(2), 171–8.

43. **Pfeiffer P, Clausen PP, Andersen K,** et al. (1996) Lack of prognostic significance of epidermal growth factor receptor and the oncoprotein p185HER-2 in patients with systemically untreated non-small-cell lung cancer: an immunohistochemical study on cryosections. *Br J Cancer* **74**(1), 86–91.

44. **Hingorani AD, Windt DA, Riley RD,** et al. (2013) Prognosis research strategy (PROGRESS) 4: stratified medicine research. *BMJ* **346**, e5793.

45. **Lassere MN, Johnson KR, Boers M**, et al. (2007) Definitions and validation criteria for biomarkers and surrogate endpoints: development and testing of a quantitative hierarchical levels of evidence schema. *J Rheumatol* **34**(3), 607–15.

46. **Moons KG** (2010) Criteria for scientific evaluation of novel markers: a perspective. *Clin Chem* **56**, 537–41.

47. **Diabetes Care** (2011) Executive summary: standards of medical care in diabetes—2011. *Diabetes Care* **34**(1), S4–10.

48. **Renehan AG, Egger M, Saunders MP**, et al. (2002) Impact on survival of intensive follow up after curative resection for colorectal cancer: systematic review and meta-analysis of randomised trials. *BMJ* **324**, 813.

49. **Pincus T, Vogel S, Burton AK**, et al. (2006) Fear avoidance and prognosis in back pain. *Arthr Rheum* **54**, 3999–4010.

50. **Iles RA, Davidson M**, and **Taylor NF** (2008) Psychosocial predictors of failure to return to work in non-chronic non-specific low back pain: a systematic review. *Occup Environ Med* **65**, 507–17.

51. **Picavet HS, Vlaeyen JW**, and **Schouten JS** (2002) Pain catastrophizing and kinesiophobia: predictors of chronic low back pain. *Am J Epidemiol* **156**, 1028–34.

52. **Fritz JM, George SZ**, and **Delitto A** (2001) The role of fear-avoidance beliefs in acute low back pain: relationships with current and future disability and work status. *Pain* **94**, 7–15.

53. **Von Korff M, Balderson BH, Saunders K**, et al. (2005) A trial of an activating intervention for chronic back pain in primary care and physical therapy settings. *Pain* **113**, 323–30.

54. **Shah A, Nicholas O, Timmis A**, et al. (2011) Threshold haemoglobin levels and the prognosis of stable coronary disease: two new cohorts and a systematic review and meta-analysis. *PLoS Med* **8**(5), e1000439.

55. **Marmarou A, Lu J, Butcher I**, et al. (2007) IMPACT database of traumatic brain injury: design and description. *J Neurotrauma* **24**(2), 239–50.

56. **Van Beek JGM, Mushkudiani NA, Steyerberg EW**, et al. (2007) Prognostic value of admission laboratory parameters in traumatic brain injury: Results from the IMPACT study. *J Neurotrauma* **24**(2), 315–328.

57. **Hayden JA, Côté P, Steenstra IA**, et al. (2008) Identifying phases of investigation helps planning, appraising, and applying the results of explanatory prognosis studies. *J Clin Epidemiol* **61**, 552–60.

58. **Wald DS, Wald NJ, Morris JK**, et al. (2006) Folic acid, homocysteine, and cardiovascular disease: judging causality in the face of inconclusive trial evidence. *BMJ* **333**, 1114–17.

59. **Maas AI, Marmarou A, Murray GD**, et al. (2007) Prognosis and clinical trial design in traumatic brain injury: the IMPACT study. *J Neurotrauma* **24**(2), 232–8.

60. **Jordan RE, Adab P, Sitch A**, et al. (2016) Targeted case finding for chronic obstructive pulmonary disease versus routine practice in primary care (TargetCOPD): a cluster-randomised controlled trial. *Lancet Respir Med* **4**(9), 720–30.

61. **Royston P, Altman DG**, and **Sauerbrei W** (2006) Dichotomizing continuous predictors in multiple regression: a bad idea. *Stat Med* **25**(1), 127–41.

62. **Hernandez AV, Eijkemans MJ**, and **Steyerberg** EW (2006) Randomized controlled trials with time-to-event outcomes: how much does prespecified covariate adjustment increase power? *Ann Epidemiol* 16, 41–8.

63. **Maas AI, Steyerberg EW, Marmarou A**, et al. (2010) IMPACT recommendations for improving the design and analysis of clinical trials in moderate to severe traumatic brain injury. *Neurotherapeutics* 7(1), 127–34.

64. **Roozenbeek B, Maas AI, Lingsma HF**, et al. (2009) Baseline characteristics and statistical power in randomized controlled trials: selection, prognostic targeting, or covariate adjustment? *Crit Care Med* 37(10), 2683–90.

65. **Hernández AV, Steyerberg EW**, and **Habbema JD** (2004) Covariate adjustment in randomized controlled trials with dichotomous outcomes increases statistical power and reduces sample size requirements. *J Clin Epidemiol* 57(5), 454–60.

66. **Robinson LD** and **Jewell NP** (1991) Some surprising results about covariate adjustment in logistic regression models. *Int Stat Rev* 58, 227–40.

67. **Abo-Zaid G, Guo B, Deeks JJ**, et al. (2013) Individual participant data meta-analyses should not ignore clustering. *J Clin Epidemiol* 66(8), 865–73, e4.

68. **Gail MH, Wieand S**, and **Piantadosi S** (1984) Biased estimates of treatment effect in randomized experiments with nonlinear regressions and omitted covariates. *Biometrika* 71, 431–44.

69. **Dupuy A** and **Simon RM** (2007) Critical review of published microarray studies for cancer outcome and guidelines on statistical analysis and reporting. *J Natl Cancer Inst* 99(2), 147–57.

70. **Tinker AV, Boussioutas A**, and **Bowtell DD** (2006) The challenges of gene expression microarrays for the study of human cancer. *Cancer Cell* 9(5), 333–9.

71. **Winzer KJ, Buchholz A, Schumacher M**, et al. (2016) Improving the prognostic ability through better use of standard clinical data—the Nottingham Prognostic Index as an example. *PLoS One* 11(3), e0149977.

72. **McShane LM, Altman DG**, and **Sauerbrei W** (2005) Identification of clinically useful cancer prognostic factors: what are we missing? *J Natl Cancer Inst* 97(14), 1023–5.

73. **Wolbers M, Babiker A, Sabin C**, et al. (2010) Pretreatment CD4 cell slope and progression to AIDS or death in HIV-infected patients initiating antiretroviral therapy—the CASCADE Collaboration: a collaboration of twenty-three cohort studies. *PLOS Med* 7(2), e1000239.

74. **Riley RD, Burchill SA, Abrams KR**, et al. (2003) A systematic review and evaluation of the use of tumour markers in paediatric oncology: Ewing's sarcoma and neuroblastoma. *Health Technol Assess* 7(5), 1–162.

75. **Abo-Zaid G, Sauerbrei W**, and **Riley RD** (2012) Individual participant data meta-analysis of prognostic factor studies: state of the art? *BMC Med Res Methodol* 12, 56.

76. **Dalerba P, Sahoo D, Paik S**, et al. (2016) CDX2 as a prognostic biomarker in stage II and stage III colon cancer. *N Engl J Med* 374(3), 211–22.

77. **Hayden JA, Cote P**, and **Bombardier** C (2006) Evaluation of the quality of prognosis studies in systematic reviews. *Ann Intern Med* 144(6), 427–37.

78. **Adab P, Fitzmaurice DA, Dickens AP**, et al. (2017) Cohort profile: the Birmingham chronic obstructive pulmonary disease (COPD) cohort study. *Int J Epidemiol* 46(1), 23.

79. **Ganna A, Reilly M, de Faire U**, et al. (2012) Risk prediction measures for case-cohort and nested case-control designs: an application to cardiovascular disease. *Am J Epidemiol* **175**(7), 715–24.

80. **Moons KG, Royston P, Vergouwe Y**, et al. (2009) Prognosis and prognostic research: what, why, and how? *BMJ* **338**, b375.

81. **Moons KG, Kengne AP, Woodward M**, et al. (2012) Risk prediction models: I. Development, internal validation, and assessing the incremental value of a new (bio) marker. *Heart* **98**(9), 683–90.

82. **Goebell PJ, Groshen S, Schmitz-Drager BJ**, et al. (2004) The International Bladder Cancer Bank: proposal for a new study concept. *Urol Oncol* **22**(4), 277–84.

83. **Qualman SJ, France M, Grizzle WE**, et al. (2004) Establishing a tumour bank: banking, informatics and ethics. *Br J Cancer* **90**(6), 1115–9.

84. **Schilsky RL, Dressler LM, Bucci D**, et al. (2002) Cooperative group tissue banks as research resources: the cancer and leukemia group B tissue repositories. *Clin Cancer Res* **8**(5), 943–8.

85. **Hayden JA, van der Windt DA, Cartwright JL**, et al. (2013) Assessing bias in studies of prognostic factors. *Ann Intern Med* **158**(4), 280–6.

86. **Whittle R, Royle K-L, Jordan KP**, et al. (2017) Prognosis research ideally should measure time-varying predictors at their intended moment of use. *Diagn Progn Res* **1**(1), 1.

87. **Fayers PM and Machin D** (1995) Sample size: how many patients are necessary? *Br J Cancer* **72**(1), 1–9.

88. **Schoenfeld DA** (1983) Sample-size formula for the proportional-hazards regression model. *Biometrics* **39**(2), 499–503.

89. **Machin D, Campbell MJ, Tan SB**, et al. (2008) Sample size tables for clinical studies (third edition). Chichester: Wiley-Blackwell.

90. **Hsieh FY and Lavori PW** (2000) Sample-size calculations for the Cox proportional hazards regression model with nonbinary covariates. *Control Clin Trials* **21**(6), 552–60.

91. **Hsieh FY** (1989) Sample size tables for logistic regression. *Stat Med* **8**(7), 795–802.

92. **Hsieh FY, Bloch DA, and Larsen MD** (1998) A simple method of sample size calculation for linear and logistic regression. *Stat Med* **17**(14), 1623–34.

93. **Schmoor C, Sauerbrei W, and Schumacher M** (2000) Sample size considerations for the evaluation of prognostic factors in survival analysis. *Stat Med* **19**(4), 441–52.

94. **Hsieh FY, Lavori PW, Cohen HJ**, et al. (2003) An overview of variance inflation factors for sample-size calculation. *Eval Health Prof* **26**(3), 239–57.

95. **Altman DG and Royston P** (2006) Statistics notes: the cost of dichotomising continuous variables. *BMJ* **332**, 1080.

96. **Hilsenbeck SG, Clark GM, and McGuire WL** (1992) Why do so many prognostic factors fail to pan out? *Breast Cancer Res Treat* **22**(3), 197–206.

97. **Royston P and Sauerbrei W** (2008) *Multivariable Model-building—a Pragmatic Approach to Regression Analysis Based on Fractional Polynomials for Modelling Continuous Variables*. Chichester: Wiley.

98. **Harrell FE, Jr.** (2015) *Regression Modeling Strategies: with Applications to Linear Models, Logistic and Ordinal Regression, and Survival Analysis* (second edition). New York: Springer.

99. **Schumacher M, Holländer N, Schwarzer G**, et al. (2012) Prognostic factor studies. In: **Crowley J, Hoering A**, eds. *Handbook of Statistics in Clinical Oncology* (third edition). Boca Raton, Florida: Chapman and Hall/CRC. pp. 415–70.

100. **Altman DG, McShane LM, Sauerbrei W**, et al. (2012) Reporting recommendations for tumor marker prognostic studies (REMARK): explanation and elaboration. *PLoS Med* **9**(5), e1001216.

101. **McShane LM, Altman DG, Sauerbrei W**, et al. (2005) Reporting recommendations for tumor marker prognostic studies (REMARK). *J Natl Cancer Inst* **97**(16), 1180–4.

102. **Groenwold RH, Moons KG, Pajouheshnia R**, et al. (2016) Explicit inclusion of treatment in prognostic modeling was recommended in observational and randomized settings. *J Clin Epidemiol* **78**, 90–100.

103. **Carroll RJ** and **Stefanski LA** (1994) Measurement error, instrumental variables and corrections for attenuation with applications to meta-analyses. *Stat Med* **13**(12), 1265–82.

104. **Crowther MJ, Lambert PC**, and **Abrams KR** (2013) Adjusting for measurement error in baseline prognostic biomarkers included in a time-to-event analysis: a joint modelling approach. *BMC Med Res Methodol* **13**, 146.

105. **Crowther MJ, Abrams KR**, and **Lambert PC** (2012) Flexible parametric joint modelling of longitudinal and survival data. *Stat Med* **31**(30), 4456–71.

106. **Lawrence Gould A, Boye ME, Crowther MJ**, et al. (2015) Joint modeling of survival and longitudinal non-survival data: current methods and issues. Report of the DIA Bayesian joint modeling working group. *Stat Med* **34**(14), 2181–95.

107. **Riley RD, Ridley G, Williams K**, et al. (2007) Prognosis research: toward evidence-based results and a Cochrane methods group. *J Clin Epidemiol* **60**(8), 863–5.

108. **Royston P** and **Lambert PC** (2011) *Flexible Parametric Survival Analysis Using Stata: Beyond the Cox Model*. Boca Raton, Florida: CRC Press.

109. **Sauerbrei W, Royston P, Bojar H**, et al. (1999) Modelling the effects of standard prognostic factors in node-positive breast cancer. German Breast Cancer Study Group (GBSG). *Br J Cancer* **79**(11–12), 1752–60.

110. **Malats N, Bustos A, Nascimento CM**, et al. (2005) P53 as a prognostic marker for bladder cancer: a meta-analysis and review. *Lancet Oncol* **6**(9), 678–86.

111. **Sekula P, Pressler JB, Sauerbrei W**, et al. (2016) Assessment of the extent of unpublished studies in prognostic factor research: a systematic review of p53 immunohistochemistry in bladder cancer as an example. *BMJ Open* **6**(8).

112. **Hlatky MA, Greenland P, Arnett DK**, et al. (2009) Criteria for evaluation of novel markers of cardiovascular risk: a scientific statement from the American Heart Association. *Circ Cardiovasc Qual Outcomes* **119**, 2408–16.

Chapter 7

Prognostic model research

Richard D Riley, Karel GM Moons,
Thomas PA Debray, Kym IE Snell,
Ewout W Steyerberg, Douglas G Altman,
and Gary S Collins

7.1 Introduction

'The Median Isn't the Message.' (1)

The holy grail of prognosis research is to improve patient outcomes by enabling a more personalized (rather than population- or group-based) approach to healthcare and risk prediction. In this regard, the scope of Chapters 5 and 6 is insufficient, as it only covers the overall (average) prognosis of individuals in in a certain population, and the identification of prognostic factors associated with differences in that overall prognosis. Though a single prognostic factor refines (stratifies) estimates of overall prognosis, it is rarely sufficient to provide accurate individualized outcome predictions. For example, Figure 6.1 shows that tumour grade is a prognostic factor in breast cancer patients, with distinct Kaplan-Meier curves for grade 1, 2 and 3. However, Figure 7.1 reveals that the individual survival times vary within each grade, and the survival distribution for each grade overlaps considerably, and some individuals with a grade 3 tumour survived far longer than those within grade 2 or even 1 (2). Thus, the overall (across all patients combined) median survival time within each grade is not useful for the individual patient. This point was famously made by Stephen Jay Gould in his essay entitled: 'The Median Isn't the Message'. (1) Dr Gould died in 2002 at the age of 60, some twenty years after his diagnosis of meso-thelioma at which he was quoted an eight-month median survival time.

In daily practice, a more individualized approach to prognosis inevitably re-quires *multiple* prognostic factors (referred to as 'predictors') to be utilized in combination, to tailor outcome predictions for each individual conditional on their unique set of observed characteristics (referred to as predictor values). To serve such practice, prognosis research needs a focus on the development, val-idation, and implementation of *multivariable* prognostic models. A prognostic

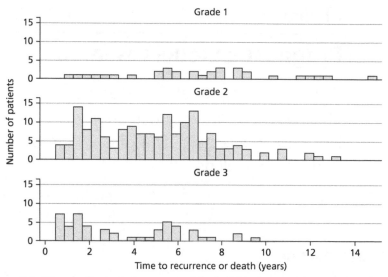

Figure 7.1 "The median isn't the message" for individual prognosis: evidence of wide and overlapping distributions of survival times across tumour grades in 246 breast cancer patients treated with tamoxifen over a possible 7 years of follow up.

Source: reproduced courtesy of Richard D. Riley, using data from Schumacher, M., et al. Randomized 2 x 2 trial evaluating hormonal treatment and the duration of chemotherapy in node-positive breast cancer patients. Journal of Clinical Oncology. 12(10), 2086-93. Copyright © 1994 American Society of Clinical Oncology

model is a formal combination of multiple predictors in order to make individualized predictions about a particular outcome (endpoint) of interest from a given state of health (startpoint) over a specified time interval. For continuous outcomes, a prognostic model predicts an individual's expected (mean) outcome value by a particular time point. For binary or time-to-event outcomes, a prognostic model predicts an individual's outcome risk (probability) by a particular time point (or time points). A well-known, simple example of a prognostic model is the Nottingham Prognostic Index (NPI) (3), which gives a score that relates to the survival probability of a woman with newly diagnosed breast cancer based on a combination of tumour grade, number of involved lymph nodes, and tumour size (Box 7.1). Thus, the NPI combines tumour grade with two other prognostic factors, to give a more individualized prediction than using tumour grade alone.

Other names for a prognostic model include risk score, risk classification tool, prognostic score or index, and clinical prediction model. The term clinical decision (or prediction) *rule* is best reserved for a simplified or categorised prediction model that explicitly incorporates one or more risk thresholds to guide clinical decisions (e.g. initiate treatment if a patient's predicted outcome risk is above 10%, and withhold the treatment otherwise) (4).

Box 7.1 The Nottingham Prognostic Index (NPI) (3)

The NPI combines tumour size, whether the cancer has spread to the lymph nodes, and the grade of the cancer to produce a risk score for women with newly diagnosed breast cancer. The formula is:

$$\text{NPI} = \left(0.2 \times \text{tumour diameter in cm}\right) + \text{lymph node stage} + \text{tumour grade}$$

where lymph node stage can be 1 (if there are no nodes affected), 2 (if up to three glands are affected) or 3 (if more than three glands are affected) and tumour grade is scored as either 1, 2, or 3.

A lower score suggests a good outcome. Haybittle et al. and Todd et al. propose three risk groups (3, 5): Good (NPI ≤ 3.4), Moderate (NPI > 3.4, NPI ≤ 5.4), and Poor (NPI > 5.4), whose five-year overall prognosis is about 90%, 70% and 20%, respectively.

Source: data from Haybittle, J.L., et al. A prognostic index in primary breast cancer. British Journal of Cancer. 45(3), 361-6. Copyright © 1982 Springer Nature.

In this chapter we explain the potential role of prognostic models in healthcare and practice, including how they support personalized (stratified or precision) medicine. (5–8) We outline a rigorous framework for prognostic model research, from model development to external validation and then impact evaluation. A range of examples are used to illustrate the messages. The scope of the field is enormous; here we focus on the key principles for good practice and major bottlenecks that can prevent progress. Other textbooks and series complement this chapter (7, 9–21).

7.2 Examples and format of prognostic models

Prognostic models are typically developed using a multivariable regression framework, which provides an equation to estimate an individual's expected outcome value (for continuous outcomes) or outcome risk (for binary or time-to-event outcomes) based on their values of multiple prognostic factors (such as age and smoking, symptoms and signs, imaging and electrophysiology results, biomarkers and genetic information). In this context, the included prognostic factors are better known as predictors, independent variables, or covariates, which are more generic terms used in regression modelling textbooks (9). We adopt the term 'predictor' for the remainder of this chapter.

Chapter 3 explained the format of a prognostic model equation based on linear, logistic, and proportional hazards (Cox or parametric) regression, which are the common frameworks for developing a model for continuous, binary, and time-to-event outcomes, respectively. These regression models involve an intercept or baseline hazard (or baseline survival) combined with multiple predictor effects (corresponding to mean differences, log odds ratios or log hazard ratios). For example, a logistic regression model is of the format,

$$\ln\left(\frac{p_i}{1-p_i}\right) = \alpha + \beta_1 X_{1i} + \beta_2 X_{2i} + \beta_3 X_{3i} + \cdots$$

where p_i is an individual's probability of developing the outcome, which is dependent on the model intercept (α), the values of included predictors (X_{1i}, X_{2i}, X_{3i}, etc.) and their corresponding log odds ratios ($\beta_1, \beta_2, \beta_3$, etc.). After estimation of a regression model's parameters, the model can be applied to a new individual by inputting their predictor values, to provide an estimate of their specific outcome value (for continuous outcomes) or their probability to develop the outcome (for dichotomous and time-to-event outcomes), conditional on the individual's specific predictor values. For example, after developing a logistic regression model, predictions of the outcome probability (risk) for new individuals are made by using:

$$\hat{p}_i = \frac{\exp(\hat{\alpha} + \hat{\beta}_1 X_{1i} + \hat{\beta}_2 X_{2i} + \hat{\beta}_3 X_{3i} + \cdots)}{1 + \exp(\hat{\alpha} + \hat{\beta}_1 X_{1i} + \hat{\beta}_2 X_{2i} + \hat{\beta}_3 X_{3i} + \cdots)}$$

Figure 7.2 illustrates individualized predictions from a prognostic model for the risk of recurrence of a venous thromboembolism within a certain time period, in patients finishing therapy for a first venous thromboembolism (22).

Sometimes prognostic models are presented without an intercept or baseline hazard term, such that they only provide a risk score based on the model's combination of predictor effects (i.e. $\hat{\beta}_1 X_{1i} + \hat{\beta}_2 X_{2i} + \hat{\beta}_3 X_{3i} + \cdots$). Such risk scores are hard to interpret directly, as they cannot provide an individual's probability or risk of the outcome since the intercept or baseline hazard is lacking (9, 10, 12). An example of such a risk score is the NPI (Box 7.1). Consider the NPI for a breast cancer patient with a 2 cm tumour diameter, with no lymph nodes affected, and a grade 1 tumour. Her NPI is: (0.2 × 2) + 1 + 1 = 2.4. This value alone is meaningless without assigning the associated measure of probability of developing the outcome of interest within a particular time interval. To this end, survival curves need to be plotted for groups of women with similar NPI scores, and then the probability of survival over time can be derived from the observed data, and reported for each group. Based on the risk grouping shown in Box 7.1 (3, 5), the prognosis for this particular patient is good, as she falls within the first risk group which has an overall five-year survival of about 90%.

However, a problem with any model that provides outcome probabilities categorized according to 'risk score groups', is that the formation of the groups is often arbitrary, and hides variation of individual risk within the same group. Two individuals with almost the same score that just happen to fall in different risk groups will be given a different prognosis and outcome risk. Consider two women with breast cancer who each have a grade 2 tumour and two lymph

---

Context: A prognostic model predicting the risk of recurrent venous thromboembolism after cessation of initial therapy following a first venous thromboembolism[22]

(a) Developed model equation

Probability of recurrence by time t is defined by $F(t) = 1 - S_0(t)^{\exp(risk\ score)}$ where

$$risk\ score = (-0.0105 \times Age) + (0.545 \times Gender:Male)$$
$$+ (1.735 \times Site:Proximal\ DVT) + (1.756 \times Site:PE)$$
$$+ (0.701 \times \log(D\text{-}dimer)) + (-0.291 \times \log(Lag\ time))$$

and $S_0(t)$ is the baseline survival available at all time points up to 4 years, e.g. $S_0(6\ months) = 0.9996$, $S_0(1\ year) = 0.9993$, and $S_0(2\ years) = 0.9988$, and the reference site is a distal deep vein thrombosis (DVT).

(b) Applying the model to produce predicted recurrence risk curves for three different patients

Values of predictors for each patient:

Predictor	Patient A	Patient B	Patient C
Age (years)	51	64	74
Gender:Male	1	1	1
Site:Proximal DVT	0	1	0
Site:Pulmonary Embolism (PE)	0	0	1
D-dimer (ng/mL)	275	417.5	747
log(D-dimer)	5.55	6.03	6.62
Lag time (days)	22	29	33
log(Lag time)	3.14	3.4	3.53

Figure 7.2 Example of prognostic model equation and individualised survival curve prediction.
Source: data from Ensor, J. et al. Prediction of risk of recurrence of venous thromboembolism following treatment for a first unprovoked venous thromboembolism: systematic review, prognostic model and clinical decision rule, and economic evaluation. Health Technology Assessment. 20(12), 1-190. Copyright © 2016 NETSCC

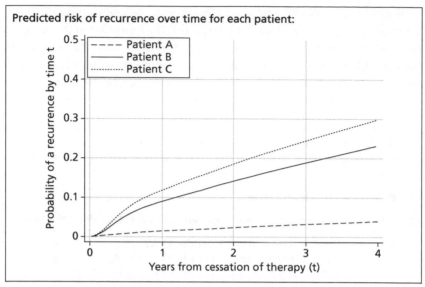

Figure 7.2 Continued

node glands affected, but one of the women has a tumour diameter of 72 mm and the other has 73 mm. These women have almost identical NPIs of 5.4 and 5.5, respectively, and yet would be assigned to two different risk groups with a wildly different overall prognosis of about 70% and 20%, respectively (3, 5).

Therefore, prognostic models should always be reported with an intercept or baseline hazard (or survival) term (as in Figure 7.2) to avoid unnecessary and misleading risk grouping, and to allow the direct estimation of the absolute outcome risks tailored to each individual rather than to a group of individuals. In this way, patients and their clinicians have an immediate and more refined picture of expected prognosis to enable more personalized healthcare decisions and counselling. This is illustrated in Figure 7.2, where a prognostic model for the risk of recurrent venous thromboembolism is reported with a baseline survival term, which allows individualized outcome risk predictions over time (22).

Prognostic models are sometimes developed using a regression model, including an intercept or baseline hazard term, but then presented in a simplified form or rule (e.g. by rounding predictor effects to whole numbers) or as a nomogram, which provides a graphical representation of the original mathematical equation from which the predicted outcome (risk) can be calculated (23). An example of a nomogram is shown in Figure 7.3. Such graphical and simplified approaches are attractive for situations where computer access is limited, but generally will lose information or increase the potential for prediction errors. For example, nomograms may not be familiar for many users and may lead to calculation mistakes. Therefore, wherever possible, it is preferable for the original model equation to be presented and embedded within

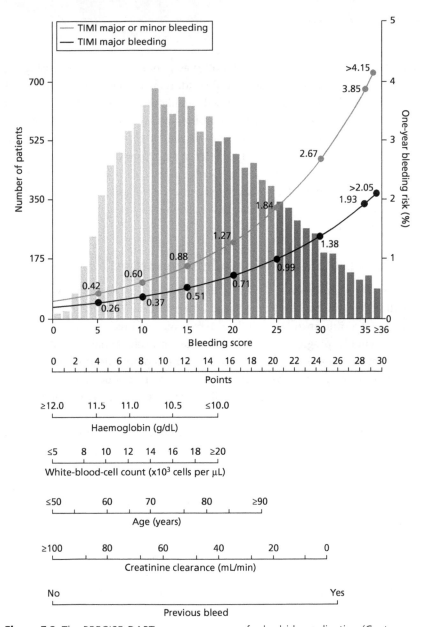

Figure 7.3 The PRECISE-DAPT score nomogram for bedside application (Costa et al., 2017).

Risk curves refer to out-of-hospital Thrombosis in Myocardial Infarction (TIMI) major or minor bleeding and TIMI major bleeding at 12 months while on-treatment with dual antiplatelet therapy (DAPT). Histogram refers to the PRECISE-DAPT score distribution in the derivation cohort, split into four shaded colors denoting (from left to right) very low risk (lightest shade), low risk, moderate risk, and high risk (darkest shade).

Source: reproduced with permission from Costa, F., et al. Derivation and validation of the predicting bleeding complications in patients undergoing stent implantation and subsequent dual antiplatelet therapy (PRECISE-DAPT) score: a pooled analysis of individual-patient datasets from clinical trials. The Lancet.389(10073), 1025-34. Copyright © 2017 Elsevier

software applications or web-based tools that automate calculations (using the full model equation behind the scenes) conditional on the user's inputted predictor values. For example, a web-based calculator for the Global Registry of Acute Cardiac Events (GRACE) (24) tool is available at www.gracescore.org, and this also provides graphical displays to help users interpret the predicted risk of myocardial infarction and mortality in patients with acute coronary syndrome. Note that in some articles, especially in the cancer field (25), the words nomogram and prognostic model are used interchangeably, and so 'nomogram' does not always indicate a graphical visualization of a prognostic model, even though it should.

7.3 Why are prognostic models important?

The use of prognostic models ties in with the strong movement towards personalized or stratified healthcare, where risk communication and treatment decisions are informed by an individual's profile of predictor values (7, 27). Fundamentally, prognostic models allow health professionals to tailor prognostic information to their patient, with clearer communication such as: "In individuals with similar characteristics to you, the risk of death by one-year is 20%; therefore, for every five patients similar to you, we expect four to be alive by one-year."

Prognostic models aim to assist (not replace) healthcare professionals with their prediction of a patient's future outcome and to enhance informed decision making together with the patient (12). In particular, they help translate the results of randomized trials examining the effect of interventions on prognosis. Considering a binary outcome, then under the common assumption that a particular treatment has a constant *relative* benefit across all patients (i.e. the risk ratio for treatment versus control is constant across the entire outcome risk range, i.e. 0 to 1), the *absolute* treatment benefit depends on a person's risk of the outcome without treatment (27); those with the highest baseline risk will have the greatest absolute reduction in risk. Expensive therapies or those with harmful potential side-effects may thus be reserved for those considered at higher risk, as estimated by a prognostic model. For example, in women with osteoporosis the effectiveness of alendronate for reducing the rate of non-vertebral fracture was, when expressed as a rate ratio, constant across subgroups defined by increasing fracture risk according to the FRAX prognostic model. However, the reduction in *absolute* rate due to alendronate increased as the baseline fracture risk increased (28), and therefore those at highest outcome risk defined by FRAX had larger potential reduction in their absolute rate (see Chapter 8 for more details).

Some prognostic models are used routinely in medical practice without being described as such, in particular the Apgar score for assessing the wellbeing of

Table 7.1 Examples of the development, validation, and impact of prognostic models.

Name of prognostic model	Development	Validation	Impact on guidelines
Nottingham Prognostic Index (NPI)	Cox regression of mortality rates in 387 women (with 62 deaths by 5 years) with primary, operable breast cancer (3, 40)	Many validation studies, including a validation study in 9149 Danish patients (41)	Cited in guidelines (e.g. NICE CG80) Survey indicated use in many centres to decide on adjuvant chemotherapy (76) Modelling study for cost-effectiveness analysis (42)
CRASH and IMPACT	6-month outcome after traumatic brain injury (n = 10,008 for CRASH; n = 8530 for IMPACT) (43)	Cross-validation of CRASH on IMPACT and vice versa (44)	Cited as source of prognostic risk estimation (36) Used to select trial participants and in the analysis of RCTs
GRACE and GRACE 2.0 score	6-month mortality, developed using registry data involving 94 hospitals in 14 countries, containing about 15000 patients (later updated using about 32000 patients)	Many external validation studies, (45) including for updated model (46, 47)	Cited in many guidelines, such as NICE CG94 (30)
Manchester Triage System	Urgency classification system by experts (29)	N = 16,735 children in 2 Dutch hospitals (48)	Widely cited in most western guidelines. Widely implemented, even before publication.

newborn babies (24). Other examples of well-used prognostic models that are implemented in clinical guidelines include the NPI (3), the Manchester Triage System to assign priority based on clinical need in patients visiting the emergency department (29), and the GRACE (24) risk score (Table 7.1). For example, the National Institute for Clinical Excellence (NICE) recommended that (30):

> 'As soon as the diagnosis of unstable angina or non ST-segment-elevation myocardial infarction (NSTEMI) is made, and aspirin and antithrombin therapy have been offered, formally assess individual risk of future adverse cardiovascular events using an established risk scoring system that predicts 6-month mortality (for example, GRACE) ... Use risk assessment to guide clinical management, and balance the benefit of a treatment against any risk of related adverse events in the light of this assessment ... Use predicted 6-month mortality to categorise the risk of future adverse cardiovascular events as follows: 1.5% or below = Lowest; > 1.5 to 3.0% = Low; > 3.0 to 6.0% = Intermediate; > 6.0 to 9.0% = High; over 9.0% = Highest.'

Some prognostic models are even more directive toward clinical decision making, for example with treatment decisions explicitly linked to whether the predicted outcome risk (or predicted risk score value) is above a chosen threshold. As mentioned previously, such models are then known as a clinical decision (or prediction) rule. For example, when using the CHA_2DS_2-VASc score for predicting the risk of a future stroke event in patients diagnosed with atrial fibrillation, it is generally advocated that anticoagulation treatment is not required for a male individual with a score of 0 (low risk), but should be considered for a male individual with a score of 1 or higher.

Besides assisting clinical decision making and improving patient counselling (addressing the 'median isn't the message' problem), prognostic models also may enhance the design and analysis of future studies, in a similar way to that described for prognostic factors in Chapter 6 (31, 32). For example, in randomized intervention trials they can be used for enabling stratified randomization strategies, to improve balance in prognosis across intervention and control groups at baseline. Furthermore, the model's predicted outcomes risks at baseline can be pre-defined as an adjustment factor in the trial analyses (31–35). For example, the CRASH and IMPACT prognostic models for adverse outcomes following a traumatic brain injury are well validated (Table 7.1) (36), but their application lies predominantly in research (37), in particular for enhancing the design and analysis of randomized intervention trials in that domain (32).

Prognostic models also help to adjust for case-mix variation in health services research (38), for example in understanding variations in patients' outcome across hospitals or countries (39), and can be considered as confounders to adjust for in observational research of potential causal factors of poor outcome.

7.4 Phases of prognostic model research

'We believe that the main reasons why doctors reject published prognostic models are lack of clinical credibility and lack of evidence that a prognostic model can support decisions about patient care (that is, evidence of accuracy, generality, and effectiveness).' (49)

Prognostic models should be viewed as a health technology and thus undergo rigorous development, validation, and impact evaluation before being rolled out. For instance, the GRACE 2.0 Risk Calculator 'app' has been defined as a medical device under the European Union Medical Device Directive 93/42/EEC. Therefore, high-quality evidence is needed to ensure prognostic models are fit for purpose. This requires phases of prognostic model research, from careful development with internal validation, to external validation in multiple studies or settings, and then evaluation of impact on health outcomes and cost-effectiveness of care. These phases are illustrated for well-known existing models in Table 7.1, and now described in detail.

7.4.1 Development and internal validation of a prognostic model

The development of prognostic models is very common (19). Development studies aim to derive a model using a particular dataset, and to quantify the model's performance (usually in the same development dataset, but sometimes also in other data). Box 7.2 summarizes good principles and

---

Box 7.2 Key recommendations for studies that develop a prognostic model

- Register the study (e.g. at clinicaltrials.gov), and publish a protocol describing data sources, patient inclusion (startpoint) criteria, predictor, and outcome definitions, and (intended) strategy for data analysis.

- Use a high-quality dataset representative of the target population. Ideally, use data from a well-designed and conducted, preferably prospective, cohort study or, if not feasible, from some other type of existing data set such as from a biobank, electronic-health records, or a completed randomized trial.

- Use clearly defined outcomes and time points (e.g. in relation to startpoint at which predictions are made, and the horizon for predicted risk estimates) that are meaningful to the targeted individuals and healthcare professionals.

- Specify appropriate eligibility criteria so that included participants reflect the case-mix variation of the targeted population and setting of interest.

- Identify relevant candidate predictors *a priori* (e.g. based on previous evidence), including any relevant treatments that are administered (in routine care) to patients at baseline.

- Use a clear definition of each predictor and outcome, and ensure they are valid and reliably measured.

- Use a statistical model appropriate to the outcome data of interest (e.g. logistic regression for a binary outcome, survival model for a time-to-event outcome), and deal with loss to follow-up appropriately (e.g. censor individuals at their drop-out time if non-informative).

Box 7.2 Continued

- ♦ Handle continuous predictors appropriately (i.e. avoid categorization), ideally by considering potential non-linear trends using, for example, restricted cubic splines or fractional polynomials.

- ♦ Handle missing data appropriately by considering methods that account for the missing data mechanism (e.g. using multiple imputation).

- ♦ Reduce the potential for overfitting (i.e. producing models that are overly tailored to the data at hand, hence yielding predictions that are too extreme in new data sets) by:

  - ensuring a sufficiently large sample size (and numbers of events)

  - reducing the number of candidate predictors in advance of predictor-outcome analysis (e.g. based on previous evidence, and by removing some predictors from a set of highly correlated predictors)

  - avoiding univariable screening to select candidate predictors for the multivariable model

  - applying penalized estimation or other shrinkage techniques (e.g. uniform shrinkage, LASSO, elastic net, ridge regression), that penalise (shrink) predictor effect estimates to reduce overfitting

  - including all candidate predictors in the final model, regardless of their statistical significance, or incorporating predictor selection within a penalization method such as LASSO or elastic net. If backwards selection is applied, use a more liberal p-value for retention (e.g. $p < 0.20$ rather than < 0.05).

- ♦ Use internal validation methods that adopt resampling techniques, such as bootstrapping or cross validation, to quantify the optimism in the model's apparent performance in terms of calibration and discrimination.

- ♦ Derive optimism-adjusted estimates of calibration and discrimination performance.

- ♦ Report the study process and findings (e.g. full regression model, model performance) according to the TRIPOD guideline.

Source: data from Thangaratinam, S., et al. Prediction of complications in early-onset pre-eclampsia (PREP): development and external multinational validation of prognostic models. BMC Medicine. 15(1), 68. Copyright © 2017 Springer Nature. Open Access.

practice for model development, and below we discuss in more detail some of the key issues, building on detailed recommendations elsewhere (9–16). A case study illustrating the main aspects of model development is given in Box 7.3.

Box 7.3 Case study of prognostic model development: prediction of adverse outcomes in pre-eclampsia (50)

Background: Thangaratinam et al. (50) developed multivariable prognostic models for providing individual risks (over time, and by hospital discharge) of adverse maternal outcomes in women with early-onset pre-eclampsia in the UK (50). A protocol for the study objectives, design, and analysis was published.

Methods: A prospective cohort study, with consecutive recruitment of women with suspected or confirmed pre-eclampsia before thirty-four weeks' gestation from December 2011 to April 2014, from fifty-three obstetric units within secondary and tertiary care hospitals in the UK. Women with confirmed early-onset pre-eclampsia contributed to model development. The outcome for prediction was defined as any maternal complication that included maternal death, neurological, hepatic, cardiorespiratory, renal or haematological complications, or delivery before thirty-four weeks. An initial list of thirty-three candidate predictors was identified from published systematic reviews and primary studies, and (*before* any data analysis) reduced to twenty-two after prioritizing their importance by a Delphi consensus among experts. The number of events was over twenty per candidate predictor. Two prognostic models were developed: a logistic regression model for any adverse outcome risk by discharge (PREP-L) and a Royston-Parmar flexible parametric survival model (Chapter 3) for adverse outcome risk over time until thirty-four weeks' gestation (PREP-S). Multiple imputation was used to deal with missing data, and a backwards selection procedure for exclusion of predictors, except with gestational age and maternal age forced to improve clinical acceptability. Non-linear trends for continuous predictors were evaluated using multivariable fractional polynomials, and bootstrapping was then used to estimate optimism in discrimination and calibration performance. Uniform shrinkage factors were applied to account for any optimism, with model intercepts re-estimated.

Results: There were 946 women included in the development dataset. About a fifth of the women suffered a complication (169/946, 18%) by forty-eight hours after diagnosis, and two-thirds (633/946, 66.9%) by postnatal discharge. The most frequent outcome was early preterm delivery before thirty-four weeks' gestation (580/946, 61.3%). After model development, the PREP-L and PREP-S model equations were penalized by applying a uniform shrinkage factor of 0.86 (derived from bootstrapping) to the predictor effect estimates, and the intercept/baseline hazard re-estimated

Box 7.3 Continued

accordingly. This produced the final PREP-L and PREP-S models. The apparent C statistic for the PREP-L model was 0.84 (95% CI 0.82, 0.87), and after bootstrap adjustment for optimism it was 0.82 (95% CI 0.80, 0.84). The apparent and optimism-adjusted Harrell's C statistic of the developed PREP-S model were 0.77 (95% CI 0.75, 0.79) and 0.75 (95% CI 0.73, 0.78), respectively.

Source: data from Thangaratinam, S., et al. Prediction of complications in early-onset pre-eclampsia (PREP): development and external multinational validation of prognostic models. BMC Medicine. 15(1), 68. Copyright © 2017 Springer Nature. Open Access.

7.4.1.1 Initiating a model development study

The decision to develop a prognostic model should be motivated by the (clinical) need for outcome prediction and the absence of reliable existing models, rather than the availability of a convenient dataset for personal academic gain (51). A systematic review of existing models (and their performance) for the intended population, outcome, and setting, is an ideal first step (see Chapter 9). There is no need to develop a new model when an existing model performs well enough, or when it can be adjusted reliably for the intended target population. For this reason, new studies should prioritize external validation of existing models (see section 7.4.2), rather than immediately aiming to develop a new model. Such validation studies help to determine whether the existing models perform adequately, and can also be used to tailor (and combine) existing models to other settings and target populations (52–54).

7.4.1.2 Obtaining a high-quality dataset

When there is justification to develop a new model, researchers need to obtain a high-quality dataset for model development: this is often referred to as the development, derivation, or training dataset. It is essential that this dataset represents the intended population (e.g. disease or health condition, setting, and population) of interest, and includes information on the relevant startpoint and outcome (and corresponding time points). Such a dataset is best obtained from a prospective (i.e. predesigned) cohort study, in order to prospectively recruit (a sample of) the relevant or targeted individuals, and define and measure the appropriate startpoint, candidate predictors and health outcomes of interest. In such prospective studies, researchers can better define the inclusion and exclusion criteria, control the desired definitions and methods of measurement used for predictors and outcomes, ensure the timing of predictor and outcome measurement is sensible (55), reduce the potential for missing data, and minimize potential biases (e.g. by using a random or, ideally, consecutive sample of participants to avoid selection bias, and ensuring measurement of predictor values are made blind to outcome classifications). Included participants should be representative of the population of interest for using the model, to ensure that case-mix variations are adequately reflected. For reasons of efficiency or cost, sampling of patients rather than using the full cohort can be applied. Examples are case-cohort and nested case-control designs (56, 57). Care is needed for such sampling strategies, as selectively choosing or omitting certain cases and non-cases may cast doubt on the representativeness of the sample for the population of interest. Furthermore, the sampling (fractions) of cases and non-cases needs to be incorporated in the model development in order to correctly estimate the proper intercept or baseline hazard, so that the model provides accurate predictions of the absolute outcome risk.

Pre-designed prospective cohort studies can be costly and time-consuming, usually requiring many years of follow-up, and may be difficult to obtain funding for. Therefore, existing data from randomized trials of interventions, from cohort studies (designed for other purposes than prognostic modeling), or from case-cohort and nested case-control studies, are an attractive alternative. A special case of existing datasets, and becoming increasingly popular in the era of big data and open access, are large, routinely collected participant data stored in registries and electronic healthcare databases, already containing many years of follow-up for thousands (often millions) of patients. However, researchers must be aware that existing data sets are often not specifically defined and collected for the purpose of developing or validating prognostic models. For example, randomized trials may have narrow eligibility criteria, and routine care datasets may not record (or may have more missing data for) predictors and outcomes of interest. Chapters 13 and 14 consider the use of existing databases for prognosis research in more detail.

7.4.1.3 The problem of overfitting and optimism in predictive performance

A prognostic model should have good predictive performance as quantified statistically in terms of discrimination (e.g. C statistic) and calibration (e.g. calibration slope), and overall measures of fit (e.g. R^2). Such measures were explained in detail in Chapter 3. When examining the predictive performance of a model in the same dataset used for its development ('apparent' peformance), the estimates of calibration and discrimination are usually misleading (optimistic), primarily due to overfitting of predictor effects to the dataset at hand. Empirical evidence for optimism is shown in Figure 7.4 (58). Here, the apparent C statistics of multivariable prediction models (in the development dataset) are compared with subsequent C statistics of the model when tested (validated) in

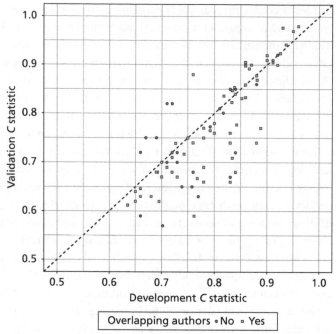

Figure 7.4 Empirical evidence of optimism in C statistic from model development compared with subsequent external validation studies.
Source: adapted from Collins, G.S., et al. External validation of multivariable prediction models: a systematic review of methodological conduct and reporting. BMC Medical Research Methodology. 14, 40. Copyright © 2014 Springer. Open Access.

other datasets. In 58 of the 88 cases (66%), the C statistics in the development dataset (mean C statistic = 0.787) are higher than those in the validation dataset (mean C statistic = 0.757), suggesting that apparent C statistics are often too large (too close to 1).

One plausible reason for this is that many developed models have poor internal validity because they do not account for overfitting; in particular, they have too small sample sizes relative to the number of predictors studied (section 7.4.1.4), do not use penalization (shrinkage) methods (Section 7.4.1.8) and do not provide optimism-corrected performance statistics (section 7.4.1.7). Differences in predictive performance may also be due to poor transportability of the model to different settings or populations than included in the model development dataset (see also section 7.4.2.1) (59).

7.4.1.4 Sample size and candidate predictors

A large sample size is important when initiating a model development study (16, 60, 61), to estimate regression coefficients precisely, whilst reducing the potential for overfitting and optimism in apparent predictive performance of a developed model. The effective sample size for a continuous outcome is determined by the total number of study participants; for binary outcomes it is the minimum of the number of events and non-events; and for time-to-event outcomes it is approximately the total number of events (9). For binary or time-to-event outcomes, a well-known rule of thumb is at least ten Events Per candidate predictor Parameter (*EPP*). This is often referred to as ten Events Per Variable (EPV) (62, 63), but this is misleading. The word 'parameter' is more accurate, as there is often more parameters than variables (predictors). For example, a predictor with four categories will require three parameters in the model (i.e. three β s are estimated). The word 'candidate' is also important, as it is not the number of parameters included eventually in the final model, but rather the total number considered in the study.

Some researchers suggest that ten is too conservative (e.g. for rare events, an *EPP* of fifty may be required) (60, 64, 65), while others suggest ten is too high (66). The differences in these recommendations are largely down to the design of the individual simulation studies from which these recommendations were made (including range in simulated true effect sizes of regression coefficients, total sample size, number of predictors), as well as the complexity and problems due to lack of convergence. Furthermore, there is growing evidence to suggest that any general *EPP* rule is too simplistic (60, 61, 67), as the required sample size depends on many intricate factors other than the number of events and candidate predictors, including the distribution of predictor values and the percentage of outcome variability explained by the predictors.

To address this, Riley et al. (building on Harrell (9)) suggest criteria to identify the *minimum* sample size needed to develop a prognostic model (68, 69). For example, for binary and time-to-event outcomes, they suggest the sample size should be at least large enough to meet three key criteria: (i) small optimism in predictor effect estimates as defined by a uniform shrinkage factor of ≥0.9; (ii) small absolute difference of ≤0.05 in the model's apparent and adjusted Nagelkerke's R^2; and (iii) precise estimation of the overall risk in the population. To be extra stringent, researchers might additionally ensure the sample size will give precise estimates of key predictor effects; this is especially important when key categorical predictors have few events in some categories, as this may substantially increase the numbers required.

Criteria (i) and (ii) aim to reduce overfitting conditional on a chosen P (i.e. the chosen number of predictor parameters to be considered). Criteria (i) will often dominate the sample size calculation, as large sample sizes are usually needed to ensure an expected shrinkage factor (S) close to 1, such as 0.9, that reflects low overfitting. To calculate the sample size (n) to meet criteria (i), a formula is presented by Riley et al. (69), derived from the heuristic shrinkage factor of Van Houwelingen and Le Cessie (70, 71), which is introduced fully in Section 7.4.1.8. The formula requires the researcher to pre-specify a lower bound for the model's anticipated Cox-Snell R^2 (proportion of variance explained by the model) and also P, the total number of predictor parameters to be considered (which excludes the intercept). It is written as:

$$n = \frac{P}{(S-1)\ln\left(1 - \frac{R^2}{S}\right)}$$

For example, when developing a logistic regression model with up to twenty predictor parameters and an anticipated R^2 of at least 0.1, then to target an expected shrinkage of 0.9, one needs a sample size of:

$$n = \frac{P}{(S-1)\ln\left(1 - \frac{R^2}{S}\right)} = \frac{20}{(0.9-1)\ln\left(1 - \frac{0.1}{0.9}\right)} = 1698$$

and thus a minimum of 1698 patients. For a binary outcome, this corresponds to $EPP = n\lambda / P$, where λ is the expected cumulative incidence of the outcome (outcome proportion). For example, if λ is 0.1 (10%) then $EPP = (1698 \times 0.1) / 20 = 8.5$. However, if λ is 0.3 (30%) then $EPP = 25.5$, much larger than the EPP = 10 rule of thumb. A case study illustrating the approach is given in Figure 7.5

Riley et al. show how to obtain realistic values of the Cox-Snell R^2 in advance of model development by using published information from existing models in the same field (68, 69). Crucially, for binary and time-to-event outcomes, the anticipated value of the Cox-Snell R^2 may be low (i.e. closer to zero than one), even for a good model, as the maximum value of R^2 is bounded at a value less than one according to the outcome prevalence or rate in the setting of interest. For futher details, we refer the reader to the publications (68, 69).

Where the minimum sample size (total events) derived is considered not achievable (e.g. due to time and cost constraints), or ultimately not obtained (e.g. due to cumulative outcome incidence being lower than anticipated), a shrinkage close to 1 (e.g. 0.9) can still be targeted by reducing the set of candidate predictors (before analysis of predictor-outcome associations in the dataset available). One might prioritize those predictors known to be prognostic factors based on previous evidence (e.g. a systematic review), exclude those predictors with high amounts of missing information, retain just one predictor from a set of highly correlated predictors, or combine related predictors where considered sensible (72).

Ensor et al. developed a prognostic model for the risk of a recurrent venous thromboembolism (VTE) following cessation of therapy for a first VTE (see Figure 7.3).[22] The model performed well on average, but the model's predicted risks did not calibrate well with the observed risks in some populations.[22] Therefore, new research is needed to update and extend this model, for example by including additional predictors. A sample size calculation is helpful for this purpose.

Let us assume that inclusion of 25 predictor parameters (P) is of interest for the new model, and that the existing model's adjusted Cox-Snell R^2 value of 0.051 is a lower bound for the expected R^2 of the new model. Then, targeting a shrinkage factor of 0.9, the formula of Riley et al.[69] gives a total sample size of,

$$n = \frac{P}{(S-1)\ln\left(1-\dfrac{R^2}{S}\right)} = \frac{25}{(0.9-1)\ln\left(1-\dfrac{0.051}{0.9}\right)} = 4285.5$$

and thus 4286 participants. This assumes the new cohort will have a similar follow-up, censoring rate, and cumulative incidence (λ) to that reported by Ensor et al., where 13.42% of individuals had a VTE recurrence by the end of follow-up. Thus, the number of events required for the new model is then $n\lambda = 4286 \times 0.1342 = 575.2$ events, which corresponds to $575.2/25 = 23$ events per predictor parameter (EPP). This is over twice the commonly used EPP of 10. Indeed, an EPP of 10 only ensures a shrinkage factor of 0.79, as shown below.

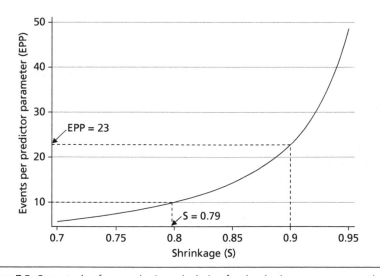

Figure 7.5 Case study of a sample size calculation for developing a new prognostic model, based on minimizing the expected shrinkage (overfitting). (68, 69)
Source: reproduced courtesy of Richard D. Riley

7.4.1.5 Consideration of treatment and dynamic modelling

'If a prognostic model aims to produce correct probabilities of the outcome in the absence of treatment, ignoring treatments that affect that outcome can lead to suboptimal model performance and incorrect treatment decisions. Explicitly, modeling treatment is recommended.' (73)

If not standardized for all patients, any treatments received at baseline should be considered as predictors, as they are themselves (potential) prognostic factors (73). This is emphasized in the REMARK (Item 10f and Item 17) and TRIPOD (item 5c) guidelines (15, 74). For example, when developing a prognostic model using data from all patients within a randomized trial where the treatment is effective, treatment should be included as a predictor in the model, otherwise predictions from the model will be miscalibrated in those with and without treatment (73).

For most prognostic models, only information at baseline (i.e. the startpoint for making predictions from) is used and therefore treatments and predictors measured *after* baseline are not included in the model itself, as this information would be unknown at the moment of application of the model. In this situation, the prognostic model will give predictions at baseline that reflect prognosis in the context of current care, in which treatments and clinical decisions change over time according to the health and symptoms of the patient (73, 75).

Where the focus is on making risk predictions in the absence of treatment, a major challenge is developing prognostic models from observational data of individuals where treatment is initiated after the startpoint; so-called "treatment drop-ins" (76). To address this, Sperrin et al. propose the use of marginal structural models that adjust for treatment drop-in, and so allow a prognostic model to predict outcome risk over time conditional on receiving no treatment during follow-up (76). In a simulation study, their novel approach led to prognostic models with larger outcome risk predictions than other modelling options that ignored treatment drop-in.

An extended idea is to update predictions over time, for example using dynamic prognostic models. This allows predictor values to be updated over time, including treatment status and the individual's medical condition. For instance, new outcome predictions may be required when an individual moves onto a new treatment, reflecting a change in condition or a new health state. For example, in the early stages of pregnancy (the startpoint) a model is needed to predict the mother's risk of pre-eclampsia. Subsequently, in those that develop pre-eclampsia (the new state), a further model is needed to predict adverse outcome risk for the mother in the context of chosen treatments. Pertinent approaches for this purpose are competing risks and multi-state models, joint modelling of longitudinal and survival data, and landmarking (77–80). Chapter 15 describes these concepts in more detail.

7.4.1.6 Statistical methods

Appropriate statistical methods and principles are needed throughout the whole development process. This includes choosing a suitable modelling framework (e.g. multivariable regression), dealing with missing data, estimating the baseline hazard, handling of continuous predictors (81), dealing with complexities such as censoring and competing risks (82, 83), selecting predictors for inclusion in the multivariable modeling, assigning weights per predictor, quantifying and adjusting optimism (e.g. due to overfitting), developing a final model (equation), and quantifying the predictive performance of the model (e.g. in terms of discrimination and calibration). Box 7.2 provides recommendations, and key issues are covered in detail in Chapters 3 and 4.

7.4.1.7 Internal validation

'*Whenever data-dependent modelling is used, the analyst should be aware that the "final" model selected is partly a result of "chance" and can have many weaknesses. Investigation of its stability should become standard practice.*' (84)

All studies that develop a prognostic model should include internal validation. This is essential to ascertain and, if necessary, reduce the optimism (due to overfitting) in a developed prognostic model (section 7.4.1.3). The goal is to ensure the model is more likely to be reliable when tested or applied in new data (a concept known as reproducibility; see section 7.4.2.1).

Split-sample approach
A common approach for internal validation is to leave out a random part of the development cohort to form a 'testing' dataset; for example 70% of the data may be used for model development and 30% reserved for validation. However this split-sample approach is statistically inefficient and methodologically weak, since no difference in time or place exists other than by chance, and thus the testing dataset is expected to show the same performance (14, 85). In small datasets the results of split-sample validation can also vary depending on the split (85–87). A variant on this approach is a non-random split-sample, where the dataset is split by some clustering factor such as geographical location, centre, study, or time (14, 15, 20, 88). This is preferable because the 'testing' dataset is then more likely to be different from the development data in some key characteristics (15). However, similar problems as with split-sample validation may arise in small samples, and so this approach is best reserved for situations when the development data remains large even after some clusters are non-randomly removed.

Resampling methods: cross-validation and bootstrapping

Usually, it is far better to use *all* the data for model development to improve stat-istical efficiency, and then apply internal validation via data resampling tech-niques such as bootstrapping or cross-validation. These approaches allow the optimism in the developed model's apparent predictive performance (in the original dataset) to be quantified, in terms of both discrimination and calibra-tion, and then 'optimism-adjusted' performance statistics and model param-eters (e.g. intercept and predictor effects) to be produced.

Leave-one-out cross-validation means leaving one participant out of the ana-lysis at a time and predicting the outcome for that individual using a model developed with n-1 patients. This is repeated n times and model performance is summarized across the n patients when excluded. However, reserving *groups* of participants for cross-validation, (for example, ten-fold cross-validation would divide the data into ten parts) is considered more accurate, especially if the number of events per group is kept fixed (9). Within each cycle, the model de-velopment process is repeated using all but one of the groups, and then model performance is estimated for the omitted group. This is repeated across all permutations of the omitted group, to obtain performance statistics for each omitted group, which are then averaged. In this way, the expected performance of the model in new patients can be quantified.

Non-parametric bootstrapping is often considered the best technique for in-ternal validation as it does not require excluding any data for internal validation, and retains the same, original sample size for model development. This is done by sampling with replacement from the original data to obtain a new sample of the same size as the original data, and this is called a bootstrap sample (89). The same model-building steps used to develop the original model are applied to each bootstrap sample, and the resulting bootstrap model is then evaluated on the same sample (to obtain apparent performance) and on the original dataset (to obtain test performance). The optimism in the bootstrap model is then cal-culated as the difference between the apparent performance in the bootstrap sample and the test performance in the original sample. This process is repeated many times (e.g. taking 1000 bootstrap samples), and the average of the (1000) optimism estimates is obtained. 'Optimism-adjusted' performance statistics can then be derived for the original model, simply by subtracting the average opti-mism estimate (as derived using bootstrapping) from the apparent performance of the original model (as derived in the original dataset) (9,10,16,21). The steps are outlined in Box 7.4. It also provides a way of estimating a uniform shrinkage factor to apply a global shrinkage of the predictor effects (see Section 7.4.1.8)

It is important that all model building steps (e.g. predictor selection) are re-played in each bootstrap sample; merely refitting the final developed model in each bootstrap sample will underestimate the optimism. Some steps of the

Box 7.4 The bootstrap procedure for internal validation of the predictive performance of a prognostic model (9, 10)

1. Develop the prognostic model using the entire original sample (size n) and determine the apparent predictive performance (e.g. calibration and discrimination) by applying the model in the very same data.

2. Generate a bootstrap sample, by sampling n individuals with replacement from the original sample.

3. Develop a model using the bootstrap sample (applying all the same modelling and predictor selection methods, as in step 1):

   a. Determine the performance (e.g. C statistic and calibration slope) of this bootstrap model on the bootstrap sample (apparent performance).

   b. Determine the performance of the bootstrap model in the original sample (test performance).

4. For each performance statistic, calculate the optimism as the difference between the estimated bootstrap performance and the estimated test performance.

5. Repeat steps 2 through 4 at least 100 times.

6. For each performance statistic, average the estimates of optimism in step 5, and subtract the value from the apparent performance obtained in step 1 to obtain an optimism-corrected estimate of performance for the original model.

Source: data from Harrell, F.E. 2015. Regression modeling strategies, with applications to linear models, logistic regression, and survival analysis.2nd Ed. New York, USA: Springer. Copyright © 2015 Springer; and Steyerberg, E.W. 2009. Clinical prediction models: a practical approach to development, validation, and updating. New York, USA: Springer. Copyright © 2009 Springer.

model building (e.g. selection of non-linear functions for continuous predictors) may not be easily implemented (automatically) in each bootstrap sample (e.g. when there is also multiple imputation of missing values) and in these instances, some compromise may be required (e.g. with a slightly reduced set of steps being replayed) or an alternative strategy should be sought.

As an example of the bootstrap approach to internal validation, consider van Diepen et al., who develop a prognostic model for one-year mortality risk in patients with diabetes starting dialysis (90). The model was developed using logistic regression, with backwards selection to choose predictors in a dataset of 394 patients with eighty-four deaths by one year. When examining the predictive performance of the model in the same dataset, the apparent calibration slope was 1 (as it should be in the development dataset) and the apparent C statistic was 0.810. Using bootstrapping, the optimism was estimated as 0.097 and 0.020 for the calibration slope and the C statistic respectively, leading to an optimism-adjusted calibration slope of 0.903 (= 1–0.097) and an optimism-adjusted C statistic of 0.790 (= 0.810–0.020). Another advantage of bootstrapping is to examine model instability across bootstrap samples, for example in terms of predictors selected and functional form of continuous predictors when using selection procedures (84, 91).

7.4.1.8 Shrinkage and penalized estimation methods

In addition to adjusting performance statistics for optimism, it is also important to adjust (penalize) predictor effect estimates of the developed model. Chapter 4 explained that the general concept of penalization is to reduce mean-square error in the model's outcome predictions, at the expense of adding some (slight) bias in the predictor effects. This is the premise of Stein's paradox (92).

There are various approaches to penalization. Perhaps the most common is to apply a uniform (linear, global) shrinkage factor (S) to all estimated predictor effects. For example, after fitting a logistic regression model using standard techniques (e.g. maximum likelihood estimation), a modified (penalised) logistic regression model with shrunken predictor effects can be obtained by:

$$ln\left(\frac{\hat{p}_i}{1-\hat{p}_i}\right) = \alpha^* + S(\hat{\beta}_1 X_{1i} + \hat{\beta}_2 X_{2i} + \hat{\beta}_3 X_{3i} + \cdots)$$

where S represents a value between 0 and 1, and corrects for overfitting. Also, α^* is the updated intercept, and is estimated after fixing S to ensure that the calibration-in-the-large is correct (i.e. that the sum of predicted probabilities equals the total number of observed events). Compared to the original (non-penalized) model, this will shrink predicted probabilities toward the overall mean (i.e. make the predicted probabilities less extreme, pulled away from zero and one). The value of S can be set equal to the optimism-adjusted calibration slope identified from bootstrapping. For example, in the aforementioned van Diepen et al. example the optimism-adjusted calibration slope of 0.903 was used as the shrinkage factor, and the revised (penalized) model is given in Table 7.2 (90). Recall that S was also used in Section 7.4.1.4 to inform sample size calculations, where a target value of >= 0.9 was recommended, to reflect low overfitting.

Closed-form solutions have also been proposed for S, including the James-Stein shrinkage estimator (93), and the heuristic shrinkage factor proposed by Van Houwelingen and le Cessie (71):

$$S = \frac{\text{model} \, \chi^2 - P}{\text{model} \, \chi^2}$$

Table 7.2 Example of uniform shrinkage applied to a prognostic model for one-year mortality risk in patients with diabetes starting dialysis.

	Developed model	Final model after adjustment for overfitting
Intercept	$\hat{\alpha}$	α^*
	1.962	1.427
Predictor	$\hat{\beta}$	$S\hat{\beta} = 0.903\,\hat{\beta}$
Age (years)	0.047	0.042
Smoking	0.631	0.570
Macrovascular complications	1.195	1.078
Duration of DM (years)	0.026	0.023
Karnofsky scale	−0.043	−0.039
Haemoglobin level (g/dl)	−0.186	−0.168
Albumin level (g/l)	−0.060	−0.054

where P is the number of estimated parameters for the predictors included in the model (excluding the intercept) and 'model χ^2' is the likelihood ratio (chi-squared) statistic for the model. Copas suggests that, for linear regression, an unbiased shrinkage factor is (70):

$$S = \frac{\text{model}\,\chi^2 - P + 2}{\text{model}\,\chi^2}$$

These suggested equations relate to a model developed without any automated predictor selection procedure, and thus P represents the number of parameters that correspond to the entire set of candidate predictors considered. Even when predictor selection procedures are used during model development, the P in these equations will be closer to that from the full model with all predictors included, than that from the final model with a reduced set of predictors.

Generally, we prefer bootstrapping to calculate S rather than a closed form solution, as bootstrapping can also incorporate any automated steps used during model development, such as backwards selection. However, other more sophisticated approaches to shrinkage (penalization) are available (94). In particular, regression approaches that directly penalize the likelihood function (rather than adopting post-hoc shrinkage) are becoming popular. A classical approach known as *ridge regression* adds a penalty factor to the likelihood function for the model (95), which shrinks predictor effects according to the variance of each predictor (95). A popular alternative is the LASSO (Least Absolute Shrinkage and Selection Operator) as it also enables predictor selection. Here, the penalty factor is defined such that it can shrink predictor effects to zero and hence allows the exclusion of some predictors (96). Another option is elastic net, which combines the penalty terms of ridge regression and LASSO, and also allows exclusion of predictors. Some authors suggest there is not much difference in the predictive performance of models developed by the various shrinkage methods (97, 98), but others argue in favour of particular approaches (99). It is an area of active research. A key recommendation is to use some form of shrinkage (penalization) method, either during or after model development.

7.4.2 **External validation of a prognostic model**

Usually, a developed prognostic model also needs its predictive performance to be examined using high-quality patient data not used in the development process. This process is known as external validation (4, 59, 100–105), and the emphasis is on accurate and precise estimation of a model's predictive performance so that meaningful conclusions can be drawn for a population of interest. A model's predictive performance upon external validation is crucial (arguably all that matters), and how a model was derived is of little importance if it performs well in new data. The validation population may or may not be similar to the population used to develop the model; indeed, it may be a deliberate intention to test the model's performance in a different setting (e.g. secondary care) than that used in model development (e.g. primary care). For this reason many external validation studies are conducted for the same model, to evaluate performance across different populations and settings. For example, the predictive performance of the NPI has been tested in many external, often large, validation studies (Table 7.1) (106). A case study of external validation is given in Figure 7.6.

7.4.2.1 Approaches to external validation

External validation does *not* mean refitting the original model and comparing how estimates of intercept and predictor effects have changed. Rather, external validation means applying the original model exactly as presented, and evaluating its predictive performance in terms of calibration and discrimination, and in terms of its net benefit (see Section 7.4.3.1). This requires large sample sizes to obtain precise estimates of performance. For prognostic models of binary or time-to-event outcomes, one hundred events is a suggested minimum effective sample size to ensure precise estimates of performance (107, 108), although ideally 200 is required to properly examine calibration (103, 108).

To improve external validation studies, Debray et al. (59) recommend that researchers should quantify the relatedness between the development and validation samples, in order to interpret external validation performance in terms of reproducibility and transportability. Reproducibility relates to when the external validation cohort is from a population and setting that is similar to that

Background: Consider again pre-eclampsia models (PREP-L and PREP-S, **Box 7.3**). To examine their predictive performance in a wider population, Thangaratinam et al. performed an external validation using an existing dataset ('PIERS') of women recruited in Canada, New Zealand, Australia and the UK.

Methods: The PIERS dataset contained 437 patients applicable to PREP-L and 339 patients with time-to-event data applicable to PREP-S. However, an issue was that the dataset did not include a few of the predictors (e.g. serum urea) included in PREP-L and PREP-S. To address this, reduced PREP-L and PREP-S models were developed in the original dataset (using the same methods as before, including optimism-adjustment) with only available predictors included. External validation could then be undertaken.

Results: For the reduced PREP-L model, this showed a C statistic of 0.81 (95% CI 0.77, 0.85) and a calibration slope of 0.93 (95% CI 0.72, 1.13) indicating good discrimination and calibration upon external validation.

For the reduced PREP-S model, the C statistic was 0.71 (95% CI 0.67, 0.75) and a calibration slope was 0.67 (95% CI 0.56, 0.79). The latter reveals miscalibration of the model's predictions, and the calibration plot below highlights that this is mainly in the high risk individuals, whose observed risk is lower than expected based on the model. When examining predictive performance up to just 48 hours, there was improvement in the C statistic (0.75, 95%CI 0.69, 0.81) and the calibration slope (0.80, 95% CI 0.62, 0.99), suggesting that the model performance deteriorates over time.

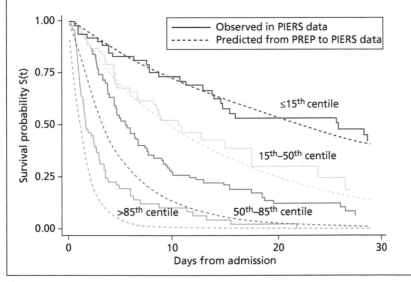

Figure 7.6 Case study in pre-eclampsia to illustrate external validation research.
Source: data from Thangaratinam, S., et al. Prediction of complications in early-onset pre-eclampsia (PREP): development and external multinational validation of prognostic models. BMC Medicine. 15(1), 68. Copyright © 2017 Springer Nature. Open Access.

used for model development. Conversely, transportability relates to validation in a different population or setting, for which model performance is often different due to changes in predictor effects and the participant case-mix compared to the original development dataset (e.g. when using a dataset from a secondary care setting to validate a model originally developed in a primary care setting).

Most external validation studies are based on local datasets, and thus only assess a prognostic model's performance in a specific setting or population. If that setting and population are identical to that used for the development dataset (i.e. same case-mix variation), then the external validation exercise rather evaluates model reproducibility (not transportability). Recall, reproducibility is also examined when applying internal validation methods (e.g. cross validation, bootstrapping) to the original development data. Indeed, other things being equal, reproducibility examined using internal validation with a large development dataset is often superior to using external validation with a small validation dataset. This is not well recognized.

Where interest lies in a model's transportability to multiple populations and settings, multiple external validation studies are often needed (59, 109–111). Then, not only is the *overall* (average) model performance of interest, but also the *heterogeneity* in performance across the different settings and populations (59). This can be addressed through data sharing and using individual participant data meta-analyses (Chapter 13) (52).

7.4.2.2 Updating, extending, and comparing prognostic models

The external validation phase may incorporate some model updating, which is often needed to improve the performance of the original prognostic model and tailor it to the validation study setting (10, 13, 112–114). In particular, some systematic miscalibration is common for predictions obtained from models in settings that differ from that of the development sample. A common updating approach is recalibration, where one or more terms in the model are changed to better fit the new setting. The simplest option is to change the model's intercept or baseline hazard term, and this can often substantially improve performance. An example of this is shown in Chapter 13 (52).

Another option is to investigate the addition of new prognostic factors, including biomarkers, to an existing model (112). The contribution of genomic, proteomic, or metabolomic measures and new imaging tests over and above established prognostic factors is a key issue in current prognosis research, and is especially useful to improve model performance across different settings and populations (115, 116). For example, a simple model for traumatic brain injury patients that included just three strong prognostic factors was extended with CT scanning results in a second stage, and laboratory test results in a third stage (44). The more extended models yielded more refined predictions and better discrimination. Often, though, the addition of new biomarkers may yield only marginal benefit (117). Because standard models generally include some very important predictors, the independent or added effects of new predictors need to be quite strong before a clinically useful improvement is achieved (118). Furthermore the measurement of new predictors, including biomarkers, carries cost implications, which need to be evaluated (115).

Though the importance of assessing the impact of new markers on the accuracy of a model is widely agreed, how best to quantify any changes in prediction is an active topic of methodological research (119–121). One could examine the improvement in model fit and discrimination performance. For example, adding hormone receptor status to the NPI, combined with more appropriate modelling of the continuous predictors of tumour size and number of lymph nodes, improves the C statistic from 0.65 to 0.71, and improves the percentage variance explained (R_D^2) from 22% to 29% (122). When linked to clinical decision making, the net reclassification improvement index has also been widely used, to quantify the overall improvement in classification (compared to existing models) across risk groups (123). However, this measure has received strong criticism, with Pepe et al. showing that it is often positive even when the new marker has no predictive information (124). Decision analytic techniques, such as the net benefit approach and decision curves, are preferable (see Section 7.4.3.1) (125). Such measures may also be improved after recalibration (126).

A particular motivation to update a prognostic model is to replace existing predictors that suffer from substantial measurement error or inter-observer variability (such as physical examination, imaging, and histopathological techniques) (127), with more reliably measured predictors. Moreover, prognostic models that include factors or markers with a causal effect on the outcome under study may be expected to better generalize. Such models are also more likely to be used, since they are linked to biological (or other) pathways that lead to the occurrence of the outcome, rather than merely based on statistical association between a predictor and outcome (100). While these suggestions are plausible, empirical evidence is lacking.

Ideally there should be an ongoing process of external validation and model updating (10, 13, 112–114). A related issue is how to compare competing prognostic models developed for the same targeted population and outcome (128). Again, this could be done by directly comparing their model fit, discrimination and calibration in new data; when linked directly to clinical decision making, net benefit and decision curve approaches are also important (see Section 7.4.3.1).

7.4.3 Evaluating the impact of a prognostic model on clinical practice and outcomes

Prognostic models can influence an individual's health outcomes or the cost-effectiveness of care only when changes in clinical management are made based on the model's predictions (e.g. of individual outcome risk) (4, 13). Therefore, when used to direct clinical decision making (e.g. as part of a decision rule), a prognostic model should also be evaluated for its overall benefit on clinical outcomes and healthcare. For example, for binary or time-to-event outcomes, if the predicted risks from a prognostic model are above a certain threshold value, then the patient and clinician may be directed to administer a particular intervention. The benefits, harms and overall impact of such directive prognostic models (rules) can be evaluated in different ways, as now described.

7.4.3.1 Net benefit and decision curves

Calibration and discrimination characterize the predictive performance of a prognostic model, but neither captures the clinical consequences of a particular level of discrimination or degree of miscalibration (129). Indeed, a model may have high discrimination and perfect calibration yet no clinical role, whereas the converse may also hold. Vickers argues this point in regard to a model to predict the outcome of prostate cancer biopsy (130):

> 'This could be because, for example, the predicted risks from the model ranged from 50% to 95%. Patients with prostate cancer tended to have higher predicted risks—leading to good discrimination—but no patient was given a probability low enough that a urologist would forgo biopsy. To put it another way, specifying that a patient with cancer is at very high risk, rather than just high risk, reflects that the model is a good one, but makes no clinical difference because the patient would be biopsied in both cases. By contrast, a model with only moderate discrimination might be useful if the clinical decision is a "toss-up" providing just enough information to push a clinical decision one way or the other.'

To examine potential clinical value, and without having to perform a new prospective long-term comparative impact study (see Section 7.4.3.3), decision analysis methods have been proposed, which use the model development or validation study data only. In particular, the overall consequences of using a prognostic model for clinical decisions can be measured using the so-called net benefit, which requires only the weighing of the benefits (e.g. improved patient outcomes) against the harms (e.g. worse patient outcomes, additional costs) (131, 132). This approach essentially puts benefits and harms on the same scale by specifying an exchange rate, a clinical judgement of the relative value of benefits and harms associated with using the model to determine clinical decisions. (131) For binary outcomes, it provides, for a chosen outcome risk threshold, the difference between the number of true-positive predictions and the number of false-positive predictions, weighted by a factor that gives the cost of a false-positive relative to a false-negative

$$\text{net benefit} = \frac{TP}{N} - \left(\frac{FP}{N} \times \frac{p_t}{1-p_t} \right) = \frac{TP - \left(FP \times \dfrac{p_t}{1-p_t} \right)}{N}$$

Here, N is the total sample size and p_t is the threshold probability used to classify patients into risk categories for medical decision making (e.g. to inform upon treatment or referral decisions). For example, a threshold value of $p_t = 0.08$ has been suggested to inform the continuation of treatment after thirty days following a first venous thromboembolism (22), such that those with a predicted risk of 0.08 or above continue treatment, but those with a risk < 0.08 stop. The threshold p_t reflects the ratio of harm to benefit, where harm is the burden of a treatment to the FP cases, and benefit refers to the gain/improvement for the TP cases. Then, for a given value of p_t, one calculates the number of patients with a 'positive' result (risk $\geq p_t$) who have the disease (true positives; TP), and the number of patients who have a 'positive' result but are disease-free (false positives; FP).

A so-called decision curve (Figure 7.7) can be used to display net benefit across a range of thresholds of predicted risk (p_t) (131–133), and to compare the utility of competing models and strategies (e.g. treat all, or treat none). The basic interpretation of a decision curve is that the model/strategy with the highest net benefit at a particular threshold probability, has the highest clinical value (131). It is wrong to use the plot to guide the choice of threshold to direct clinical decisions, as other factors such as costs must be considered (135). Rather, the graph should be interpreted as a sensitivity analysis over a range over plausible decision thresholds. Kerr et al. recommend that: '*a decision curve is best interpreted by reading vertically: given a chosen risk threshold, the curve displays the net benefit of using the risk model with that risk threshold, assuming that the risk threshold accurately summarizes the costs and benefits of intervention*' (135).

Lamain-de Ruiter et al. (136) perform external validation and direct head-to-head comparison of published first trimester prognostic models for developing gestational diabetes mellitus in pregnant women, in one independent cohort. For each of the four prognostic models with a C statistic of at least 0.75, decision curves were derived to examine the net benefit of initiating intervention (including lifestyle changes) above particular thresholds of predicted risk

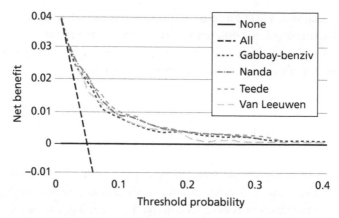

None = net benefit when all pregnant women are considered as not having the outcome (gestational diabetes mellitus); All = net benefit when all pregnant women are considered as having the outcome. The preferred model is the model with the highest net benefit at any given threshold, where threshold = risk probability above which a woman is considered as having the outcome

Figure 7.7 Decision curve analysis of four prognostic models for risk of gestational diabetes mellitus.

Source: reproduced with permission from Lamain-de Ruiter M, Kwee A, Naaktgeboren CA, et al. External validation of prognostic models to predict risk of gestational diabetes mellitus in one Dutch cohort: prospective multicentre cohort study. BMJ.354:i4338. Copyright © 2016 BMJ Publishing Group Ltd

(Figure 7.7). These showed a positive net benefit for thresholds between 0% and 40%, with very little difference between the four models, but with noticeable improvement over the comparison options of 'treat all' and 'treat none'.

7.4.3.2 Decision-analytical (cost-effectiveness) modelling

The (cost-)effectiveness of using a prognostic model can also be evaluated using decision-analytical or health economic modelling techniques, again without having to perform a new prospective comparative impact study (see Section 7.4.3.3) (13, 20, 115, 137). For example, Ensor et al. performed an evaluation of a prognostic model for cessation of anticoagulation therapy after a first unprovoked venous thromboembolism based on different thresholds of predicted risk from their model shown in Figure 7.2 (22). Using a decision-analytic (Markov) model, hypothetical patients from a population were allowed to follow various possible outcome pathways once they have suffered a first unprovoked venous thromboembolism, including remaining event free, having another venous thromboembolism (either a deep vein thrombosis or a pulmonary embolism), having a major bleed and dying from a clinical event or other causes.

The approach assigns probabilities for initial pathways utilizing the risk predictions from the prognostic model shown in Figure 7.2; these are then modified to take into account if a patient is on therapy or not, and risks of further clinical events are determined by their therapy status and population-level evidence. In addition, if events occur then the therapy status of a patient is allowed to change. The whole process allows the risk of a further venous thromboembolism off therapy to be weighed against the risk of bleeding on therapy, by attaching costs, impact on quality of life and survival to both therapy and clinical events. These costs and outcomes, in quality-adjusted life years (QALYs), are then compared between strategies to determine the most cost-effective strategy. Assuming willingness to pay up to £20,000/QALY gained, Ensor et al. conclude that thresholds of 8% (or greater) are cost-effective (compared with treating no one, i.e. usual care), such that only those with a predicted risk below 8% by the end of the first year should stop therapy (22). That would suggest patients B and C in Figure 7.2 should remain on therapy, but patient A should stop.

7.4.3.3 Comparative studies examining the impact of a prognostic model

Convincing evidence for the impact, positive or negative, of using prognostic models on patient outcome is hard to come by (Table 7.1) (13, 20, 115). Full assessment of the impact of a model on decision making and individual health outcomes requires a comparative follow-up study (4, 13, 20, 115). Here two groups (cohorts) need to be compared, one in which usual care is provided without the use of the model's predictions, and another group in which model predictions are made available to doctors and other health professionals to guide treatment decisions.

This comparison is scientifically strongest in a (cluster) randomized trial (perhaps with a stepped-wedge design) (13, 20, 115, 138), and would ideally show some overall benefit on clinical outcomes (e.g. as measured by a mean difference, risk ratio, odds ratio or hazard ratio comparing the index group using the model with the control group receiving standard care). An example from the musculoskeletal domain is the STarTBack trial in which primary care patients with back pain were randomized to receive either stratified care based on their risk of future disability or non-stratified current best care. The results showed a significantly larger reduction in disability as well as more cost savings in the group receiving treatment matched to their prognostic risk compared to the control group (139).

Randomized trials are expensive and time-consuming, and other approaches are possible. One can compare clinicians' decision making and patient outcomes observed in a time period before the model was introduced versus a time period after which it was available (13, 20, 115). An example of such a before-after impact study is an investigation of the effect of using the NPI on the decision to treat women with adjuvant chemotherapy, resulting in modest effects on survival following implementation (140). Potential time effects, such as change in treatments and differences in case-mix (confounding factors), should always be considered in the interpretation of before-after designs (13, 20, 115). It is therefore desirable to include control practices which continue to deliver usual care in the time period following implementation.

Alternative designs are necessary when there is a long time lag between the moment of prognostic assessment (use of the model) and patient outcome, or when outcomes are relatively rare. Decision analytic modelling (Section 7.4.3.2) could then rather be used. Another option is a 'cross sectional' study with physicians' decisions as the primary outcome (13, 20, 115). Clinicians or patients are randomized to either have or not have access to predictions from the prognostic model, and their therapeutic or other management decisions are compared. In another design, clinicians can be asked to decide on treatment or patient management before and after being provided with a model's predicted probabilities. This design has been used to assess the effect of using an additional test on medical decision making, for example FDG-PET scanning to guide decisions on brain surgery (141). If decisions do not change by the model, there can be no impact on clinical outcomes.

7.5 **Reporting a prognostic model research study**

Reviews have shown that the reporting of prognostic model studies is poor, with basic information often missing on the sample size, number of outcome events, number of candidate predictors, handling of continuous predictors, amount of missing data, and so on (142–144). Sometimes the model equation is omitted or only partially reported, for example without an intercept or baseline hazard (survival) term, even though the full equation is needed for making new predictions and undertaking external validation. Poor reporting prevents an objective evaluation of the model, and limits systematic reviews, by hindering assessments of risk of bias and the extraction of relevant results for meta-analysis (see Chapter 9). To prevent this, the TRIPOD (Transparent Reporting of a multivariable prediction model for Individual Prognosis Or Diagnosis) statement should be adhered to, which provides a checklist of twenty-two items for reporting of studies developing, validating, or updating a prediction model, whether for diagnostic or prognostic purposes (15, 16). The items were produced following a consensus process amongst experts, and provide a minimum set of information that authors should report (Table 7.3).

Table 7.3 The TRIPOD checklist of items to include when reporting a study developing (D) or validating (V) a multivariable prediction model for diagnosis or prognosis (15, 16).

Section/topic	No.		Checklist item
Title and abstract			
Title	1	D,V	Identify the study as developing and/or validating a multivariable prediction model, the target population, and the outcome to be predicted.
Abstract	2	D,V	Provide a summary of objectives, study design, setting, participants, sample size, predictors, outcome, statistical analysis, results, and conclusions.
Introduction			
Background and objectives	3a	D,V	Explain the medical context (including whether diagnostic or prognostic) and rationale for developing or validating the multivariable prediction model, including references to existing models.
	3b	D,V	Specify the objectives, including whether the study describes the development or validation of the model or both.
Methods			
Source of data	4a	D,V	Describe the study design or source of data (e.g. randomized trial, cohort, or registry data), separately for the development and validation datasets, if applicable.
	4b	D,V	Specify the key study dates, including start of accrual, end of accrual, and if applicable end of follow-up.
Participants	5a	D,V	Specify key elements of the study setting (e.g. primary care, secondary care, general population) including number and location of centres.
	5b	D,V	Describe eligibility criteria for participants.
	5c	D,V	Give details of treatments received, if relevant.
Outcome	6a	D,V	Clearly define the outcome that is predicted by the prediction model, including how and when assessed.
	6b	D,V	Report any actions to blind assessment of the outcome to be predicted.
Predictors	7a	D,V	Clearly define all predictors used in developing the multivariable prediction model, including how and when they were measured.
	7b	D,V	Report any actions to blind assessment of predictors for the outcome and other predictors.
Sample size	8	D,V	Explain how the study size was arrived at.

(continued)

Table 7.3 Continued

Section/topic	No.		Checklist item
Missing data	9	D,V	Describe how missing data were handled (e.g. complete-case analysis, single imputation, multiple imputation) with details of any imputation method.
Statistical analysis methods	10a	D	Describe how predictors were handled in the analyses.
	10b	D	Specify type of model, all model-building procedures (including any predictor selection), and method for internal validation.
	10c	V	For validation, describe how the predictions were calculated.
	10d	D,V	Specify all measures used to assess model performance and, if relevant, to compare multiple models.
	10e	V	Describe any model-updating (e.g. recalibration) arising from the validation, if done.
Risk groups	11	D,V	Provide details on how risk groups were created, if done.
Development versus validation	12	V	For validation, identify any differences from the development data in setting, eligibility criteria, outcome, and predictors.
Results			
Participants	13a	D,V	Describe the flow of participants through the study, including the number of participants with and without the outcome and, if applicable, a summary of the follow-up time. A diagram may be helpful.
	13b	D,V	Describe the characteristics of the participants (basic demographics, clinical features, available predictors), including the number of participants with missing data for predictors and outcome.
	13c	V	For validation, show a comparison with the development data of the distribution of important variables (demographics, predictors, and outcome).
Model development	14a	D	Specify the number of participants and outcome events in each analysis.
	14b	D	If done, report the unadjusted association between each candidate predictor and outcome.
Model specification	15a	D	Present the full prediction model to allow predictions for individuals (i.e. all regression coefficients, and model intercept or baseline survival at a given time point).
	15b	D	Explain how to the use the prediction model.
Model performance	16	D,V	Report performance measures (with confidence intervals) for the prediction model.

Table 7.3 Continued

Section/topic	No.		Checklist item
Model updating	17	V	If done, report the results from any model-updating (i.e. model specification, model performance)
Discussion			
Limitations	18	D,V	Discuss any limitations of the study (such as non-representative sample, few events per predictor, missing data).
Interpretation	19a	V	For validation, discuss the results with reference to performance in the development data, and any other validation data.
	19b	D,V	Give an overall interpretation of the results considering objectives, limitations, results from similar studies, and other relevant evidence.
Implications	20	D,V	Discuss the potential clinical use of the model and implications for future research.
Other information			
Supplementary information	21	D, V	Provide information about the availability of supplementary resources, such as study protocol, web calculator, and datasets.
Funding	22	D, V	Give the source of funding and the role of the funders for the present study.

Adapted with permission from Collins, G.S., et al. Transparent Reporting of a multivariable prediction model for Individual Prognosis Or Diagnosis (TRIPOD): explanation and elaboration. Annals of Internal Medicine.162(1), 55–63. Copyright © 2015 American College of Physicians.

Illustrations of good reporting are provided in the accompanying explanation and elaboration article (16).

7.6 **Barriers to clinical use of a prognostic model**

Many prognostic models fail to be used in healthcare. Fundamentally, there should be a clinical need for the model in the first place (130), with good predictive performance upon validation, and evidence of a positive impact on healthcare. Even then barriers may remain (145), especially a lack of support by leading professionals in the field of application, and the model's predictors being expensive and not routinely available. Other barriers may include the complexity of the model, the format of the model, the ease of the model's use in the consulting room, the need to consider the other outcomes not predicted by the model (e.g. harms *and* benefits), and the fear of cook-book medicine or medico-legal consequences with undue reliance on model-based predictions and decisions (146).

To help catalogue and potentially ease the use of prognostic models, various registries and libraries have been initiated, such as the Tufts PACE Clinical Predictive Model (http://pace.tuftsmedicalcenter.org/cpm) (147), Evidencio (https://www.evidencio.com/), and the Cleveland clinical risk calculator library (http://riskcalc.org/). It is likely that prognostic models and associated risk calculators will be housed within the Electronic Medical Record, so that health professionals and their patients have more timely access to outcome (risk) predictions at the point of care.

7.7 Regression versus machine learning

An alternative to regression-based prognostic models are those based on machine learning techniques, such as random forests and neural networks (148). Extremely large datasets are needed for machine learning techniques, which are often not encountered in medical research. For example, for binary outcomes, van der Ploeg et al. conclude that machine learning techniques 'may need over 10 times as many events per variable to achieve a stable C statistic and a small optimism than classical modelling techniques such as logistic regression', and 'showed instability and a high optimism even with > 200 events per variable' (150). Therefore, machine learning methods require truly 'big data' to be competitive with traditional approaches. In such situations, they may indeed have an advantage for dealing with highly non-linear relationships and complex interactions. Harrell notes that 'machine learning algorithms do seem to have unique advantages in high signal:noise ratio situations such as image and sound pattern recognition problems', but that 'medical diagnosis and outcome prediction problems involve a low signal:noise ratio' (151). Indeed, in our experience, regression models (including penalization approaches) perform at least as well as machine learners (149), and are preferable given that they are founded on well-established statistical theory, and provide a clear model equation that facilitates transparent implementation, validation, and graphical displays. A broader discussion of machine learning methods for prognosis research is given in Chapter 16.

7.8 Summary

Prognostic model studies are abundant in the medical literature, with hundreds if not thousands published each year. However, many current published models are not fit for purpose, with evidence often lacking about their reproducibility, transportability, impact, and cost-effectiveness. This chapter has described how to undertake high-quality prognostic model research from development, to validation and then impact evaluation. Subsequent chapters will consider prognostic model research using additional methods such as systematic reviews (Chapter 9), meta-analysis of individual participant data (Chapter 13), electronic healthcare databases (Chapter 14), and modern methods (Chapters 15 and 16). A summary of the key messages from this chapter is now provided.

7.8.1 **Summary points**

- Prognostic models utilize multiple prognostic factors (predictors) in combination to predict the (risk of) future outcomes or health states in individuals.

- A useful prognostic model provides accurate predictions that inform individuals and their caregivers, allows for better informed decisions to improve the individual's health outcomes, and supports clinical decision making.

- Predictions from a prognostic model can also be used to improve the design and analysis of randomized trials and observational studies of interventions.

- Prognostic model research has three main phases: model development (including internal validation), external validation (potentially including model updating), and investigations of its impact on decision making and individual health outcomes.

- Datasets used for model development and (external) validation should be sufficiently large, high-quality, and representative of the intended populations (e.g. their case mix, how predictors and outcomes are defined and measured).

- When developing a prognostic model, the potential for overfitting should be reduced by identifying potentially relevant predictors *a priori* (e.g. based on previous evidence); having a large number of participants and events per predictor; by using penalized (shrinkage) estimation techniques; avoiding predictor selection (e.g. based on *p*-values) from univariable analyses; and using internal validation via data resampling approaches (such as bootstrapping) to identify and adjust for optimism in the model performance estimates.

- For binary and time-to-event outcomes, a prognostic model's predictive performance should at least be quantified in terms of discrimination (how well it separates participants who do and do not have the outcome of interest) and calibration (whether predicted risks agree with the observed risks across the entire risk spectrum).

- External validation examines a prognostic model's performance in data not used to develop the model; ideally this data should be from a different source, and for binary or time-to-event outcomes have over one hundred events, and preferably over 200.

♦ When a validated prognostic model is then linked to clinical decisions based on a chosen threshold of predicted risk (e.g. treat if predicted risk is > 10%, and withhold treatment otherwise), the net benefit of the model (in terms of benefits versus harms) can be estimated (without requiring individual follow-up data) to reveal whether the model has potential to do more good than harm when using that threshold.

♦ Prospective comparative studies are needed to examine whether the actual use of a (validated) model to guide treatment decisions (as compared to not using that model), impacts clinical decision making and subsequently individuals' health outcomes and healthcare costs.

♦ The predictive performance and impact of a prognostic model is likely to differ between settings and populations, due to changes in outcome occurrence, differences in patient spectrum (case-mix) or differences in predictor effects. Both may also change over time, for example because diagnosis or treatments change.

♦ Rather than developing a new prognostic model, it is preferable that investigators first validate existing models available for the setting, population, and outcomes of interest; in case of poor validation, simple model tailoring or updating, such as recalibration (e.g. of the intercept or baseline hazard) or adding novel predictors (e.g. new biomarkers), may lead to acceptable improvement.

♦ The TRIPOD statement aims to guide complete reporting on all aspects of a prognostic model study, and covers development, validation, and updating studies.

References

1. Gould S (1985) The median isn't the message. *Discover magazine* 1985.
2. Schumacher M, Bastert G, Bojar H, et al. (1994) Randomized 2 × 2 trial evaluating hormonal treatment and the duration of chemotherapy in node-positive breast cancer patients. German Breast Cancer Study Group. *Journal of Clinical Oncology: Official Journal of the American Society of Clinical Oncology* 12(10), 2086–93.
3. Haybittle JL, Blamey RW, Elston CW, et al. (1982) A prognostic index in primary breast cancer. *Br J Cancer* 45(3), 361–6.
4. Reilly BM and Evans AT (2006) Translating clinical research into clinical practice: impact of using prediction rules to make decisions. *Ann Intern Med* 144(3), 201–9.
5. Todd JH, Dowle C, Williams MR, et al. (1987) Confirmation of a prognostic index in primary breast cancer. *Br J Cancer* 56(4), 489–92.

6. **Ciardiello F, Arnold D, Casali PG,** et al. (2014) Delivering precision medicine in oncology today and in future-the promise and challenges of personalised cancer medicine: a position paper by the European Society for Medical Oncology (ESMO). *Ann Onc* (Official Journal of the European Society for Medical Oncolog) /ESMO 25(9), 1673–8.

7. **Hingorani AD, Windt DA, Riley RD,** et al. (2013) Prognosis research strategy (PROGRESS) 4: stratified medicine research. *BMJ* **346**, e5793.

8. **Trusheim MR, Berndt ER,** and **Douglas FL** (2007) Stratified medicine: strategic and economic implications of combining drugs and clinical biomarkers. *Nat Rev Drug Discov* 287–93.

9. **Harrell FE, Jr.** (2015) *Regression Modeling Strategies: with Applications to Linear Models, Logistic and Ordinal Regression, and Survival Analysis* (second edition). New York: Springer.

10. **Steyerberg EW** (2009) *Clinical Prediction Models: a Practical Approach to Development, Validation, and Updating.* New York: Springer.

11. **Royston P, Moons KGM, Altman DG,** et al. (2009) Prognosis and prognostic research: developing a prognostic model. *British Medical Journal* **338**, b604 (1373–77).

12. **Moons KG, Royston P, Vergouwe Y,** et al. (2009) Prognosis and prognostic research: what, why, and how? *BMJ* **338**, b375.

13. **Moons KG, Altman DG, Vergouwe Y,** et al. (2009) Prognosis and prognostic research: application and impact of prognostic models in clinical practice. *BMJ* **338**, b606.

14. **Altman DG, Vergouwe Y, Royston P,** et al. (2009) Prognosis and prognostic research: validating a prognostic model. *BMJ* **338**, b605.

15. **Collins GS, Reitsma JB, Altman DG,** et al. (2015) Transparent Reporting of a multivariable prediction model for Individual Prognosis Or Diagnosis (TRIPOD): The TRIPOD Statement. *Ann Intern Med* **162**, 55–63.

16. **Moons KG, Altman DG, Reitsma JB,** et al. (2015) Transparent Reporting of a multivariable prediction model for Individual Prognosis Or Diagnosis (TRIPOD): explanation and elaboration. *Ann Intern Med* **162**(1), W1–73.

17. **Hemingway H, Croft P, Perel P,** et al. (2013) Prognosis research strategy (PROGRESS) 1: a framework for researching clinical outcomes. *BMJ* **346**, e5595.

18. **Riley RD, Hayden JA, Steyerberg EW,** et al. (2013) Prognosis Research Strategy (PROGRESS) 2: prognostic factor research. *PLoS Med* **10**(2), e1001380.

19. **Steyerberg EW, Moons KG, van der Windt DA,** et al. (2013) Prognosis Research Strategy (PROGRESS) 3: prognostic model research. *PLoS Med* **10**(2), e1001381.

20. **Moons KG, Kengne AP, Grobbee DE,** et al. (2012) Risk prediction models: II. External validation, model updating, and impact assessment. *Heart* **98**(9), 691–8.

21. **Moons KG, Kengne AP, Woodward M,** et al. (2012) Risk prediction models: I. Development, internal validation, and assessing the incremental value of a new (bio) marker. *Heart* **98**(9), 683–90.

22. **Ensor J, Riley RD, Jowett S,** et al. (2016) Prediction of risk of recurrence of venous thromboembolism following treatment for a first unprovoked venous thromboembolism: systematic review, prognostic model and clinical decision rule, and economic evaluation. *Health Technol Assess* **20**(12), i-xxxiii, 1–190.

23. **Iasonos A, Schrag D, Raj GV,** et al. (2008) How to build and interpret a nomogram for cancer prognosis. *Journal of Clinical Oncology: Official Journal of the American Society of Clinical Oncology* **26**(8), 1364–70.

24. **Eagle KA, Lim MJ, Dabbous OH**, et al. (2004) A validated prediction model for all forms of acute coronary syndrome: estimating the risk of 6-month postdischarge death in an international registry. *JAMA* **291**(22), 2727–33.

25. **Kattan MW** (2008) Should I use this nomogram? *BJU Int* **102**(4), 421–2.

26. **Costa F, van Klaveren D, James S**, et al. (2017) Derivation and validation of the predicting bleeding complications in patients undergoing stent implantation and subsequent dual antiplatelet therapy (PRECISE-DAPT) score: a pooled analysis of individual-patient datasets from clinical trials. *Lancet* **389**(10073), 1025–34.

27. **Kent DM and Hayward RA** (2007) Limitations of applying summary results of clinical trials to individual patients: the need for risk stratification. *JAMA* **298**(10), 1209–12.

28. **Donaldson MG, Palermo L, Ensrud KE**, et al. (2012) Effect of alendronate for reducing fracture by FRAX score and femoral neck bone mineral density: the Fracture Intervention Trial. *J Bone Miner Res* **27**(8), 1804–10.

29. **Mackway-Jones K** (1997) *Emergency Triage.* London: BMJ Publishing.

30. **NICE** (2010) NICE Clinical Guideline 94: Unstable angina and NSTEMI: early management. nice.org.uk/guidance/cg94.

31. **Hernández AV, Steyerberg EW**, and **Habbema JD** (2004) Covariate adjustment in randomized controlled trials with dichotomous outcomes increases statistical power and reduces sample size requirements. *J Clin Epidemiol* **57**(5), 454–60.

32. **Roozenbeek B, Maas AI, Lingsma HF**, et al. (2009) Baseline characteristics and statistical power in randomized controlled trials: selection, prognostic targeting, or covariate adjustment? *Crit Care Med* **37**(10), 2683–90.

33. **Steyerberg EW, Bossuyt PM**, and **Lee KL** (2000) Clinical trials in acute myocardial infarction: should we adjust for baseline characteristics? *Am Heart J* **139**(5), 745–51.

34. **Hernandez AV, Eijkemans MJ**, and **Steyerberg EW** (2006) Randomized controlled trials with time-to-event outcomes: how much does prespecified covariate adjustment increase power? *Ann Epidemiol* **16**, 41–8.

35. **Robinson LD** and **Jewell NP** (1991) Some surprising results about covariate adjustment in logistic regression models. *Int Stat Rev* **58**, 227–40.

36. **Perel P, Arango M, Clayton T**, et al. (2008) Predicting outcome after traumatic brain injury: practical prognostic models based on large cohort of international patients. *BMJ* **336**(7641), 425–9.

37. **De Silva MJ, Roberts I, Perel P**, et al. (2009) Patient outcome after traumatic brain injury in high, middle and low-income countries: analysis of data on 8927 patients in 46 countries. *Int J Epidemiol* **38**(2), 452–58.

38. **Jarman B, Pieter D, van der Veen AA**, et al. (2010) The hospital standardised mortality ratio: a powerful tool for Dutch hospitals to assess their quality of care? *Quality & Safety in Health Care* **19**(1), 9–13.

39. **Lingsma HF, Roozenbeek B, Li B**, et al. (2011) Large between-center differences in outcome after moderate and severe traumatic brain injury in the international mission on prognosis and clinical trial design in traumatic brain injury (IMPACT) study. *Neurosurgery* **68**(3), 601–7.

40. **Galea MH, Blamey RW, Elston CE**, et al. (1992) The Nottingham Prognostic Index in primary breast cancer. *Breast Cancer Res Treat* **22**(3), 207–19.

41. **Balslev I, Axelsson CK, Zedeler K**, et al. (1994) The Nottingham Prognostic Index applied to 9149 patients from the studies of the Danish Breast Cancer Cooperative Group (DBCG). *Breast Cancer Res Treat* **32**(3), 281–90.

42. **Williams C, Brunskill S, Altman D**, et al. (2006) Cost-effectiveness of using prognostic information to select women with breast cancer for adjuvant systemic therapy. *Health Technol Assess* **10**(34), 1–217.

43. **Steyerberg EW, Mushkudiani N, Perel P**, et al. (2008) Predicting outcome after traumatic brain injury: development and international validation of prognostic scores based on admission characteristics. *PLoS Medicine* **5**(8), 1251–61.

44. **Steyerberg EW, Mushkudiani N, Perel P**, et al. (2008) Predicting outcome after traumatic brain injury: development and international validation of prognostic scores based on admission characteristics. *PLoS Med* **5**(8), e165.

45. **Bradshaw PJ, Ko DT, Newman AM**, et al. (2006) Validity of the GRACE (Global Registry of Acute Coronary Events) acute coronary syndrome prediction model for six month post-discharge death in an independent data set. *Heart* **92**(7), 905–9.

46. **Huang W, FitzGerald G, Goldberg RJ**, et al. (2016) Performance of the GRACE risk score 2.0 simplified algorithm for predicting 1-year death after hospitalization for an acute coronary syndrome in a contemporary multiracial cohort. *Am J Cardiol* **118**(8), 1105–10.

47. **Fox KA, Fitzgerald G, Puymirat E**, et al. (2014) Should patients with acute coronary disease be stratified for management according to their risk? Derivation, external validation and outcomes using the updated GRACE risk score. *BMJ Open* **4**(2), e004425.

48. **van Veen M, Steyerberg EW, Ruige M**, et al. (2008) Manchester triage system in paediatric emergency care: prospective observational study. *BMJ* **337**, a1501.

49. **Wyatt J** and **Altman DG** (1995) Commentary: Prognostic models: clinically useful or quickly forgotten? *BMJ* **311**, 1539–41.

50. **Thangaratinam S, Allotey J, Marlin N**, et al. (2017) Prediction of complications in early-onset pre-eclampsia (PREP): development and external multinational validation of prognostic models. *BMC Medicine* **15**(1), 68.

51. **Hemingway H, Riley RD**, and **Altman DG** (2009) Ten steps towards improving prognosis research. *BMJ* **339**, b4184.

52. **Riley RD, Ensor J, Snell KI**, et al. (2016) External validation of clinical prediction models using big datasets from e-health records or IPD meta-analysis: opportunities and challenges. *BMJ* **353**, i3140.

53. **Debray TP, Koffijberg H, Nieboer D**, et al. (2014) Meta-analysis and aggregation of multiple published prediction models. *Stat Med* **33**(14), 2341–62.

54. **Debray TP, Koffijberg H, Vergouwe Y**, et al. (2012) Aggregating published prediction models with individual participant data: a comparison of different approaches. *Stat Med* **31**(23), 2697–712.

55. **Whittle R, Royle K-L, Jordan KP**, et al. (2017) Prognosis research ideally should measure time-varying predictors at their intended moment of use. *Diagnostic and Prognostic Research* **1**(1), 1.

56. **Sanderson J, Thompson SG, White IR**, et al. (2013) Derivation and assessment of risk prediction models using case-cohort data. *BMC Med Res Methodol* **13**, 113.

57. **Ganna A, Reilly M, de Faire U,** et al. (2012) Risk prediction measures for case-cohort and nested case-control designs: an application to cardiovascular disease. *Am J Epidemiol* **175**(7), 715–24.

58. **Collins GS, de Groot JA, Dutton S,** et al. (2014) External validation of multivariable prediction models: a systematic review of methodological conduct and reporting. *BMC Med Res Methodol* **14**, 40.

59. **Debray TP, Vergouwe Y, Koffijberg H,** et al. (2015) A new framework to enhance the interpretation of external validation studies of clinical prediction models. *J Clin Epidemiol* **68**(3), 279–89.

60. **Ogundimu EO, Altman DG,** and **Collins GS** (2016) Adequate sample size for developing prediction models is not simply related to events per variable. *J Clin Epidemiol* **76**, 175–82.

61. **van Smeden M, de Groot JA, Moons KG,** et al. (2016) No rationale for 1 variable per 10 events criterion for binary logistic regression analysis. *BMC Med Res Methodol* **16**(1), 163.

62. **Peduzzi P, Concato J, Feinstein AR,** et al. (1995) Importance of events per independent variable in proportional hazards regression analysis. II. Accuracy and precision of regression estimates. *J Clin Epidemiol* **48**(12), 1503–10.

63. **Peduzzi PN, Concato J, Kemper E,** et al. (1996) A simulation study of the number of events per variable in logistic regression analysis. *J Clin Epidemiol* **49**(12), 1373–79.

64. **Austin PC** and **Steyerberg EW** (2017) Events per variable (EPV) and the relative performance of different strategies for estimating the out-of-sample validity of logistic regression models. *Stat Methods Med Res* **26**(2), 796–808.

65. **Wynants L, Bouwmeester W, Moons KG,** et al. (2015) A simulation study of sample size demonstrated the importance of the number of events per variable to develop prediction models in clustered data. *J Clin Epidemiol* **68**(12), 1406–14.

66. **Vittinghoff E** and **McCulloch CE** (2007) Relaxing the rule of ten events per variable in logistic and Cox regression. *Am J Epidemiol* **165**(6), 710–8.

67. **Courvoisier DS, Combescure C, Agoritsas T,** et al. (2011) Performance of logistic regression modeling: beyond the number of events per variable, the role of data structure. *J Clin Epidemiol* **64**(9), 993–1000.

68. **Riley RD, Snell KIE, Ensor J,** et al. (2018) Minimum sample size for developing a multivariable prediction model: PART I—continuous outcomes. *Stat Med* (in press).

69. **Riley RD, Snell KIE, Ensor J,** et al. (2018) Minimum sample size for developing a multivariable prediction model: PART II—binary and time-to-event outcomes. *Stat Med* (in press).

70. **Copas JB** (1983) Regression, prediction, and shrinkage. *Journal of the Royal Statistical Society Series B (Methodological)* **45**(3), 311–54.

71. **Van Houwelingen JC** and **Le Cessie S** (1990) Predictive value of statistical models. *Stat Med* **9**(11),1303–25.

72. **Steyerberg EW, Balmaña J, Stockwell DH,** et al. (2007) Data reduction for prediction: a case study on robust coding of age and family history for the risk of having a genetic mutation. *Statistics in Medicine* **26**(30), 5545–56.

73. **Groenwold RH, Moons KG, Pajouheshnia R,** et al. (2016) Explicit inclusion of treatment in prognostic modeling was recommended in observational and randomized settings. *J Clin Epidemiol* **78**, 90–100.

74. **Altman DG, McShane LM, Sauerbrei W**, et al. (2012) Reporting Recommendations for Tumor Marker Prognostic Studies (REMARK): explanation and elaboration. *PLoS Med* **9**(5), e1001216.

75. **Pajouheshnia R, Peelen LM, Moons KGM**, et al. (2017) Accounting for treatment use when validating a prognostic model: a simulation study. *BMC Medical Research Methodology* **17**(1), 103.

76. **Sperrin M, Martin GP, Pate A**, et al. (2018) Using marginal structural models to adjust for treatment drop-in when developing clinical prediction models. *Stat Med* (in press).

77. **Lawrence Gould A, Boye ME, Crowther MJ**, et al. (2015) Joint modeling of survival and longitudinal non-survival data: current methods and issues. Report of the DIA Bayesian joint modeling working group. *Stat Med* **34**(14), 2181–95.

78. **Crowther MJ, Abrams KR,** and **Lambert PC** (2012) Flexible parametric joint modelling of longitudinal and survival data. *Stat Med* **31**(30), 4456–71.

79. **van Houwelingen HC** and **Putter H** (2008) Dynamic predicting by landmarking as an alternative for multi-state modeling: an application to acute lymphoid leukemia data. *Lifetime Data Anal* **14**(4), 447–63.

80. **Nicolaie MA, van Houwelingen JC, de Witte TM**, et al. (2013) Dynamic prediction by landmarking in competing risks. *Stat Med* **32**(12), 2031–47.

81. **Collins GS, Ogundimu EO, Cook JA**, et al. (2016) Quantifying the impact of different approaches for handling continuous predictors on the performance of a prognostic model. *Stat Med* **35**(23), 4124–35.

82. **Wolbers M, Blanche P, Koller MT**, et al. (2014) Concordance for prognostic models with competing risks. *Biostatistics* **15**(3), 526–39.

83. **Wolbers M, Koller MT, Witteman JCM**, et al. (2009) Prognostic models with competing risks methods and application to coronary risk prediction. *Epidemiology* **20**, 555–61.

84. **Sauerbrei W, Royston P,** and **Binder H** (2007) Selection of important variables and determination of functional form for continuous predictors in multivariable model building. *Stat Med* **26**(30), 5512–28.

85. **Steyerberg EW, Harrell FE, Jr., Borsboom GJ**, et al. (2001) Internal validation of predictive models: efficiency of some procedures for logistic regression analysis. *J Clin Epidemiol* **54**(8), 774–81.

86. **Steyerberg EW, Bleeker SE, Moll HA**, et al. (2003) Internal and external validation of predictive models: a simulation study of bias and precision in small samples. *J Clin Epidemiol* **56**(5), 441–7.

87. **Steyerberg EW, Eijkemans MJ, Harrell FE, Jr.**, et al. (2001) Prognostic modeling with logistic regression analysis: in search of a sensible strategy in small data sets. *Med Decis Making* **21**(1), 45–56.

88. **Altman DG** and **Royston P** (2000) What do we mean by validating a prognostic model? *Stat Med* **19**(4), 453–73.

89. **Efron B** (1979) Bootstrap methods: another look at the jackknife. *Ann Statistics* **7**(1), 1–26.

90. **van Diepen M, Schroijen MA, Dekkers OM**, et al. (2014) Predicting mortality in patients with diabetes starting dialysis. *PLoS One* **9**(3), e89744.

91. **Sauerbrei W** and **Schumacher M** (1992) A bootstrap resampling procedure for model building: application to the Cox regression model. *Stat Med* **11**(16), 2093–109.

92. **Stein C** (1956) Inadmissibility of the usual estimator of the mean of a multivariate normal distribution. *Proceedings of the Third Berkeley Symposium on Mathematical Statistics and Probability* **1**, 197–206.

93. **James W** and **Stein C** (1962) Estimation with quadratic loss. *Proceeding of the Fourth Berkeley Symposium* **1**, 361–73.

94. **Van Houwelingen JC** (2001) Shrinkage and penalized likelihood as methods to improve predictive accuracy. *Statistica Neerlandica* **55**, 17–34.

95. **Hoerl AE** and **Kennard RW** (1970) Ridge regression: applications to nonorthogonal problems. *Technometrics* **12**(1), 69–82.

96. **Tibshirani R** (1996) Regression shrinkage and selection via the lasso. *J Royal Statist Soc B* **58**, 267–88.

97. **Janssen KJ, Siccama I, Vergouwe Y**, et al. (2012) Development and validation of clinical prediction models: marginal differences between logistic regression, penalized maximum likelihood estimation, and genetic programming. *J Clin Epidemiol* **65**(4), 404–12.

98. **Steyerberg EW, Eijkemans WJC, Harrell FE**, et al. (2000) Prognostic modelling with logistic regression analysis: a comparison of selection and estimation methods in small data sets. *Stat Med* **19**, 1059–79.

99. **Pavlou M, Ambler G, Seaman SR**, et al. (2015) How to develop a more accurate risk prediction model when there are few events. *BMJ* **351**, h3868.

100. **Altman DG, Vergouwe Y, Royston P**, et al. (2009) Prognosis and prognostic research: validating a prognostic model. *BMJ* **338**, b605.

101. **Justice AC, Covinsky KE**, and **Berlin JA** (1999) Assessing the generalizability of prognostic information. *Ann Intern Med* **130**(6), 515–24.

102. **Toll DB, Janssen KJ, Vergouwe Y**, et al. (2008) Validation, updating and impact of clinical prediction rules: a review. *J Clin Epidemiol* **61**(11), 1085–94.

103. **Van Calster B, Nieboer D, Vergouwe Y**, et al. (2016) A calibration hierarchy for risk models was defined: from utopia to empirical data. *J Clin Epidemiol* **74**, 167–76.

104. **Royston P** and **Altman DG** (2013) External validation of a Cox prognostic model: principles and methods. *BMC Med Res Methodol* **13**, 33.

105. **Bleeker SE, Moll HA, Steyerberg EW**, et al. (2003) External validation is necessary in prediction research: a clinical example. *Journal of Clinical Epidemiology* **56**(9), 826–32.

106. **Altman DG** (2009) Prognostic models: a methodological framework and review of models for breast cancer. *Cancer Invest* **27**(3), 235–43.

107. **Vergouwe Y, Steyerberg EW, Eijkemans MJ**, et al. (2005) Substantial effective sample sizes were required for external validation studies of predictive logistic regression models. *J Clin Epidemiol* **58**(5), 475–83.

108. **Collins GS, Ogundimu EO**, and **Altman DG** (2016) Sample size considerations for the external validation of a multivariable prognostic model: a resampling study. *Stat Med* **35**(2), 214–26.

109. **Pennells L, Kaptoge S, White IR**, et al. (2014) Assessing risk prediction models using individual participant data from multiple studies. *Am J Epidemiol* **179**(5), 621–32.

110. **Royston P, Parmar MKB**, and **Sylvester R** (2004) Construction and validation of a prognostic model across several studies, with an application in superficial bladder cancer. *Statistics in Medicine* **23**, 907–26.

111. **Vergouwe Y, Moons KG,** and **Steyerberg EW** (2010) External validity of risk models: use of benchmark values to disentangle a case-mix effect from incorrect coefficients. *Am J Epidemiol* **172**(8), 971–80.

112. **Steyerberg EW, Borsboom GJ, van Houwelingen HC,** et al. (2004) Validation and updating of predictive logistic regression models: a study on sample size and shrinkage. *Stat Med* **23**(16), 2567–86.

113. **van Houwelingen HC** and **Thorogood J** (1995) Construction, validation, and updating of a prognostic model for kidney graft survival. *Stat Med* **14**(18), 1999–2008.

114. **Janssen KJ, Moons KG, Kalkman CJ,** et al. (2008) Updating methods improved the performance of a clinical prediction model in new patients. *Journal of Clinical Epidemiology* **61**, 76–86.

115. **Moons KG** (2010) Criteria for scientific evaluation of novel markers: a perspective. *Clin Chem* **56**, 537–41.

116. **Hlatky MA, Greenland P, Arnett DK,** et al. (2009) Criteria for evaluation of novel markers of cardiovascular risk: a scientific statement from the American Heart Association. *Circ Cardiovasc Qual Outcomes* **119**(17), 2408–16.

117. **Melander O, Newton-Cheh C, Almgren P,** et al. (2009) Novel and conventional biomarkers for prediction of incident cardiovascular events in the community. *JAMA* **302**(1), 49–57.

118. **Pepe MS, Janes H, Longton G,** et al. (2004) Limitations of the odds ratio in gauging the performance of a diagnostic, prognostic, or screening marker. *Am J Epidemiol* **159**(9), 882–90.

119. **Pencina MJ, D'Agostino RB, Sr., D'Agostino RB, Jr.,** et al. (2008) Evaluating the added predictive ability of a new marker: from area under the ROC curve to reclassification and beyond. *Stat Med* **27**(2), 157–72.

120. **Steyerberg EW, Vickers AJ, Cook NR,** et al. (2010) Assessing the performance of prediction models: a framework for traditional and novel measures. *Epidemiology* **21**(1), 128–38.

121. **Vickers AJ** and **Cronin AM** (2010) Traditional statistical methods for evaluating prediction models are uninformative as to clinical value: towards a decision analytic framework. *Semin Oncol* **37**(1), 31–8.

122. **Winzer KJ, Buchholz A, Schumacher M,** et al. (2016) Improving the prognostic ability through better use of standard clinical data—the Nottingham prognostic index as an example. *PLoS One* **11**(3), e0149977.

123. **Pencina MJ, D'Agostino SRB, D'Agostino JRB,** et al. (2008) Evaluating the added predictive ability of a new marker: from area under the ROC curve to reclassification and beyond. *Statistics in Medicine* **27**, 157–72.

124. **Pepe MS, Fan J, Feng Z,** et al. (2015) The net reclassification index (NRI): a misleading measure of prediction improvement even with independent test data sets. *Statistics in Biosciences* **7**(2), 282–95.

125. **Baker SG, Schuit E, Steyerberg EW,** et al. (2014) How to interpret a small increase in AUC with an additional risk prediction marker: decision analysis comes through. *Stat Med* **33**(22), 3946–59.

126. **Calster BV** and **Vickers AJ** (2015) Calibration of risk prediction models: impact on decision-analytic performance. *Medical Decision Making* **35**(2), 162–9.

127. **Marchevsky AM** and **Gupta R** (2010) Interobserver diagnostic variability at 'moderate' agreement levels could significantly change the prognostic estimates of clinicopathologic studies: evaluation of the problem using evidence from patients with diffuse lung disease. *Ann Diag Path* **14**(2), 88–93.

128. **Collins GS** and **Moons KG** (2012) Comparing risk prediction models. *BMJ* **344**, e3186.

129. **Localio A** and **Goodman S** (2012) Beyond the usual prediction accuracy metrics: Reporting results for clinical decision making. *Ann Intern Med* **157**(4), 294–95.

130. **Vickers AJ** and **Cronin AM** (2010) Everything you always wanted to know about evaluating prediction models (but were too afraid to ask). *Urology* **76**(6), 1298–301.

131. **Vickers AJ, Van Calster B,** and **Steyerberg EW** (2016) Net benefit approaches to the evaluation of prediction models, molecular markers, and diagnostic tests. *BMJ* **352**, i6.

132. **Vickers AJ** and **Elkin EB** (2006) Decision curve analysis: a novel method for evaluating prediction models. *Med Decis Making* **26**(6), 565–74.

133. **Vickers AJ, Cronin AM, Elkin EB,** et al. (2008) Extensions to decision curve analysis, a novel method for evaluating diagnostic tests, prediction models and molecular markers. *BMC Med Inform Decis Mak* **8**, 53.

134. **Steyerberg EW** and **Vickers AJ** (2008) Decision curve analysis: a discussion. *Med Decis Making* **28**(1), 146–9.

135. **Kerr KF, Brown MD, Zhu K,** et al. (2016) Assessing the clinical impact of risk prediction models with decision curves: guidance for correct interpretation and appropriate use. *Journal of Clinical Oncology: Official Journal of the American Society of Clinical Oncology* **34**(21), 2534–40.

136. **Lamain-de Ruiter M, Kwee A, Naaktgeboren CA,** et al. (2016) External validation of prognostic models to predict risk of gestational diabetes mellitus in one Dutch cohort: prospective multicentre cohort study. *BMJ* **354**, i4338.

137. **Dahabreh IJ, Trikalinos TA, Balk EM,** et al. (2016) Recommendations for the conduct and reporting of modeling and simulation studies in health technology assessment. *Ann Intern Med* **165**(8), 575–81.

138. **Poldervaart JM, Reitsma JB, Koffijberg H,** et al. (2013) The impact of the HEART risk score in the early assessment of patients with acute chest pain: design of a stepped wedge, cluster randomised trial. *BMC Cardiovascular Disorders* **13**, 77.

139. **Hill JC, Whitehurst DG, Lewis M,** et al. (2011) Comparison of stratified primary care management for low back pain with current best practice (STarT Back): a randomised controlled trial. *Lancet* **378**(9802), 1560–71.

140. **Feldman M, Stanford R, Catcheside A,** et al. (2002) The use of a prognostic table to aid decision making on adjuvant therapy for women with early breast cancer. *Eur J Surg Oncol* **28**(6), 615–19.

141. **Uijl SG, Leijten FS, Arends JB,** et al. (2007) The added value of [18F]-fluoro-D-deoxyglucose positron emission tomography in screening for temporal lobe epilepsy surgery. *Epilepsia* **48**(11), 2121–29.

142. **Collins GS, Omar O, Shanyinde M,** et al. (2013) A systematic review finds prediction models for chronic kidney disease were poorly reported and often developed using inappropriate methods. *J Clin Epidemiol* **66**(3), 268–77.

143. **Bouwmeester W, Zuithoff NP, Mallett S**, et al. (2012) Reporting and methods in clinical prediction research: a systematic review. *PLoS Med* **9**(5), 1–12.

144. **Mallett S, Royston P, Waters R**, et al. (2010) Reporting performance of prognostic models in cancer: a review. *BMC Medicine* **8**, 21.

145. **Kappen TH, van Loon K, Kappen MA**, et al. (2016) Barriers and facilitators perceived by physicians when using prediction models in practice. *J Clin Epidemiol* **70**, 136–45.

146. **Black L, Knoppers BM, Avard D**, et al. (2012) Legal liability and the uncertain nature of risk prediction: the case of breast cancer risk prediction models. *Public Health Genomics* **15**(6), 335–40.

147. **Wessler BS, Paulus J, Lundquist CM**, et al. (2017) Tufts PACE clinical predictive model registry: update 1990 through 2015. *Diagnostic and Prognostic Research* **1**(1), 20.

148. **Hastie T, Tibshirani R**, and **Friedman J** (2009) The *Elements of Statistical Learning: Data Mining, Inference, and Prediction* (second edition). New York: Springer.

149. **Steyerberg EW, van der Ploeg T**, and **Van Calster B** (2014) Risk prediction with machine learning and regression methods. *Biom J* **56**(4), 601–6.

150. **van der Ploeg T, Austin PC**, and **Steyerberg EW** (2014) Modern modelling techniques are data hungry: a simulation study for predicting dichotomous endpoints. *BMC Medical Research Methodology* **14**(1), 137.

151. **Harrell FE, Jr.** (2018) how can machine learning be reliable when the sample is adequate for only one feature? http://www.fharrell.com/post/ml-sample-size/.

Chapter 8

Predictors of treatment effect

Danielle A van der Windt, Richard D Riley,
Aroon Hingorani, and Karel GM Moons

8.1 Introduction

The previous chapters described research into prognostic factors and prognostic models, aimed at improving our understanding and prediction of the future course of a disease or health condition in the context of the care provided.
These types of prognosis research generally do not focus on the potential effects
of treatment on prognosis, and typically only describe the treatment or treatments received by study participants; use treatment as a prognostic factor; and/
or adjust associations between prognostic factors and outcome for the potential
influence of treatment. Although most treatments are expected to have beneficial effects on average, the magnitude of this effect, as well as the risk of harm
(adverse effects from treatment) can potentially vary widely between individuals. Healthcare providers and patients thus aim to make optimal treatment
decisions, increasing the likelihood of a positive outcome for individuals, while
minimizing the risk of harm. Such decisions require not just information on
overall prognosis and the average effects of available treatments for the population of interest, but also estimates of the individual's probability of responding to
(or experiencing harm from) specific treatments. These questions have become
more urgent and complex, with more and more people in ageing populations
being exposed to treatment (including self-management), and an increasing
emphasis on preventive interventions. Given this, and the need to optimize the
use of limited healthcare resources, it is desirable to target treatment to those
people who are likely to benefit most or experience least harm (1).

This has stimulated the development of models of stratified care based on
predictors of benefit or harm from treatment, also referred to as 'stratified
medicine', 'precision medicine', 'targeted treatment', or 'personalized medicine', historically driven by the identification of genetic variations, proteins,
and other biomarkers that were perceived as potential predictors of treatment
effect. In this chapter, we will explain the difference between prognostic factors

(as introduced in Chapter 6, type II prognosis research) and predictors of treatment effect (type IV prognosis research); discuss the study designs used to investigate predictors of treatment effect; and highlight some of the methodological challenges encountered in this field. Specific attention will be given to the importance of research aimed at developing and evaluating models of stratified care based on predictors of treatment effect, and how this may impact on clinical decision making, patient outcomes, and costs of care. Throughout the chapter we use the term treatment, but this could refer to any type of intervention, including self-management, lifestyle interventions, drugs, exercise programmes, or surgical procedures.

8.2 Predictors of treatment effect

8.2.1 Prognostic factors, predictors, and mediators

A predictor of treatment effect can be any type of factor (patient characteristic, symptom, sign, biomarker)—or even a combination of factors—that is associated with the response (benefit or harm) to a specific intervention. This means that these predictors need to meet a different requirement compared to the prognostic factors or prognostic models discussed in the two previous chapters. That is, predictors of treatment effect should be able to discriminate between individuals who experience larger effects of, or less harm from, a specific treatment compared to another type of treatment, or compared with no treatment. Prognostic factors can also be predictors of treatment effect. For example, among people with atrial fibrillation, age influences the risk of stroke in the absence of treatment, as well as the effectiveness of treatment with anticoagulants. Here, age is both a prognostic factor and a factor that predicts treatment effect (2). However, most prognostic factors do not also predict the effect of treatment. For example, symptoms of distress strongly predict future levels of disability in patients with back pain, but were not associated with differences in treatment effect in several trials comparing different treatments for back pain (3, 4). Conversely, some factors (such as those that influence the metabolism or elimination of a specific drug) can predict treatment effect, but may not be identified as a prognostic factor in the absence of treatment.

Predictors of treatment effect can reflect any characteristic of the patient, or their underlying disease or health problem, which may include features that are relatively static, such as age, sex, educational attainment, imaging results, or genetic information. Such baseline predictors can help to understand who is likely to benefit from a treatment. Researchers, however, are increasingly interested in factors that change over time and can potentially be modified by intervention. For example, fear of movement is associated with an increased risk of poor outcome in people with back pain. Fear of movement may be targeted by specific treatment (e.g. graded activity or cognitive behavioural approaches), and if treatment indeed leads to a reduction in the levels of fear, and subsequently, to better patient outcome, this also helps to explain how a treatment works, not just who it works for (5). In this situation, the factor is not merely considered a predictor of treatment effect, but is also a mediator or intermediate factor, part of the underlying causal mechanism that explains the response to treatment. Mediation analysis requires a longitudinal study design, with repeated measurements of the potential mediator as well as the outcome, and the use of suitable analysis approaches (causal inference methods, structural equation, or latent growth models). This is outside the scope of this book.

8.2.2 Analysis and interpretation of predictors of treatment effect

Across research disciplines and clinical fields, different terms are used to refer to predictors of treatment effect. In epidemiological research these variables are usually referred to as *effect modifiers*, in psychology the term *moderators* is commonly used, whereas statisticians tend to use the term *treatment-covariate interactions*, as it is the interaction of the predictor with treatment that generates the additional effect on outcome over and above that of the predictor and treatment alone.

The impact of a predictor of treatment effect will vary depending on the baseline risk or probability of the outcome in the individual patient (i.e. prognosis). People with the highest absolute risk are likely to achieve the largest absolute benefit from a treatment, or the greatest reduction in harm, *even when the treatment effect expressed as a risk ratio or rate ratio is the same across individuals*. For example, in a large trial of women with low bone mineral density (osteoporosis), prescription of bisphosphonates (in this case alendronate) significantly reduced the incidence of non-vertebral fracture (incidence rate ratio (IRR) 0.86; 95% CI, 0.75–0.99) in the total trial sample (6). Fracture risk at baseline was estimated using the FRAX model (www.sheffield.ac.uk/FRAX), a prognostic model designed to estimate ten-year fracture risk for individual patients (independently from treatment) based on a set of twelve clinical characteristics. The effect of alendronate, when expressed as a rate ratio, was constant across subgroups with increasing fracture rate, and there was no evidence of interaction between the effect of alendronate and fracture risk (p = 0.61).

However, Table 8.1 shows that the absolute benefit of alendronate appeared to be larger among women with increasing risk of fracture, with the difference in fracture rate being estimated at 0.34, 0.41 and 0.91 per hundred person-years among those with low, medium, or high fracture risk according to the FRAX

Table 8.1 Example of the effect of treatment with alendronate across subgroups of women with osteoporosis at increasing risk of fracture according to the FRAX tool plus bone mineral density (BMD) (i.e. varying prognosis), expressed in terms of incidence rate ratio (IRR) and absolute difference in fracture rate (rate difference, RD), with rate calculated as fractures per hundred person years.

FRAX with BMD (tertiles)	Alendronate			Placebo			IRR (95% CI)	RD (95% CI)
	person-years	events	rate	person-years	events	rate		
4.8–22.0	4119	91	2.21	4081	104	2.55	0.87 (0.65–1.15)	−0.34 (−1.0–0.33)
22.1–34.1	3883	129	3.32	3750	140	3.73	0.89 (1.70–1.13)	−0.41 (−1.3–0.49)
34.2–85.4	3453	164	4.75	3483	197	5.66	0.84 (0.68–1.03)	−0.91 (−2.0–0.17)

FRAX = World Health Organisation Fracture Risk Assessment Tool.

Source: data from Donaldson MG, et al. (2012) Effect of alendronate for reducing fracture by FRAX score and femoral neck bone mineral density: the Fracture Intervention Trial. *Journal of Bone and Mineral Research* 27(8), 1804–10. Copyright © 2012 John Wiley & Sons, Inc.

model, respectively. In such situations, alternative statistical tests can be used to assess whether there is excess risk or benefit due to interaction on an additive rather than a multiplicative (ratio) scale between the predictor and treatment outcome (7, 8). The clinical implication is that, based on a judgement of the balance of benefits, costs, and potential harms, the treatment may be restricted to those who will benefit the most in terms of their absolute risk reduction, given their absolute risk at the startpoint (i.e. their prognosis).

When the effect of treatment as measured by a risk ratio, odds ratio, or hazard ratio varies across patient subgroups, in statistical terms there is interaction on a multiplicative (ratio) scale, and in biological terms there may be an underlying mechanism explaining the difference in treatment effect between subgroups. So when investigating the influence of a candidate predictor of treatment effect (e.g. sex) on a binary outcome (e.g. fracture) in individuals (denoted by i) using a logistic regression analysis, the model will have the following form (see also Chapter 3: Fundamental statistical concepts and methods):

$$\ln\left(\frac{p_i}{1-p_i}\right) = \alpha + \beta_1\, sex_i + \beta_2\, treatment_i + \beta_3\left(sex_i \times treatment_i\right)$$

where p_i is the outcome probability; sex and treatment equals 1 for males and those treated, respectively, and 0 otherwise; β_1 is the change in log odds of the outcome for men compared to others (i.e. the prognostic effect of male sex); β_2 represents the effect of treatment on outcome for women; and β_3 the difference in the effect of treatment between men and women. Thus, after fitting the model, of key importance is the magnitude, direction, and precision of the estimate of β_3, as this quantifies whether the factor (here sex) is a predictor of treatment effect (see Figure 8.1 for a graphical presentation of the interaction effect). The $\exp(\beta_3)$ represents a ratio of odds ratios (i.e. the treatment effect for men compared to women). When the predictor concerns a binary or categorical variable (e.g. sex), the analysis can subsequently be stratified to present treatment effects separately for subgroups defined using the predictor (here, men and women).

However, some caution is needed when comparing odds ratios across subgroups to identify potential predictors of treatment effect. The dependence of treatment effect on baseline risk is stronger when effect estimates are expressed as odds ratios, with estimates diverting more from the risk

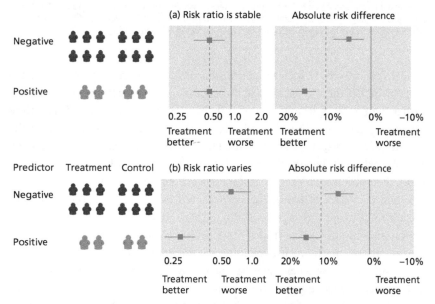

Figure 8.1 Estimated absolute effect of treatment (expressed as absolute risk difference) in the situation where the treatment effect expressed as a ratio is (a) stable or (b) varies across subgroups defined based on a predictor of treatment effect. The prevalence of the predictor is arbitrarily shown as 25%. The dotted vertical line shows the overall treatment effect.

Source: adapted with permission from (Hingorani, A.D., et al. Prognosis research strategy (PROGRESS) 4: Stratified medicine research. BMJ. 2013 (346), 5793. Copyright © 2013 BMJ Publishing Group Ltd.

ratio as the baseline risk increases. This means that differences in treatment effect between subgroups (relative odds ratio is unequal to 1) may emerge if subgroups have been defined based on a prognostic factor, even when there is no genuine difference in treatment effect when measured by a risk ratio (RR=1.0, see section 4.6) (9).

Examples of factors where there is evidence of interaction in terms of both relative and absolute benefit from treatment include HER-2 status in women with breast cancer treated with trastuzumab, where the risk ratio for mortality or disease progression was significantly larger in HER-2 positive women compared to women negative for HER-2 (10). Another example concerns the treatment of lung cancer, where epidermal growth factor receptor mutations were found to significantly interact with the effectiveness of gefitinib (11). An example of identifying subgroups based on increased risk of harm from treatment includes the antiretroviral drug abacavir, where HLA typing helps identify patients at high risk of abacavir toxicity (12). Here, the clinical implication is that, depending on the status (or value) of the predictor, decisions can be made between specific types of treatment based on the observed differences in treatment effect or harm across subgroups.

8.3 Identifying and testing predictors of treatment effect

Although stratified care based on predictors of treatment effect is often heralded as the new standard for clinical practice and research, the actual identification, validation, and successful implementation of such predictors is rare. In 2013 the European Medicines Agency (EMA) found that the proportion of licensed drugs for which biomarkers were used to predict benefit (an indication) or harm (a contra-indication) was still very small relative to the total number of drugs licensed (see Figure 8.2) (13). This is because genuine predictors of treatment effect are rare, but also because the methods used to identify them are often substandard.

8.3.1 Study design: treatment-only designs

Robust studies to quantify the effect of candidate predictors of treatment effect are ideally designed as part of experimental research, that is, nested in randomized trials comparing the effectiveness of the treatment of interest with that of a control or a different, active treatment. Hypotheses regarding potential predictors of treatment effect, however, are often generated in observational research such as clinical cohorts or single treatment arms within trials (see Figure 8.3), where all patients receive a similar type of treatment (which

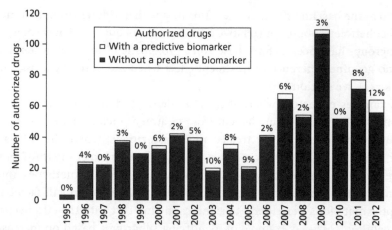

Figure 8.2 New drugs authorized each year by the European Medicines Agency with and without a biomarker as indication or contraindication (excludes biomarkers added after the drug was initially licensed). Percentages shown are the percentage of the total number of authorised drugs that contain a biomarker as an indication or contraindication.
Source: reproduced from Malottki, K. et al., Stratified medicine in European Medicines Agency licensing: a systematic review of predictive biomarkers. BMJ Open. 4(1). Copyright © 2014 BMJ Publishing Group Ltd.

may be a control treatment or usual care), and associations between patient characteristics and outcomes are investigated. Such research is important, but should be considered as generating exploratory information only, with the need for further testing of candidate predictors in future trials being highlighted. Unfortunately, data from treatment-only designs are regularly used to draw strong conclusions regarding predictors of treatment effect, which

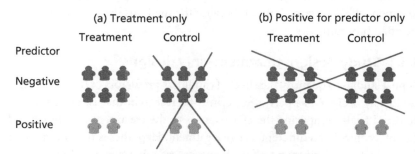

Figure 8.3 Designs that do not adequately identify or test predictors of treatment effect: (a) Treatment-only designs, (b) Factor positive or enrichment designs.
Source: reproduced courtesy of Danielle van der Windt

leads to incorrect inferences about the potential value of such predictors for selecting appropriate treatment.

For example, patients with rheumatoid arthritis are often treated with 'biologic' medicines that target pivotal mediators in the inflammatory process. However, of all patients receiving such treatment, 30–40% do not respond to the prescribed biologic. Furthermore these treatments are expensive and associated with possible serious adverse effects. To identify individuals most likely to benefit, a large number of biomarkers have been evaluated as candidate predictors of treatment effect, but mainly using treatment-only cohort designs. The results of these studies show that biomarkers are rarely replicated in other cohorts, and do not consistently or substantially improve the prediction of response to biologics (14). More importantly, the use of the treatment-only design means that the effects of biologics cannot be estimated against a control intervention, and treatment-predictor interactions cannot be tested. Therefore, any of the associations found between a biomarker and outcome could merely represent the biomarker being a prognostic factor (i.e. it is associated with outcome regardless of treatment offered), and not being a predictor of the treatment effect of biologics in individuals.

8.3.2 Study design: test-positive only designs

Trials are often being undertaken exclusively among individuals who test positive for a potential, but as yet untested, predictor of treatment effect (test-positive only trials), or in patients who are assumed to benefit most, based on other known or untested predictors (enrichment trials). One of the early randomized trials investigating the efficacy and safety of trastuzumab was conducted only in women with metastatic breast cancer who tested positive for HER2 (15). The addition of trastuzumab to chemotherapy was associated with a longer time to disease progression (median, 7.4 vs. 4.6 months; $P < 0.001$), and a 20% reduction in the risk of death compared to chemotherapy only. This trial on its own does not tell us whether or not the over-expression of HER2 is a predictor of differential treatment effect, as the study only included test-positives (women classified with over-expression of HER2). The treatment could potentially have been effective more widely across the spectrum of this genetic marker. Test-positive only or enrichment trials therefore cannot investigate to what extent a prognostic factor (baseline patient or disease characteristic) predicts differences in treatment effect across all patients with the disease or health condition. The clinical implication is that patients may miss out on receiving a treatment that is potentially of benefit, or alternatively that the effect of treatment is disappointingly low when the treatment is rolled out more widely across the entire spectrum of patients without adequate testing.

8.3.3 **Study design: non-randomized comparative studies**

Clinical observational cohorts in which patients with the same startpoint are offered several treatments are sometimes used to identify or test predictors of treatment effect. Such research has the advantage of investigating predictors in the entire target population, without the strict selection criteria often used in trials, and provide 'real-life' estimates. However, bias and confounding cannot be ignored in observational research. A retrospective cohort study was conducted to investigate the effects of twelve months of statin therapy (compared to no statins) on the rate of all-cause mortality (the endpoint) in patients newly diagnosed with severe pulmonary hypertension in the USA (the startpoint), and assessed whether the effect of statin therapy varied between patients with or without chronic obstructive pulmonary disease (COPD) (16). The study investigated a candidate predictor of treatment effect. Propensity score matching was used to account for potential confounding by indication. No significant interaction was found between the presence of COPD and the effects of statins, but residual confounding could not be excluded in this non-randomized design. The authors recommend that findings should be confirmed in large randomized trials.

8.3.4 **Sample size, precision, and risk of spurious results**

As explained in Section 8.2, investigation of a candidate predictor of treatment effect should involve estimation of an interaction between predictor and treatment effect. However, as interaction effects are often small, most randomized trials are not designed with sufficient statistical power to detect genuine interactions and thus may miss potentially important predictors (false-negative findings or type 2 error) (17). This is not surprising, as an adequately powered analysis to test for treatment-predictor interaction would usually require at least four times the sample size required to test the overall treatment effect (18), making funding of such trials difficult to achieve. In order to increase precision and reduce the risk of false-negative findings, meta-analyses based on individual participant data (IPD) from multiple trials are recommended to summarize interactions and examine predictors of treatment effect (1). This requires adequate processes to facilitate sharing of data, and consistent definition and measurement of candidate predictors and core outcomes across trials. Chapter 13 discusses the role of IPD meta-analysis in detail.

When analysing candidate predictors of treatment effect, appropriate statistical approaches should be used similar to those described for prognostic factor research (see Chapters 3, 4, and 6), avoiding, for example, categorizing predictors or outcomes that are measured on a continuous scale and by considering non-linear relationships. Categorization of continuous outcomes should be avoided to prevent loss of precision when estimating associations with treatment effect, but also to avoid misclassification of individuals as either responders or non-responders. Small differences in outcome values may represent measurement error rather than true differences in treatment effect. Moreover, as Senn (19) noted: 'If in a trial 70% of participants respond, one common interpretation is that the treatment works for 70% of patients 100% of the time and for 30% of the patients 0% of the time. However, nothing in the data forbids a radically different interpretation—namely, that the treatment works in 100% of the patients 70% of the time.' This highlights the importance of careful analysis and interpretation of results, especially when defining treatment response. In the situation where subgroups need to be defined to facilitate treatment decision making, thresholds can be defined in later stages of the analysis, when designing the stratified care intervention (see Section 8.4.2).

Existing guidance for the analysis of subgroup effects in randomized trials (20, 21) also holds for analysis of predictors of differential treatment response. This includes avoiding the analysis of a large number of candidate predictors, and potential correction for multiple statistical testing in order to reduce the risk of chance findings (false-positive findings or type 1 error). More importantly, newly identified interactions should be interpreted as hypothesis-generating, with replication sought in new trials or IPD meta-analyses. In order to avoid reporting bias, results for all interactions and subgroups considered should be reported regardless of their statistical significance, in accordance with CONSORT reporting guidelines for trials.

Identification of predictors of treatment effect should ideally be guided by biological reasoning and hypotheses regarding the expected working mechanism of the treatment (21, 22). The term 'mechanism' should be interpreted in a broad sense, since psychological, behavioural, or sociocultural factors may contribute to causal pathways and to explanations of variability in treatment effects (1). The following criteria have been proposed to assess the quality of subgroup analysis in trials or investigation of treatment-predictor interactions (20–22):

- A priori defined hypotheses regarding treatment-predictor interactions (including direction of association), based on biological plausibility or a mechanism driven by theory or evidence.
- Candidate predictors are measured prior to randomization in trials (prior to the start of treatment of interest).
- Small number of predictors; correction for multiple testing of associations.
- Use of valid and reliable measures for predictors and outcomes.

- Adequate sample size.
- Suitable estimate and confidence interval for treatment-covariate interaction.
- Reporting of all tested predictors, and for all analysed outcomes.
- Replication of identified interactions in other trials or datasets.

8.4 **Stratified care based on predictors of treatment effect**

Stratified care seeks to optimize benefit, reduce harm, and/or increase efficiency of care by offering the right treatment to the right person, ideally as early as possible in a disease process (1). In Chapter 7, we highlighted the potential for stratified care based on the probability that an individual will experience a particular outcome, as generated from a prognostic model, regardless or in the absence of treatment. Here, we rather focus on the potential for stratified care based on an individual's likely response to a specific type of treatment. One of the most convincing and early examples of stratified care based on a predictor of treatment effect concerns the treatment of breast cancer, where human epidermal growth factor receptor 2 (HER-2) status was discovered as an important prognostic factor. Over-expression (amplification) of this genetic variation was found in 10–34% of breast cancer patients, and is strongly associated with a decrease in survival (23). Over-expression of HER-2 status was subsequently used as a specific target for administration of a treatment called trastuzumab, which was evaluated for effectiveness in a series of trials. Subgroup analysis carried out in one of these trials demonstrated significant differences in the effects of trastuzumab between women positive versus negative for HER-2 status (10). These findings implied that trastuzumab would best be offered to women with HER-2 positive breast cancer only, optimizing the effects of treatment, while preventing harm in those unlikely to benefit. Health economic modelling demonstrated that implementation of stratified care based on HER-2 status was cost-effective (24), and was included in UK NICE guidance in 2006. This example illustrates the different phases of research that preceded successful implementation of stratified care for breast cancer (Figure 8.4).

The strong move towards stratified care based on predictors of treatment effect, initiated in cancer and cardiovascular research, is gaining a strong foothold in other clinical areas, including musculoskeletal disease and trauma (see Chapters 10 and 12 for discussion of these clinical examples). In order for a stratified care intervention to be potentially successful, evidence is needed to demonstrate: (1) variability in treatment effect between individuals; (2) high

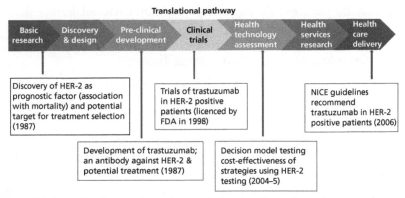

Figure 8.4 Example of research on the translational pathway from discovery of a potential predictor of treatment effect to implementation of stratified care.
Source: adapted with permission from (Hingorani, A.D., et al. Prognosis research strategy (PROGRESS) 4: Stratified medicine research. BMJ. 2013 (346), 5793. Copyright © 2013 BMJ Publishing Group Ltd.

costs, impact on resources, or risk of harm from treatment that warrant targeting of treatment to subgroups only; and (3) predictors of treatment effect that accurately identify individuals with important changes in their expected treatment effect. Figure 8.5 describes the phases of research that may be involved in the development and evaluation of stratified care interventions, from identifying

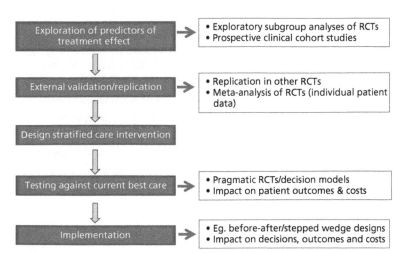

Figure 8.5 Framework for stratified care research, highlighting the phases and study designs from exploration of predictors of treatment response through to investigation of cost-effectiveness of stratified care.
Source: reproduced courtesy of Danielle van der Windt

and validating predictors through to large pragmatic trials and decision models to determine the clinical and cost-effectiveness of such interventions.

8.4.1 Developing and testing stratification

Candidate predictors of treatment effect may originate from exploratory subgroup analyses in trials or even from observational clinical cohorts, yet external validation (in new data) of their predictive value is essential in order to verify whether they do indeed explain variability in treatment effect. An early example of a series of studies designed to develop and test an approach to stratification for matched treatment concerns the effectiveness of manual therapy for low back pain. In 2002, Flynn et al. (25) used a small clinical cohort (n = 71) to derive a prediction rule (combination of candidate predictors of treatment effect) for identification of patients with high probability of responding well to a standardized manual therapy intervention. Participants scoring positive on at least four out of five clinical predictors had a 95% probability of reducing their disability scores by at least 50%. In a subsequent RCT (26), in which the effectiveness of manual therapy was compared to exercise therapy, participants scoring positive on the rule were found to have greater benefit from manual therapy compared to exercise, while the difference was smaller for participants scoring negative on the rule. The test for interaction (between prediction rule and treatment) was statistically significant, indicating potential value for using the rule to target manual therapy to patients likely to experience most benefit. However, this interaction could not be replicated in another trial of manual therapy conducted by a different research team, which showed similar outcomes for all participants scoring positive on the rule regardless of treatment, indicating that the identified predictors acted as prognostic factors rather than predictors of treatment effect (27). This was not an ideal replication study, as there were considerable differences in study design (definition of startpoint, manual therapy protocol, control intervention, and endpoint), but this example highlights the importance of replication and the potential for heterogeneity of predictive performance across populations and settings. It also confirms the importance of publishing study protocols, sharing data, and achieving agreement regarding definition of core outcomes and candidate predictors of treatment effect, in order to facilitate replication.

8.4.2 Investigating the impact of stratified care interventions

Even if there is robust evidence for a predictor of treatment effect explaining all or part of the variability in effect among trial participants, this does not necessarily guarantee that using the predictor to target specific treatments to patient subgroups will actually lead to increased patient benefit, reduced harm, or more efficient use of healthcare resources, compared with usual or best current clinical care. Similar to investigating the costs, benefits, and harms of using a prognostic model to inform clinical decision making (see Section 7.5), this requires robustly designed impact analysis studies.

As real-life treatment decisions may often be 'binary', with treatments being offered or not to individuals, the first phase of impact analysis will often require the selection of optimal thresholds to inform decisions, for example based on the probability of a favourable outcome versus risk of harm for specific treatments. Such studies may use decision curve analysis methods, as described in Section 7.5, in which the net benefit of offering the treatment is displayed against different thresholds of probability of the outcome (28). These methods will help to quantify the potential impact of treatment decisions, although the process of selecting thresholds for treatment decision making may also require consensus studies to incorporate expertise and opinions of clinicians, healthcare commissioners, and patient representatives, regarding the balance of benefits and harms, costs, and practical implications of treatment decisions. Consensus studies may include the use of qualitative research methods (Delphi approaches, nominal group techniques) to arrive at a stratified care intervention that is feasible and acceptable in routine healthcare.

Stratified care interventions, where treatment options are matched to patient subgroups derived from predictors of treatment effect, can subsequently be compared with current care in order to estimate clinical and cost-effectiveness. A range of study designs have been proposed for such impact analysis studies, including large, pragmatic, multi-centre randomized trials, sometimes requiring cluster-randomization to prevent contamination in situations where clinicians or services need to change their approach to decision making when offering the new stratified care intervention.

Stratified care trials need to be designed carefully, not only in terms of the method of randomization, but also in terms of sample size estimation (e.g. whether or not the trial will be powered to test differences of treatment effects across predictor subgroups); whether or not to use equal randomization or randomize a larger number of patients to the stratified care arm; the need for training of healthcare professionals regarding delivery of the stratified care intervention; and selection of optimal outcomes (at the level of the individual patient and/or successful delivery of stratified care). Examples of impact studies include the STarT Back Trial, which evaluated a model of stratified primary care for low back pain, showing larger improvements of stratified care on patient-reported outcomes (disability) as well as lower healthcare costs (29) (see also Chapter 10). In the MINDACT trial, women with early-stage breast cancer were stratified based on their clinical risk (using a modified version of Adjuvant! Online) as well as genomic risk (using a 70-gene signature), showing that approximately 46% of women with breast cancer classified as high clinical risk might not require chemotherapy (30).

Large, pragmatic randomized trials are complex and costly, and alternative designs may be necessary, especially when the outcome is rare, or expected time to the outcome is long. In such situations, decision analytic modelling can be used to combine information on predictors of differential treatment response from existing randomized trials or meta-analyses (using intermediate or sur-rogate outcomes where necessary) with information on long-term outcomes and adverse events obtained from observational cohorts or routinely collected healthcare data, in order to estimate the potential impact of implementing stratified care on rare or long-term outcomes.

8.4.3 Health economic evaluation in the design and evaluation of stratified care interventions

Health economic considerations are important throughout the process of developing and evaluating stratified care interventions, from analysing the costs of current care, through to deciding on treatment thresholds, and estimating cost-effectiveness. The cost-effectiveness or cost-utility of a stratified care inter-vention can be investigated using trial-based health economic evaluations, in which data on costs (related to delivery of the stratified care intervention, add-itional healthcare resource use, productivity losses, etc.) are collected alongside data on clinical outcomes. However, trial-based health economic evaluations are specific to the setting in which the trial has been conducted. They are mainly suitable when outcomes are expected to occur soon after treatment has been offered, and few changes in outcomes and costs are expected in the long-term.

Health economic decision models are often used to estimate cost-effectiveness over longer time periods, across different patient groups or different healthcare contexts. Decision models offer the flexibility to compare multiple clinically relevant scenarios, although they require valid estimations of prognosis for each of these scenarios from existing cohorts, trials or meta-analyses. For example, Zhao et al. (2) estimated the cost-effectiveness of using novel oral anticoagulants for stroke prevention in patients with atrial fibrillation, investigating whether effect estimates for different types of medication varied across age groups. The authors used effect estimates from a network meta-analysis involving over 800,000 patients from randomized controlled trials and cohorts in a Markov decision model, which projected cost and health outcomes over a lifetime in a cohort of patients with atrial fibrillation, separately for people aged 65–74 and ≥75 years old. The results showed that whilst novel oral anti-coagulants were cost-effective in the younger age group compared with warfarin, their benefits appeared to be offset by worsened risk profiles in the older age group.

The complexities of estimating the cost-effectiveness of stratified care interventions have been recognized, and a framework to guide the use of subgroup analysis in health economic evaluation has been proposed (31). The framework addresses questions related to the identification and selection of subgroups based on predictors of differential treatment response, and importantly, recognizes the uncertainty of parameters of health economic decision models and potential consequences of resulting errors in decision making. The authors propose the use of value-of-information methods to quantify the expected health that might be gained if uncertainty surrounding decisions about coverage or reimbursement of new health technologies were resolved, and to identify areas where further research is needed to resolve uncertainties and optimally explain variability in costs and outcomes (31).

8.4.4 Clinical utility

Successful design and implementation of stratified care may not only require high-quality evidence regarding its impact on patient outcomes, potential harms, and costs of treatment, but also depend on the practical consequences of delivering a more complex service, with potential additional burden to clinicians and patients. A systematic review and survey among general practitioners regarding the clinical usefulness of clinical prediction rules developed for a wide range of health conditions highlighted the importance of a clear clinical need for improvement to successfully drive implementation. When considering the use of several prediction rules, many healthcare professionals indicated a preference for their own clinical judgement, or perceived the prediction rule to be unnecessary for decision making (32).

Policymakers, healthcare professionals, and patients will also want to consider the unintended consequences of introducing new tests, markers, or tools to guide treatment decision making. These may potentially include increased healthcare-seeking behaviour and overdiagnosis or overtreatment in low-risk patients. Research clearly needs to establish the added value of introducing new predictors of treatment effect over and beyond currently available clinical information and expertise, and show a positive impact on the processes and outcomes of clinical care.

8.5 Summary

Stratified care refers to matching of pharmacological or non-pharmacological treatment according to information regarding a patient's prognosis or likely response to treatment, with the aim to optimize patient outcome, reduce harm, and/or increase the efficiency of healthcare. There is scope for developing successful stratified care interventions when there is wide variability in overall prognosis or response to treatment, and when decisions regarding treatment have important consequences in terms of healthcare costs, patient burden, or potential harm. Stratified care interventions can be developed based on prognostic stratification (as described in Chapter 7), where a prognostic model may be used to identify patients at high risk of poor outcome, who may be targeted for more intensive treatment (or conversely, to identify those at low risk who may be reassured regarding their likely favourable disease course). In this chapter, we have focused on stratified care based on predictors of treatment effect, often referred to as effect modifiers or treatment moderators, which appear to have a clear and potentially causal association with the outcome (benefit or harm) of a specific type of treatment. Genuine predictors of treatment effect are rare, although much sought after. Candidate predictors may be identified from exploratory analyses of trials and cohort studies, but external validation within randomized trials and IPD meta-analyses is needed to confirm whether a predictor is genuinely explaining variation in treatment effect. Even then, additional research is subsequently needed to investigate the clinical and cost-effectiveness of using the predictor to inform clinical decisions and target treatment accordingly. Rigorous evaluation of the impact of such stratified care interventions compared to usual care may involve large pragmatic randomized trials, health economic decision models, and implementation studies.

8.5.1 Summary points

- A predictor of treatment effect can be any type of factor (patient characteristic, symptom, sign, test, or biomarker result) or combination of factors associated with the effect (benefit or harm) of a specific treatment.

- A change in the value (or category) of the predictor (or combination of predictors) is associated with a difference in treatment effect.

- Various terms are used across disciplines to refer to prediction of treatment effect: treatment-predictor or treatment-covariate interaction, effect modification, moderation, or biological synergy. Predictors of treatment effect are sometimes, notably in the cancer field, referred to as predictive markers or treatment selection factors.

- Candidate predictors of treatment effect may originate from exploratory subgroup analyses in trials or observational clinical cohorts.

- Pre-specified analyses in randomized trials provide the most robust evidence to estimate treatment-predictor interactions, but replication using data from multiple randomized trials is usually needed to improve power and validate findings beyond a single study.

◆ Predictors of treatment effect can form the basis of stratified care, where treatments are matched to individuals or subgroups according to one or more factors that predict benefit or harm from treatment, ideally as early as possible in the disease process.

◆ Successful implementation of stratified care based on predictors of treatment effect generally requires a series of studies, to (1) identify and confirm factors that accurately predict treatment effect, and (2) evaluate whether matching treatment to individuals or subgroups based on such factors indeed leads to better outcomes and/or increased efficiency of care, compared to usual non-stratified care.

◆ Impact analysis studies (e.g. large pragmatic randomized trials, health economic decision models, comparative implementation studies) are needed to investigate the clinical effectiveness and cost-effectiveness of stratified care approaches.

References

1. **Hingorani AD, van der Windt DA, Riley RD**, et al. (2013) Prognosis research strategy (PROGRESS) 4: stratified medicine research. *BMJ* **346**, e5793. doi: 10.1136/bmj.e5793.

2. **Zhao YJ, Lin L, Zhou HJ**, et al. (2016) Cost-effectiveness modelling of novel oral anticoagulants incorporating real-world elderly patients with atrial fibrillation. *Int J Cardiol* **220**, 794–801. doi: 10.1016/j.ijcard.2016.06.087.

3. **Hay EM, Mullis R, Lewis M**, et al. (2005) Comparison of physical treatments versus a brief pain-management programme for back pain in primary care: a randomised clinical trial in physiotherapy practice. *Lancet* **365**(9476), 2024–30. doi: 10.1016/S0140-6736(05)66696-2.

4. **Jellema P, van der Windt DA, van der Horst HE**, et al. (2005) Should treatment of (sub) acute low back pain be aimed at psychosocial prognostic factors? Cluster randomised clinical trial in general practice. *BMJ* **331**(7508), 84. doi: 10.1136/bmj.38495.686736.E0.

5. **Mansell G, Hall A,** and **Toomey E** (2016) Behaviour change and self-management interventions in persistent low back pain. *Best Pract Res Clin Rheumatol* **30**(6), 994–1002. doi: 10.1016/j.berh.2017.07.004.

6. **Donaldson MG, Palermo L, Ensrud KE**, et al. (2012) Effect of alendronate for reducing fracture by FRAX score and femoral neck bone mineral density: the Fracture Intervention Trial. *J Bone Miner Res* **27**(8), 1804–10. doi: 10.1002/jbmr.1625.

7. **Knol MJ, VanderWeele TJ, Groenwold RH**, et al. (2011) Estimating measures of interaction on an additive scale for preventive exposures. *Eur J Epidemiol* **26**(6), 433–8. doi: 10.1007/s10654-011-9554-9.

8. **VanderWeele TJ** and **Vansteelandt S** (2014) Invited commentary: some advantages of the relative excess risk due to interaction (RERI)—towards better estimators of additive

interaction. *Am J Epidemiol* **179**(6), 670–1. doi: 10.1093/aje/kwt316 (published Online First: 2014/02/04).

9. **Shrier I** and **Pang M** (2015) Confounding, effect modification, and the odds ratio: common misinterpretations. *J Clin Epidemiol* **68**(4), 470–4. doi: 10.1016/j.jclinepi.2014.12.012 (published Online First: 2015/02/11).

10. **Williams C, Brunskill S, Altman D**, et al. (2006) Cost-effectiveness of using prognostic information to select women with breast cancer for adjuvant systemic therapy. *Health Technol Assess* **10**(34), iii–iv, ix–xi, 1–204.

11. **Mok TS, Wu YL, Thongprasert S**, et al. (2009) Gefitinib or carboplatin-paclitaxel in pulmonary adenocarcinoma. *N Engl J Med* **361**(10), 947–57. doi: 10.1056/NEJMoa0810699.

12. **Mallal S, Nolan D, Witt C**, et al. (2002) Association between presence of HLA-B*5701, HLA-DR7, and HLA-DQ3 and hypersensitivity to HIV-1 reverse-transcriptase inhibitor abacavir. *Lancet* **359**(9308), 727–32.

13. **Malottki K, Biswas M, Deeks JJ**, et al. (2014) Stratified medicine in European Medicines Agency licensing: a systematic review of predictive biomarkers. *BMJ Open* **4**(1), e004188. doi: 10.1136/bmjopen-2013-004188.

14. **Cuppen BV, Welsing PM, Sprengers JJ**, et al. (2016) Personalized biological treatment for rheumatoid arthritis: a systematic review with a focus on clinical applicability. *Rheumatology* (Oxford) **55**(5):826–39. doi: 10.1093/rheumatology/kev421.

15. **Slamon DJ, Leyland-Jones B, Shak S**, et al. (2001) Use of chemotherapy plus a monoclonal antibody against HER2 for metastatic breast cancer that overexpresses HER2. *N Engl J Med* **344**(11), 783–92. doi: 10.1056/NEJM200103153441101.

16. **Holzhauser L, Hovnanians N, Eshtehardi P**, et al. (2017) Statin therapy improves survival in patients with severe pulmonary hypertension: a propensity score matching study. *Heart Vessels* **32**(8), 969–76. doi: 10.1007/s00380-017-0957-8.

17. **Alosh M, Huque MF**, and **Koch GG** (2015) Statistical perspectives on subgroup analysis: testing for heterogeneity and evaluating error rate for the complementary subgroup. *J Biopharm Stat* **25**(6), 1161–78. doi: 10.1080/10543406.2014.971169.

18. **Brookes ST, Whitely E, Egger M**, et al. (2004) Subgroup analyses in randomized trials: risks of subgroup-specific analyses; power and sample size for the interaction test. *J Clin Epidemiol* **57**(3), 229–36. doi: 10.1016/j.jclinepi.2003.08.009.

19. **Senn S** (2004) Individual response to treatment: is it a valid assumption? *BMJ* **329**(7472), 966–8. doi: 10.1136/bmj.329.7472.966.

20. **Fayers PM** and **King MT** (2009) How to guarantee finding a statistically significant difference: the use and abuse of subgroup analyses. *Qual Life Res* **18**(5), 527–30. doi: 10.1007/s11136-009-9473-3 (published Online First: 2009/04/04).

21. **Sun X, Briel M, Walter SD**, et al. (2010) Is a subgroup effect believable? Updating criteria to evaluate the credibility of subgroup analyses. *BMJ* **340**, c117. doi: 10.1136/bmj.c117.

22. **Pincus T, Miles C, Froud R**, et al. (2011) Methodological criteria for the assessment of moderators in systematic reviews of randomised controlled trials: a consensus study. *BMC Med Res Methodol* **11**, 14. doi: 10.1186/1471-2288-11-14.

23. **Ross JS** and **Fletcher JA** (1998) The HER-2/neu oncogene in breast cancer: prognostic factor, predictive factor, and target for therapy. *Oncologist* **3**(4), 237–52. (published Online First: 1999/07/01).

24. **Elkin EB, Weinstein MC, Winer EP**, et al. (2004) HER-2 testing and trastuzumab therapy for metastatic breast cancer: a cost-effectiveness analysis. *J Clin Oncol* **22**(5), 854–63. doi: 10.1200/JCO.2004.04.158.

25. **Flynn T, Fritz J, Whitman J**, et al. (2002) A clinical prediction rule for classifying patients with low back pain who demonstrate short-term improvement with spinal manipulation. *Spine (Phila Pa 1976)* **27**(24), 2835–43. doi: 10.1097/01.BRS.0000035681.33747.8D.

26. **Childs JD, Fritz JM, Flynn TW**, et al. (2004) A clinical prediction rule to identify patients with low back pain most likely to benefit from spinal manipulation: a validation study. *Ann Intern Med* **141**(12), 920–8.

27. **Hancock MJ, Maher CG, Latimer J**, et al. (2008) Independent evaluation of a clinical prediction rule for spinal manipulative therapy: a randomised controlled trial. *Eur Spine J* **17**(7), 936–43. doi: 10.1007/s00586-008-0679-9.

28. **Vickers AJ, Van Calster B**, and **Steyerberg EW** (2016) Net benefit approaches to the evaluation of prediction models, molecular markers, and diagnostic tests. *BMJ* **352**, i6. doi: 10.1136/bmj.i6.

29. **Hill JC, Whitehurst DG, Lewis M**, et al. (2011) Comparison of stratified primary care management for low back pain with current best practice (STarT Back): a randomised controlled trial. *Lancet* **378**(9802), :1560–71. doi: 10.1016/S0140-6736(11)60937-9.

30. **Cardoso F, van't Veer LJ, Bogaerts J**, et al. (2016) 70-gene signature as an aid to treatment decisions in early-stage breast cancer. *N Engl J Med* **375**(8), 717–29. doi: 10.1056/NEJMoa1602253.

31. **Espinoza MA, Manca A, Claxton K**, et al. (2014) The value of heterogeneity for cost-effectiveness subgroup analysis: conceptual framework and application. *Med Decis Making* **34**(8), 951–64. doi: 10.1177/0272989X14538705.

32. **Pluddemann A, Wallace E, Bankhead C**, et al. (2014) Clinical prediction rules in practice: review of clinical guidelines and survey of GPs. *Br J Gen Pract* **64**(621), e233–42. doi: 10.3399/bjgp14X677860 (published Online First: 2014/04/02).

Chapter 9

Systematic reviews and meta-analysis of prognosis research studies

Richard D Riley, Karel GM Moons,
Thomas PA Debray, Douglas G Altman,
and Gary S Collins

9.1 Introduction

Healthcare should be evidence-based, such that decisions are founded on all the existing evidence, rather than a single study or subjective opinion. To this end, the last thirty years have seen a dramatic rise in evidence synthesis, involving specific research methods to identify and combine existing evidence. Two universally accepted approaches are a systematic review and meta-analysis. After defining a research (review) aim, *systematic reviews* provide a framework for the identification, collection, data extraction, critical appraisal, quantitative and qualitative summary, and reporting of evidence from existing studies. Systematic reviews aim to answer the pre-defined research question objectively, using explicit methods that make the review transparent and reproducible. If appropriate, a *meta-analysis* can be performed at the end of a systematic review. Meta-analysis is a statistical approach that combines the quantitative evidence from identified studies (or from the subset of better quality studies), usually to calculate overall summary results. Systematic reviews and meta-analyses of randomized trials are common in the medical literature, to summarize the benefit of one or more treatments for a particular condition. These form the cornerstone of Cochrane, an internationally renowned organization that specializes in gathering and summarizing the best evidence about available treatments (1). In recent years, Cochrane has expanded to include systematic reviews and meta-analyses of diagnostic test accuracy studies and, more recently, prognosis studies (2).

Systematic reviews and meta-analyses are essential in the prognosis field. Prognosis research evidence accumulates over time, for example about the prognostic value of a particular factor or model, and is typically presented across multiple studies. When considered as a whole, these multiple studies should provide a clearer picture and lead to more genuine (and generalizable) findings compared to a single study, which usually has a more select population and small sample size, and is more prone to the play of chance. However, compared to well-rehearsed topic areas such as treatment effects and diagnostic tests, systematic reviews and meta-analyses of prognosis studies face unique challenges and require specific methods for identifying, appraising, and synthesizing the evidence. In this chapter, we detail the key aspects of a systematic review and meta-analysis of prognosis studies, covering each of four prognosis research themes. We highlight key checklists, risk of bias tools, and methodology guidance for conducting reviews and meta-analyses of prognosis studies.

9.2 Key components of a systematic review and meta-analysis of prognosis studies

A systematic review of prognosis studies should ideally be registered in advance, for example in PROSPERO, the international prospective register of systematic reviews (http://www.crd.york.ac.uk/PROSPERO/), and the planned process for conducting the review should be detailed, ideally within a published protocol. Various journals, such as *BMC Diagnostic & Prognostic Research* and *Systematic Reviews*, advocate the publication of such protocols. They should outline the rationale, objectives, eligibility criteria, data extraction, critical appraisal, statistical methods, and reporting guidelines to be used (3). We describe these key components of the review process, from defining the research question and identifying relevant studies, to appraising study quality, extracting data, summarizing, and (if appropriate) meta-analysing and reporting study results.

9.2.1 Defining the review question

The first and most fundamental task is to define the review question(s). Though this sounds obvious, we discussed in Chapter 2 how the PROGRESS framework was initiated to address confusion about primary prognosis research questions (4–7). Therefore, reviewers should begin by establishing which of the four PROGRESS types they are interested in. Some review aims may span two or more types (Box 9.1).

Though rare, systematic reviews of overall prognosis (PROGRESS type I) may be needed. For example, in patients with Barrett's oesophagus, Yousef et al. (8) review the incidence of oesophageal cancer and high-grade dysplasia

Box 9.1 Possible objectives and aims of a systematic review (without or with a quantitative meta-analysis) of prognostic model studies (adapted from Moons et al. (13))

◆ To review all existing prognostic models for a particular condition or outcome(s):

- for example, Perel et al. (14) systematically review existing prognostic models in traumatic brain injury to describe their characteristics and quality.

◆ To summarize the predictive performance of a particular prognostic model:

- for example, Siregar et al. (15) review the performance of the original EuroSCORE model for predicting risk of operative mortality following cardiac surgery, and conclude that it generally overestimates mortality risk.

◆ To review comparisons of the predictive performance of competing prognostic models:

- for example, Warnell et al. (16) review models for predicting perioperative mortality after oesophagectomy, and identify a few studies that compare different models, of which the P-POSSUM model appears best.

◆ To summarize the value of updating (e.g. recalibration) or modifying (e.g. adding a new predictor to) an existing prognostic model:

- for example, in their protocol for a systematic review of prognostic models for chronic lymphocytic leukaemia, Skoetz et al. (19) note they will extract information, in the presence of poor validation, about whether models were 'adjusted or updated (e.g. intercept recalibrated, predictor effects adjusted, or new predictors added)'.

◆ To review studies which examine the impact of using a prognostic model in clinical practice, for example on subsequent patient outcomes:

- usually such reviews only identify a few impact studies, as they are rare. For example, a review of models for the early care of trauma patients did not find any impact studies (20) whilst a review of clinical prediction rules for physical therapy in low back pain identified only three impact studies (21).

Source: data from Moons, KG., et al. Critical appraisal and data extraction for systematic reviews of prediction modelling studies: the CHARMS checklist. *PLoS Medicine*.11(10), e1001744. Copyright © 2014 PLoS. Open Access.

per 1000 person years, to inform whether a surveillance programme is war-ranted due to high cancer risk. In patients with severe symptomatic aortic sten-osis after surgical replacement of an aortic valve with a bioprosthetic valve, Foroutan et al. (9) review the rate of subsequent outcomes, including mortality, stroke, and atrial fibrillation, to examine if their overall prognosis is comparable to that of the general population of a similar age.

Systematic reviews of prognostic factor studies are far more common, and are a growing industry, especially in cancer research. A crude search of PubMed for articles using the string 'systematic review' or 'meta-analysis' and 'prognostic factor' or 'prognostic marker' in the title or abstract identifies over one hundred per year since 2014. Most appear to have a meta-analysis as the ultimate goal, to summarize a factor's prognostic effect (e.g. a summary hazard ratio) for a certain outcome in certain individuals (patients) and to quantify the between-study het-erogeneity in this effect. Some reviews focus on one or a few prognostic factors for a specific outcome; for example Hemingway et al. review the evidence for C-reactive protein as a prognostic factor for fatal and non-fatal events in patients with stable coronary disease (10). Other reviews are broad; for example Riley et al. aim to identify *any* prognostic factor for overall and disease-free survival in children with neuroblastoma or Ewing's sarcoma (11). A guide to systematic re-views and meta-analysis of prognostic factor studies is given by Riley et al. (12).

Also growing in popularity are systematic reviews of prognostic models. Box 9.1 highlights possible objectives and aims of such reviews, with examples (13–16, 19–21). The most common aim is to identify and summarize the available models for a particular condition, and qualitatively summarize their (predictive) performance. If multiple external validation studies of a specific model are identified, meta-analysis may be a goal to formally combine and summarize the predictive performance estimates of that model (see Section 9.2.5). A guide to systematic reviews and meta-analysis of prognostic models is given by Debray et al. (17), including an empirical example of a review and meta-analysis of the additive European system for cardiac operative risk evalu-ation (EuroSCORE). The EuroSCORE is a prognostic model that aims to pre-dict thirty-day mortality in patients undergoing any type of cardiac surgery. It was developed by a European steering group in 1999 using logistic regres-sion in a dataset from 13,302 adult patients undergoing cardiac surgery under cardiopulmonary bypass. Its predictive performance has been examined (ex-ternally validated) many times, and recently reviewed and summarized (15). Debray et al. identify, appraise and summarize the validation performance of EuroSCORE in terms of thirty-day all-cause mortality amongst patients undergoing coronary artery bypass grafting (CABG) (17). We will use this em-pirical example also as a case study throughout the chapter.

Reviews falling within the fourth PROGRESS type aim to identify evidence for predictors of treatment effect. Such a review typically involves a systematic review of randomized trials, with the goal of meta-analysing estimates of *differences* in intervention effects (treatment-covariate interactions) defined by changes in predictor values. This remit is often specified as a secondary objective within reviews of the overall effect of a particular intervention. For example, most Cochrane reviews of randomized trials will summarize intervention effects for particular subgroups of patients, alongside the overall effects (18).

The CHARMS (CHecklist for critical Appraisal and data extraction for systematic Reviews of prediction Modelling Studies) provides guidance for formulating a prognostic model review question and for extracting data and critically appraising the primary studies included (13, 17). Although this checklist is focused on systematic reviews of prognostic model studies, an extension for reviews of prognostic factor studies is also available (CHARMS-PF) (12). Moreover, the guidance in these two checklists can help define the review questions for the other three prognosis study types. The CHARMS checklist addresses the key items for framing the review aim and provides a modification (called PICOTS) of the traditional PICO system (population, index, comparison, and outcome) used in systematic reviews of therapeutic intervention studies, and additionally considers Timing (that is, the time point and time period of interest for prognosis) and Setting (as it is well known that the predictive ability of prognostic models changes across healthcare settings). A summary of the PICOTS system is given in Box 9.2.

9.2.2 Searching for eligible studies

A focused review question enables researchers to define eligible studies based on particular inclusion and exclusion criteria, and to develop a tailored search strategy. Unfortunately, it is more difficult to identify prognosis research studies by literature searching than randomized trials of interventions. Prognosis studies do not tend to be indexed ('tagged') as such, most likely because a taxonomy of prognosis research is not widely recognized. Therefore many search strategies for prognosis research are quite broad, for fear of missing something important, but this comes at the expense of retrieving many irrelevant records. For example, for their review of all prognostic models for the early care of trauma patients, a broad search strategy by Rehn et al. (20) led to screening of 4939 records, of which only fourteen (0.3%) were considered relevant. When a more focused question is of interest, for example relating to *one* particular outcome or a single prognostic model, the search terms can be more specific. In the review of Siregar et al. (Box 9.1 and Box 9.2) (15), the focus was on one particular model (EuroSCORE) and so the search string included the terms 'EuroSCORE' and 'Euro SCORE'. This yielded 686 articles, a manageable number, with an additional study identified through a cross-reference check.

Box 9.2 Six key items to help define the question for reviews of prognosis studies, abbreviated as PICOTS and illustrated using the Debray et al. review (20) of the predictive performance of the EuroSCORE model to predict short term mortality in patients who underwent coronary artery bypass grafting (CABG).

◆ Population: define the target population in which the overall prognosis, prognostic factor, prognostic model, or predictor of differential intervention effect will be used.

  • In our example study, the population of interest comprised patients undergoing CABG.

◆ Index: define the prognostic factor(s), model(s) or treatment-covariate interaction(s) under review.

  • In our example, the index model was the prognostic EuroSCORE model.

◆ Comparator: if applicable, one can compare the index and review more than one factor, model or treatment-covariate interaction for the target population under review.

  • In our example, no alternative prognostic models were considered. So there is no comparator.

◆ Outcome: define the exact prognosis outcome(s) of interest for which the overall prognosis is reviewed, or for which the factor, model or treatment-covariate interaction under review is supposed to (help) predict.

  • In our example, the outcome was defined as all-cause mortality. Papers validating the EuroSCORE model to predict other outcomes such as cardiovascular mortality were excluded.

◆ Timing: define (i) the time-point of the prognostication and (ii) over what time period the outcome(s) are predicted.

  • In our example, the focus was on all-cause mortality at thirty days.

◆ Setting: define the intended setting of the overall prognosis, prognostic factor, prognostic model or predictor of intervention effect under review.

  • In our example, the originally intended use of the EuroSCORE model was to perform preoperative risk stratification in patients scheduled for cardiac surgery to predict short-term all-cause mortality.

Source: reproduced courtesy of Richard D. Riley

Geersing et al. (22) validated previous search filters and updated them with a generic search filter for identifying studies of prognostic models, which was also examined for its ability to find prognostic factor studies (Box 9.3) (23–25). When tested in two existing reviews of models, it had a number needed to read (NNR) to identify one relevant article of 68 and 125. When tested in a single review of prognostic factors, it had an NNR of 569, emphasising the extra difficulty in targeting prognostic factor articles. However, the NNR can be considerably reduced in situations where specific models, factors, outcomes, or populations are of interest, as then these terms should be added to the filter. Care is still needed to be inclusive, as some factors have multiple names, for example biomarker MYCN (a prognostic factor in neuroblastoma) is also referred to as n-myc, nmyc and bHLHe37 amongst others (11). Once the search is complete, each potentially relevant study must be screened for eligibility, ideally by two researchers independently. Any discrepancies should be resolved through discussion, and potentially with a third reviewer.

9.2.3 Data extraction

A crucial task for reviewers is to extract key information from identified studies. Ideally, this is done independently by at least two reviewers, to minimize errors. Data extraction enables reviewers to examine the applicability of the primary

---

Box 9.3 Generic search string to help in identifying prognostic factor and model studies, as proposed by Geersing et al. (23)

(Validat$ OR Predict$.ti. OR Rule$)

OR (Predict$ AND (Outcome$ OR Risk$ OR Model$))

OR ((History OR Variable$ OR Criteria OR Scor$ OR Characteristic$ OR Finding$ OR Factor$) AND (Predict$ OR Model$ OR Decision$ OR Identif$ OR Prognos$))

OR (Decision$ AND (Model$ OR Clinical$ OR Logistic Models/))

OR (Prognostic AND (History OR Variable$ OR Criteria OR Scor$ OR Characteristic$ OR Finding$ OR Factor$ OR Model$))

OR (Stratification OR "ROC Curve"[Mesh] OR Discrimination OR Discriminate OR "c-statistic" OR "*C* statistic" OR "Area under the curve" OR AUC OR Calibration OR Indices OR Algorithm OR Multivariable)

Source: data from Geersing Geersing, GJ., et al. Search filters for finding prognostic and diagnostic prediction studies in Medline to enhance systematic reviews. PLoS One. 7(2), e32844.Copyright © 2012 PLoS. Open Access.

study for the aim of the review, enables assessment of the risk of bias of the identified studies, provides the necessary descriptive data of the included studies, and ultimately allows a qualitative, and possibly quantitative (meta-analysis), summary of their findings.

For all types of prognosis studies, reviewers should extract fundamental information, such as the year(s) of patient recruitment and follow-up, setting(s), study design, definitions (e.g. participant selection criteria, outcomes, and prognostic factors), baseline characteristics (case mix), treatments received, number of participants, number of events, total (and median) follow-up time, study attrition (missing data), and analysis methods. However, especially for review questions relating to PROGRESS types II to IV, more specific details are often needed, particularly to facilitate assessments of risk of bias. For example, to complete the risk of bias tools QUIPS and PROBAST (see Section 9.2.4) for reviews of prognostic factors and models, respectively, data extraction should include the sampling of study participants (study design), the methods used to measure the prognostic factors and outcomes, the statistical models used (e.g. regression approach), the handling of continuous prognostic factors and of missing data, and model-building strategies.

For data extraction of prognostic model studies, CHARMS provides an explicit checklist of items that need to be extracted from the primary studies to enhance the assessment of study applicability and risk of bias, and the qualitative and quantitative summary of the study data (Table 9.1) (13). Although this checklist focuses on data extraction from prognostic model studies, almost all items can also be used as a starting point for systematic reviews of overall prognosis, except that the items on model development, performance, and evaluation can be deleted as these are not relevant for overall prognosis studies. Recently an extension of CHARMS for reviews of prognostic factor studies is presented (CHARMS-PF) (12). For data extraction from studies of predictors of treatment effect (PROGRESS framework type IV), data extraction guidelines outlined in the Cochrane Handbook for randomized trials should rather be considered (1).

To enable a quantitative meta-analysis, reviewers need to extract estimates of statistics that address the review question of interest, together with a measure of their uncertainty (standard errors, variances, or confidence intervals). Relevant statistics for the most common prognosis review questions are shown in Table 9.2. For overall prognosis they include the overall mean value as a continuous outcome (e.g. mean pain score), the overall risk (cumulative incidence) of a binary outcome by one or more time points, or the overall event rate of a time-to-event outcome across the whole study period. Kaplan-Meier curves of survival (or event) probabilities over time may be relevant. Unfortunately, numerical results presented in overall prognosis studies may vary in format and completeness—for example survival proportions may be

Table 9.1 Items to be extracted from primary studies of prognostic models as listed in the CHARMS checklist (19)

Source of data	Source of data (e.g. cohort, case-control, randomized trial participants, or registry data)
Participants	Partcipant eligibility and recruitment method (e.g. consecutive participants, location, number of centres, setting, inclusion and exclusion criteria)
	Participant description
	Details of treatments received, if relevant
	Study dates
Outcome(s) to be predicted	Definition and method for measurement of outcome
	Was the same outcome definition (and method for measurement) used in all patients?
	Type of outcome (e.g. single or combined endpoints)
	Was the outcome assessed without knowledge of the candidate predictors (i.e. blinded)?
	Were candidate predictors part of the outcome (e.g. in panel or consensus diagnosis)?
	Time of outcome occurrence or summary of duration of follow-up
Candidate predictors (or index tests)	Number and type of predictors (e.g. demographics, patient history, physical examination, additional testing, disease characteristics)
	Definition and method for measurement of candidate predictors
	Timing of predictor measurement (e.g. at patient presentation, at diagnosis, at treatment initiation)
	Were predictors assessed blinded for outcome, and for each other (if relevant)?
	Handling of predictors in the modelling (e.g. continuous, linear, non-linear transformations, or categorized)
Sample size	Number of participants and number of outcomes/events
	Number of outcomes/events in relation to the number of candidate predictors (events per variable)
Missing data	Number of participants with any missing value (include predictors and outcomes)
	Number of participants with missing data for each predictor
	Handling of missing data (e.g. complete-case analysis, imputation, or other methods)

Table 9.1 Continued

Model development	Modelling method (e.g. logistic, survival, neural network, or machine learning techniques)
	Modelling assumptions satisfied
	Method for selection of predictors for inclusion in multivariable modelling (e.g. all candidate predictors, pre-selection based on unadjusted association with the outcome)
	Method for selection of predictors *during multivariable modelling* (e.g. full-model approach, backward or forward selection) and criteria used (e.g. *p*-value, Akaike Information Criterion)
	Shrinkage of predictor weights or regression coefficients (e.g. no shrinkage, uniform shrinkage, penalized estimation)
Model performance	Calibration (calibration plot, calibration slope, Hosmer-Lemeshow test) and discrimination (*C* statistic, D-statistic, log-rank) measures with confidence intervals
	Classification measures (e.g. sensitivity, specificity, predictive values, net reclassification improvement) and whether a priori cut points were used
Model evaluation	Method used for testing model performance: development dataset only (random split of data, resampling methods, e.g. bootstrap or cross-validation, none) or separate external validation (e.g. temporal, geographical, different setting, different investigators)
	In case of poor validation, whether model was adjusted or updated (e.g. intercept recalibrated, predictor effects adjusted, or new predictors added)
Results	Final and other multivariable models (e.g. basic, extended, simplified) presented, including predictor weights or regression coefficients, intercept, baseline survival, model performance measures (with standard errors or confidence intervals
	Any alternative presentation of the final prediction models, e.g. sum score, nomogram, score chart, predictions for specific risk subgroups with performance)
	Comparison of the distribution of predictors (including missing data) for development and validation datasets
Interpretation and discussion	Interpretation of presented models (confirmatory, i.e. model useful for practice versus exploratory, i.e. more research needed)
	Comparison with other studies, discussion of generalizability, strengths, and limitations.

Source: data from Moons, KG., et al. Critical appraisal and data extraction for systematic reviews of prediction modelling studies: the CHARMS checklist. *PLoS Medicine*.11(10), e1001744. Copyright © 2014 PLoS. Open Access.

Table 9.2 Relevant statistics to be extracted to perform meta-analysis of prognosis studies, and the scale to use when performing a random effects meta-analysis

Research question	Relevant statistics	Appropriate scale for meta-analysis
1. Overall prognosis		
What is the overall outcome value (score) by a particular follow-up time point?	(Standardized) Mean	original
What is the overall survival probability by a particular follow-up time point?	probability*	logit
What is the overall outcome risk by a particular follow-up time point?	1 - survival probability*	logit
What is the overall outcome rate over the whole follow-up period?	Incidence rate (total events and person-years of follow-up)	ln
2. Prognostic factors		
What is the association between a particular factor and the outcome value or score at a particular time point?	(Standardized) Mean difference	original
What is the association between a particular factor and outcome risk at a particular time point?	Risk ratio	ln
	Odds ratio	ln
What is the association between a particular factor and outcome rate over the whole follow-up period?	Hazard (rate) ratio	ln
3. Prognostic models†		
What is the calibration performance of a particular model?	Calibration slope	original
	Calibration-in-the-large	original
	E/O or O/E ratio	ln
What is the discrimination performance of a particular model?	C statistic	logit
	Royston's D statistic	original
What is the net benefit of a particular model?	Net benefit	Fisher z
	Number of patients with the outcome, and, at each threshold, the number of true positives and true negatives	original (see (41))
What is the benefit on patient outcomes of incorporating the model within clinical decision making compared to current practice?	(Standardized) Mean difference	original
	Risk ratio	ln
	Odds ratio	ln
	Hazard (rate) ratio	ln

Table 9.2 Continued

Research question	Relevant statistics	Appropriate scale for meta-analysis
4. Predictors (subgroups) of differential treatment effect		
What is the association (interaction) between a particular factor and treatment effect by a particular time-point?[+]	Difference in (standardized) mean differences	original
	Ratio of risk ratios	ln
	Ratio of odds ratios	ln
What is the association (interaction) between a particular factor and treatment effect over the whole follow-up period?[+]	Ratio of hazard (rate) ratios	ln

* for example, as obtained from a Kaplan-Meier curve

[+] these statistics may be derived over the whole follow-up period, or for (by) a particular time point as relevant

[+]the change in the treatment effect for a 1-unit change in the factor (or difference in treatment effect between two subgroups)

Source: reproduced courtesy of Richard D. Riley

given for different time points, Kaplan-Meier curves may not always be presented, and even total numbers of events and total person years of follow-up may be omitted (26–28).

For prognostic factor studies, the key statistics are estimates of prognostic effect for each factor of interest, for example a risk ratio, odds ratio, hazard ratio, or mean difference (Table 9.2). As studies with binary outcomes will almost always have different follow-up lengths and include censored observations, hazard ratios are the most suitable effect measure. Chapter 6 emphasized that *adjusted* prognostic effect estimates are needed, as they quantify the independent prognostic value of a factor after adjusting for other (established) prognostic factors. Unadjusted results are less informative. It is important to extract the set of adjustment factors used, the length of follow-up, the handling of continuous factors (and choice of any cut points), and prevalence of 'positive' patients for binary (or dichotomized) factors (12).

Unfortunately, many reports of prognostic factor studies fail to provide prognostic effect estimates, especially for factors which were not statistically significant (27), or fail to give their variances, standard errors, or even confidence intervals. To address this, Parmar et al. (29) and Tierney et al. (30) describe how to obtain unadjusted hazard ratio estimates (and their variances) when they are not reported directly. For example, under assumptions, one can use the number of outcomes (events) and an available p-value (e.g. from a log-rank test or Cox regression) to indirectly estimate the hazard ratio between two groups defined by a particular factor (e.g. 'positive' versus 'negative' levels). Perneger et al. (31) suggest how to derive hazard ratios from survival proportions. Even with such indirect estimation methods, not all results will be obtainable. For example, in a systematic review of 575 studies investigating prognostic factors in neuroblastoma (27), the methods of Parmar et al. were used to obtain 204 hazard ratio estimates and their confidence intervals, but this represented only 35.5% of the potential evidence.

Indirect estimation methods mainly help retrieve *unadjusted* prognostic factor effects, and adjusted results may remain unavailable. If multiple studies do provide adjusted results, then the set of adjustment factors will usually differ across studies. This complicates the interpretation of subsequent meta-analysis results. It may help to pre-define a core set of adjustment factors that would represent the minimal adjustment needed for inclusion, such as gender, age, disease stage, and key co-morbidities.

For prognostic model studies, meta-analysis is often used to summarize estimates of a particular model's predictive performance. Therefore, data extraction should include estimates of calibration and discrimination of that model as reported in the included (external) validation studies for that model (Table 9.1 and Table 9.2) (13, 17). This may include measures such as the calibration slope, calibration-in-the-large, expected-to-observed number of events (E/O ratio), C statistic, and Royston's D statistic (see Chapters 3 and 7). Such results are often not given (notably calibration estimates) or are provided without confidence intervals (32, 33), and so Debray et al. (17, 34) provide guidance for extracting indirect estimates of the C statistic and E/O from other reported study information. Such methods are implemented in the R package 'metamisc' (https://CRAN.R-project.org/package=metamisc). Jinks et al. suggest how to approximate a C statistic from Royston's D statistic (35). An added complexity for models predicting risks over time is that model performance statistics (and calibration plots) may be available at multiple time points, as well as over all times. There are different methods to derive a C statistic for time-to-event data (36–38), which may introduce some between-study heterogeneity. If interest is in summarizing the impact of a prognostic model on decision making and health outcomes, then specific measures are required for extraction (Table 9.2), such as the model's estimated net-benefit at particular thresholds of predicted risk (39–41), or the estimated relative reduction in outcome risk when incorporating the model within clinical decision making compared to current practice (42).

For type IV prognosis studies, the key statistic to extract is the treatment-covariate interaction estimate; that is, the estimated difference in treatment effect according to changes in a particular predictor (covariate), such as a one-unit increase in age (Table 9.2). For example, an estimate of the difference in mean differences for continuous outcomes, the difference in log odds ratios (or ratio of odds ratios) for binary outcomes, or the difference in log hazard ratios (or ratio of hazard ratios) for time-to-event outcomes. Unfortunately, such estimates are often not reported, especially when they are not statistically significant. Sometimes the treatment effects in particular predictor subgroups (e.g. positive and negative biomarker levels) may be available, from which their difference can be derived (43).

Standardization of extracted estimates may be required, to ensure they all relate to the same scale and direction in each included study (Table 9.2). For example, overall prognosis studies are likely to report a mixture of survival percentages and death percentages, and so conversion from the survival to the death scale will often be necessary (or vice versa). For continuous outcomes a standardized scale may be preferred, for example in terms of units of standard deviation of the outcome. For prognostic factor studies, the direction of comparison for the extracted prognostic effect estimates (e.g. hazard ratios) may need standardizing, for example one study may compare the hazard rate in the 'positive' group versus the 'negative' group, whereas another study may compare the hazard rate in the 'negative' group versus the 'positive' group. For prognostic model studies, validation studies may report a mixture of E/O and O/E ratios. For type IV prognosis studies, the difference in treatment effect between two subgroups may relate to group A versus group B in some studies, but group B versus group A in other studies. Considerable care and attention to detail of extracted measures will therefore be necessary.

9.2.4 Evaluating the applicability and risk of bias of prognosis studies

Once eligible studies have been identified and their relevant data extracted, an important next step is to assess their *applicability*, which refers to the extent to which an eligible study matches the prognosis review question in terms of the PICOTS (Box 9.2). Just because a study is eligible for inclusion does not mean it is free from applicability concerns. For example, the PROBAST tool (Prediction model Risk Of Bias ASsessment Tool) includes three signalling topics for applicability (44):

> *Concern that the included participants and setting do not match the review question.*
> *Concern that the definition, assessment, or timing of predictors in the model do not match the review question.*
> *Concern that the outcome, its definition, timing, or determination do not match the review question.*

A study may be applicable in some aspects (e.g. correct prognostic factor or model) but not others (e.g. target population or outcomes), such as a study that externally validates a relevant prognostic model but in a setting different from that of the review question. For example Siregar et al. review the performance of the EuroSCORE model for all types of surgery (15), and therefore have a broader set of applicable studies than the review of Debray et al. (17), who examine EuroSCORE only in those patients undergoing CABG.

All eligible primary studies should be evaluated for their risk of bias (quality). *Risk of bias* refers to the extent to which flaws in the study design or analysis methods may lead to bias in, for example, estimates of overall prognosis, prognostic factor effects, prognostic model performance, or differential treatment effects. Growing empirical evidence from systematic reviews examining methodology quality shows that many prognosis studies will be at high risk of bias due to problems in their design, data quality, statistical methods, and reporting (27, 32, 33, 45–52).

Prognosis studies of types I–III typically have a non-randomized study design, although sometimes data from randomized trials are also used. For assessing the risk of bias of prognostic factor studies, Hayden et al. (53) developed the QUIPS checklist for examining risk of bias across six domains: study participation, study attrition, prognostic factor measurement, outcome measurement, adjustment for other factors, and statistical analysis and reporting. Table 9.3 shows the signalling items within these domains, to help guide reviewers toward low, moderate, or high risk of bias classifications. Items within domains 1, 2, and 4 are highly relevant for examining risk of bias for studies of overall prognosis.

Table 9.3 Assessing Quality in Prognostic Factor (PF) Studies: the QUIPS tool (53), with wording slightly adapted

Domains	Signalling items	Ratings
1. Study participation	a. Adequate participation in the study by eligible persons b. Description of the source population or population of interest c. Description of the baseline study sample d. Adequate description of the sampling frame and recruitment e. Adequate description of the period and place of recruitment f. Adequate description of inclusion and exclusion criteria	**High bias:** the relationship between the PF and outcome is very likely to be different for participants and eligible non-participants **Moderate**: the relationship between the PF and outcome may be different for participants and eligible non-participants **Low bias**: the relationship between the PF and outcome is unlikely to be different for participants and eligible non-participants

(Continued)

Table 9.3 Continued

Domains	Signalling items	Ratings
2. Study attrition	a. Adequate response rate for study participants b. Description of attempts to collect information on participants who dropped out c. Reasons for loss to follow-up are provided d. Adequate description of participants lost to follow-up e. There are no important differences between participants who completed the study and those who did not	**High bias**: the relationship between the PF and outcome is very likely to be different for completing and non-completing participants **Moderate**: the relationship between the PF and outcome may be different for completing and non-completing participants **Low bias**: the relationship between the PF and outcome is unlikely to be different for completing and non-completing participants
3. Prognostic factor measurement	a. A clear definition or description of the PF is provided b. Method of PF measurement is adequately valid and reliable c. Continuous variables are reported or appropriate cut points are used d. The method and setting of measurement of PF is the same for all study participants e. Adequate proportion of the study sample has complete data for the PF f. Appropriate methods of imputation are used for missing PF data	**High bias**: the measurement of the PF is very likely to be different for different levels of the outcome of interest **Moderate**: the measurement of the PF may be different for different levels of the outcome of interest **Low bias**: the measurement of the PF is unlikely to be different for different levels of the outcome of interest
4. Outcome measurement	a. A clear definition of the outcome is provided b. Method of outcome measurement used is adequately valid and reliable c. The method and setting of outcome measurement is the same for all study participants	**High bias**: the measurement of the outcome is very likely to be different related to the baseline level of the PF **Moderate**: the measurement of the outcome may be different related to the baseline level of the PF **Low bias**: the measurement of the outcome is unlikely to be different related to the baseline level of the PF

(Continued)

Table 9.3 Continued

Domains	Signalling items	Ratings
5. Adjustment for other factors	a. All other important PFs are measured b. Clear definitions of the important PFs measured are provided c. Measurement of all important PFs is adequately valid and reliable d. The method and setting of PF measurement are the same for all study participants e. Appropriate methods are used to deal with missing values of PFs, such as multiple imputation f. Important PFs are accounted for in the study design g. Important PFs are accounted for in the analysis	**High bias:** the observed effect of the PF on the outcome is very likely to be distorted by another factor related to PF and outcome **Moderate:** the observed effect of the PF on outcome may be distorted by another factor related to PF and outcome **Low bias:** the observed effect of the PF on the outcome is unlikely to be distorted by another factor related to PF and outcome
6. Statistical analysis and reporting	a. Sufficient presentation of data to assess the adequacy of the analytic strategy b. Strategy for model building is appropriate and is based on a conceptual framework or model c. The selected statistical model is adequate for the design of the study d. There is no selective reporting of results	**High bias**: the reported results are very likely to be spurious or biased related to analysis or reporting **Moderate**: the reported results may be spurious or biased related to analysis or reporting **Low bias**: the reported results are unlikely to be spurious or biased related to analysis or reporting

Source: data from Hayden, JA., et al. Assessing bias in studies of prognostic factors. Annals of Internal Medicine. 158(4), 280-6. Copyright © 2013 American College of Physicians.

As well as covering applicability, PROBAST provides a checklist for examining risk of bias in studies that either develop, validate, or update a prognostic model (44). This includes four domains: participants, predictors, outcome, and analysis (Table 9.4), which contain signalling questions to help reviewers decide on a low, high or unclear risk of bias. In this context, *risk of bias* refers to the likelihood that a prognostic model study leads to a distorted estimate of predictive performance (e.g. in terms of calibration and discrimination) for its intended use in the targeted individuals. For example, a study is at high risk of bias when it reports a model developed using approaches that lead to overfitting and optimism in performance (such as automated variable selection procedures, few events per candidate predictors, etc.), without optimism adjustment

Table 9.4 Domains and signalling questions within the PROBAST tool (Prediction model study Risk Of Bias ASsessment Tool) (44)

Domain 1: participants		Dev	Val
1.1	Were appropriate data sources used, e.g. cohort, RCT, or nested case-control study data?		
1.2	Were all inclusions and exclusions of participants appropriate?		
Domain 2: predictors			
2.1	Were predictors defined and assessed in a similar way for all participants?		
2.2	Were predictor assessments made without knowledge of outcome data?		
2.3	Are all predictors available at the time the model is intended to be used?		
Domain 3: outcome			
3.1	Was the outcome determined appropriately?		
3.2	Was a pre-specified or standard outcome definition used?		
3.3	Were predictors excluded from the outcome definition?		
3.4	Was the outcome defined and determined in a similar way for all participants?		
3.5	Was the outcome determined without knowledge of predictor information?		
3.6	Was the time interval between predictor assessment and outcome determination appropriate?		
Domain 4: analysis			
4.1	Were there a reasonable number of participants with the outcome?		
4.2	Were continuous and categorical predictors handled appropriately?		
4.3	Were all enrolled participants included in the analysis?		
4.4	Were participants with missing data handled appropriately?		
4.5	Was selection of predictors based on univariable analysis avoided?		
4.6	Were complexities in the data (e.g. censoring, competing risks, sampling of controls) accounted for appropriately?		
4.7	Were relevant model performance measures evaluated appropriately (e.g. calibration, discrimination and classification)?		
4.8	Was model overfitting and optimism in model performance accounted for?		
4.9	Do predictors and their assigned weights in the final model correspond to the results from multivariable analysis?		

'Dev' = model development study; 'Val' = external validation study; Shaded boxes indicate that the signalling question does not apply

Source: data from Moons, KGM., et al. PROBAST: a tool to assess risk of bias and applicability concerns of prediction model studies - explanation and elaboration. In publication.

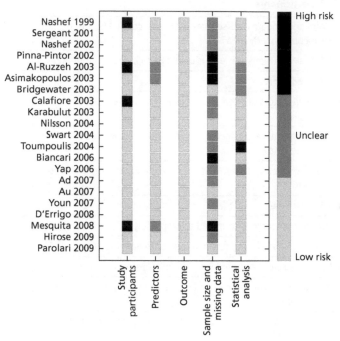

NB There are two validations within the Nashef 2002 study

Figure 9.1 Summary of the quality appraisal of validation studies of the EuroSCORE, based on a preliminary version of the PROBAST tool.

Source: reproduced with permission from Debray, TAP., et al. A guide to systematic review and meta-analysis of prediction model performance. BMJ. 356, e6460. Copyright © 2017 BMJ Publishing Group Ltd.

or external validation (see Chapter 7). All signalling questions in PROBAST are phrased so that 'yes' indicates absence of bias (Table 9.4). Debray et al. applied a preliminary version of PROBAST to their systematic review of the EuroSCORE model, including twenty-two validations of its predictive performance across twenty-one studies (17). Fourteen of the studies were classed at low or unclear risk of bias (Figure 9.1). A common concern was that only a complete-case analysis was performed (rather than multiple imputation; see Chapter 4) or the methods for handling missing data were not reported.

For reviews of type IV prognosis questions, included studies will generally be randomized trials, and therefore the Cochrane risk of bias tool will be relevant (1, 54). However, as the focus will be on predictors of treatment effect, additional criteria should be considered, such as whether the analysis was pre-planned or part of secondary data exploration; whether continuous predictors were kept as continuous or dichotomized; and whether estimated differences in treatment effects (treatment-covariate interactions) were provided (i.e. not just results for each subgroup separately) and whether estimates were adjusted for confounders (55). Sun et al. (56) and Pincus et al. (57) provide guidelines for examining the reliability of evidence for subgroup effects and interactions, which may be useful for risk of bias classifications for type IV studies.

Each primary study should ideally be assessed on its risk of bias and applicability by two people, independently, with any discrepancies resolved upon consensus by a third person.

9.2.5 **Meta-analysis**

Meta-analysis is an option when the identified studies are considered sufficiently robust and comparable, such that meta-analysis results are interpretable (and thus have potential impact) for healthcare. Sometimes, meta-analysis is restricted to those studies at low risk of bias. It requires there to be at least two estimates of the same statistic across studies. Here we focus on obtaining such estimates from study publications or study authors. An alternative, and potentially more successful, approach is a meta-analysis of individual participant data, where the raw data are obtained and synthesized. Availability of the original data allows the meta-analysts to standardize statistical methods across studies and obtain information that was otherwise unavailable (58); however, it is time-consuming and may not necessarily resolve all the issues. This topic is considered further in Chapter 13.

For meta-analyses based on extracted estimates (aggregate data) there are many potential barriers, and sometimes it may be that (a quantitative) meta-analysis should not be performed. Aside from missing estimates of prognostic effects or performance (which was discussed earlier), the most common issues facing meta-analysis of prognosis studies are: (1) different types of estimates (e.g. odds ratios or hazard ratios from prognostic factor studies; R^2, C, or D statistics for prognostic model validation studies); (2) estimates without standard errors, a problem as standard meta-analysis methods weight each study by (a function) of their standard error; (3) estimates relating to different time-points; (4) different methods of measurement, for example for a particular factor or outcome of interest; (5) a mixture of unadjusted and adjusted prognostic factor effect estimates; (6) different sets of adjustment factors; and (7) different handling of continuous factors. Many of these issues lead to substantial heterogeneity in the estimate, such that summary meta-analysis results then have no direct interpretation. Take, for example, the issue of different methods for handling a continuous prognostic factor. Some studies may consider non-linear trends, others just a linear trend, and some a trend across chosen categories of the factor. But the majority of studies will use a cut point to dichotomize the factor into two groups, even though this is not recommended (see Chapter 4), and the choice of cut point will vary across studies. In this situation, a meta-analysis is still possible, comparing 'positive' and 'negative' prognostic factor values, but how do we then interpret the summary meta-analysis result? Patients with the same values would be 'positive' in some studies and 'negative' in others. Furthermore, some studies will use a cut point that minimises the p-value associated with the prognostic effect of interest, which will lead to meta-analysis results biased toward larger prognostic effects. Even if all studies analyse a continuous factor assuming a prognostic effect, the measurement of the factor may differ across studies, such that a one-unit increase in the factor has a different interpretation across studies. In this situation, transforming the prognostic effect estimates to all corresponding to a one standard deviation increase in the factor may be helpful.

If meta-analysis is performed, a random effects approach is essential to allow for unexplained heterogeneity across studies, for all four PROGRESS types. The overall prognosis of the outcome is expected to vary across settings, due to different standards of care and administered treatment strategies, and different startpoints (e.g. earlier diagnosis of disease in some populations due to a screening programme) (4). Prognostic factor studies are heterogeneous in many aspects, causing the true prognostic effect of a factor to vary from study to study. Similarly, the performance of a prognostic model will vary across settings. A major reason is different case-mix variation, which refers to the distribution of predictor values, other relevant participant or setting characteristics (such as treatment received), and the outcome incidence (overall prognosis). Case-mix variation leads to genuine differences in the performance of a prediction model, even when the true (underlying) effects of prognostic factors in the model are consistent (59). It is, for instance, well known that the performance of models developed in secondary care is usually different when they are applied in a primary care setting, as the outcome incidence or distribution of predictor values will be very different (6, 17, 42, 60). The magnitude of prognostic factor effects may also change according to the case mix and, as mentioned, study differences in methods, again leading to heterogeneity.

A standard random effects meta-analysis combines the study estimates of the statistic of interest (e.g. the prognostic effect estimate, or estimate of predictive performance) in order to estimate the average value (denoted by μ) and the standard deviation of the parameter values (denoted by τ) across studies. If Y_i and $var(Y_i)$ denote the estimate and its variance in study i, then a general random effects meta-analysis model can be specified as:

$$Y_i \sim N(\mu, var(Y_i) + \tau^2) \text{ (model 1)}$$

Most researchers use either restricted maximum likelihood or the approach of DerSimonian and Laird to estimate this model (61), but other options are available including a Bayesian approach (62). Of key interest is the summary (average) estimate, $\hat{\mu}$. Confidence intervals for μ should ideally account for uncertainty in estimated variances (in particular τ) (63), and we have found the approach of Hartung-Knapp to be generally robust for this purpose given heterogeneity (63–65). When τ is zero, there is no between-study heterogeneity in the statistic of interest, and the random effects model then reduces to a fixed (common) effect model, which denotes that the true value of the statistic is the same (fixed) in all studies.

Table 9.2 summarizes the best scale to use for meta-analysis of statistics commonly pooled from prognosis review questions. For example, a meta-analysis of C statistics is best done on the logit scale (i.e. $\ln(C/(1-C))$ (66), so that the random effects model can be written as:

$$\mathrm{logit}(C_i) \sim N(\mu, \mathrm{var}(\mathrm{logit}(C_i)) + \tau^2),$$

where $\mathrm{logit}(C_i)$ is the logit of the C statistic in the ith study, and $\mathrm{var}(\mathrm{logit}(C_i))$ is its variance, which is assumed to be known. The estimate, $\hat{\mu}$, then provides the summary (average) logit C statistic, which can then be back-transformed to the C statistic scale. Similarly, confidence intervals are derived for μ, and then back-transformed to the C scale.

When the raw numbers of events and patients (or person years) are available, a meta-analysis with more exact within-study distributional assumptions (e.g. binomial or Poisson) may be possible (67, 68), for example for the overall incidence rate, or the E/O statistic (69). This may be preferable when the outcome proportion (or rate) is low and/or studies are small, to avoid assuming normality and known variances of estimates from each study. Advanced multivariate meta-analysis methods have been proposed for synthesis of prognosis studies, in order to handle multiple cut-points (70), multiple methods of measurement (70), or different adjustment factors in prognostic factor studies (71), or to combine discrimination and calibration jointly in prognostic model studies (72). However, heterogeneity is likely to persist even in such approaches.

For meta-analyses examining predictors of treatment effect, it is inappropriate to perform separate meta-analyses for each subgroup defined by predictor categories, and then indirectly compare their summary results. This approach breaks the randomization within each trial, and can introduce between-study confounding. Rather a predictor's effect should be summarized by a meta-analysis of the interaction estimates (difference in treatment effect for a one-unit change in the predictor) from each study. This issue is illustrated in a case study in Figure 9.2.

9.2.6 **Quantifying heterogeneity**

Although the summary result ($\hat{\mu}$) is usually the main focus of a meta-analysis, this reflects an average across studies and it may be hard to translate to clinical practice, when there is large between-study heterogeneity. Indeed, in such situations the major finding is the amount of heterogeneity, and the need for further research to identify the causes. A case study is given in Figure 9.3, where a review identifies substantial heterogeneity in the incidence of fatigue after a stroke, motivating the need to identify prognostic factors for this outcome.

In situations of large heterogeneity, it may be better to refrain from meta-analysis entirely, and to display the variability in estimates on a forest plot

Webber et al.[71] systematically review the evidence for microsatellite instability status (MSI) as a predictor of differential response to treatment with 5FU-based chemotherapy in colorectal cancer patients. In particular, they considered whether the treatment effect on survival was better for patients with MSI-H status (instability in two or more markers) than for those considered microsatellite stable (MSS). Fourteen relevant studies were identified, and most included both rectal and colon cancer patients.

Six studies gave disease-free (DFS) results for both marker status groups. A random effects meta-analysis of just the MSS group gives a summary hazard ratio (HR) of 0.62 (95% CI: 0.54 to 0.71), indicating strong evidence that *patients who received 5FU treatment had longer DFS than patients who did not*. In a random effects meta-analysis of just the MSI-H group, the summary hazard ratio was 0.84 and the confidence interval was wide (95% CI: 0.53 to 1.32). Hence, the MSS group had a statistically significant summary treatment effect, but the MSI-H group did not.

However, this analysis does not necessarily imply that MSI is a predictor of differential treatment response. To examine this question directly, the within-study differences in treatment effect between MSI groups should be synthesised. In other words, the difference in log HR between MSI-H and MSS groups should be estimated in each trial (i.e. the interaction estimate calculated), and these values synthesised in a random effects meta-analysis. The results are shown in the forest plot below, converted back to the ratio of HRs scale, such that values above 1 indicate that the treatment is less effective in the MSI-H group than the MSS group. The results provide no conclusive evidence of a difference in treatment effect between groups (for either DFS or overall survival, OS), with confidence intervals containing a HR ratio of 1.

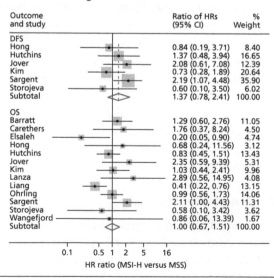

Figure 9.2 Case study illustrating the importance of a meta-analysis of interaction estimates, rather than separate meta-analyses of each subgroup, when examining predictors of treatment response.

Source: reproduced courtesy of Richard D. Riley, using data from Webber, EM., et al. Systematic review of the predictive effect of MSI status in colorectal cancer patients undergoing 5FU-based chemotherapy. BMC Cancer.2015(15), 156.

Cumming et al.[72] perform a systematic review and meta-analysis to examine the incidence of fatigue after stroke. They define fatigue as "a subjective lack of physical or mental energy (or both) that is perceived by the individual to interfere with usual or desired activities." A literature search yielded 921 studies, and following exclusion of duplicates and ineligible studies, 49 studies (containing 7475 patients) remained. Many different fatigue scales were used, with the Fatigue Severity Scale (FSS) the most common (24 studies). Results from a critical appraisal showed that 20 of these 24 studies satisfied at least three of four quality criteria; the most commonly failed criterion was consecutive recruitment (10 studies), which raises a concern of selection bias.

Twenty-two of the 24 studies reported (or provided after being contacted) fatigue incidence numbers based on a cut-off of either ≥ 4 or >4 to define fatigue. These cut-offs were deemed similar enough to be pooled together, and so a meta-analysis of these 22 studies (containing 3491 patients) was conducted. The summary estimate of fatigue incidence was 50% (95% CI 44% to 57%), and was relatively stable across time points after stroke: within one month of stroke (n = 3 studies, 55% fatigued), one month to six months (n = 7 studies, 46% fatigued), and beyond six months (n = 12 studies, 53% fatigued).

Cumming et al. note that the summary incidence estimate "should be treated with caution" due to large between-study heterogeneity (I^2 = 94%)". To help express this more clearly, we re-performed their random effects meta-analysis and subsequently derived an approximate 95% prediction interval, to give a 95% predicted range for the true incidence in a new population. This interval was remarkably wide (22% to 78%), and motivates further research to explain the heterogeneity, in order "to identify the factors contributing to it and to develop effective intervention strategies to prevent the occurrence of fatigueness that can be applied in stroke care settings."

Study	No. patients	Time	Country	Prevalence % (95% CI)	% Weight
Badaru (2013)	65	0 to >4 y	Nigeria	46.2 (34.1, 58.3)	4.39
Chestnut (2010)	13	Mean 8 d	UK	84.6 (65.0, 100.0)	3.62
Choi-Kwon (2005)	220	Mean 15 m (range 3–27)	S Korea	57.0 (50.5, 63.5)	4.84
Crosby (2012)	64	Mean 4.9 m	UK	48.0 (35.8, 60.2)	4.38
Ghotbi (2013)	83	Mean 30.9 m	Iran	45.8 (35.1, 56.5)	4.52
Harbison (2009)	69	1 to 6 m	Ireland	51.0 (39.2, 62.8)	4.42
Hoang (2012)	32	Mean 40 m	France	65.6 (49.1, 82.1)	3.95
Lerdal (2011)	115	Mean 4.6 d	Norway	57.4 (48.4, 66.4)	4.66
Michael (2007)	79	Mean 10 m (range 6–120)	USA	42.0 (31.1, 52.9)	4.51
Miller (2013)	77	>6 m	USA	66.0 (55.4, 76.6)	4.53
Mills (2012)	282	Mean 17.2 m	UK	62.4 (56.7, 68.1)	4.89
Naess (2005)	192	Mean 6.0 y (range 1.4–12.3)	Norway	51.3 (44.2, 58.4)	4.81
Naess (2012)	333	Mean 382 d (range 185–756)	Norway	60.1 (54.8, 65.4)	4.92
Park (2009)	40	Mean 32.7 m	S Korea	30.0 (15.8, 44.2)	4.19
Radman (2012)	109	6 m	Switzerland	30.3 (21.7, 38.9)	4.70
Robinson (2011)	50	Mean 85.0 m	USA	48.0 (34.2, 61.8)	4.22
Suh (2014)	282	Mean 6.7 d	S Korea	26.3 (21.2, 31.4)	4.92
Tang (2013)	500	3 m	Hong Kong	25.0 (21.2, 28.8)	4.98
Valko (2008)	235	Mean 1.2 y	Switzerland	49.0 (42.6, 55.4)	4.85
Vuletic (2011)	35	3 m	Croatia	45.0 (28.5, 61.5)	3.95
Van de Port (2012)	250	3 m	Netherlands	57.2 (51.1, 63.3)	4.87
Van de Port et al. (2007)	223	6 m	Netherlands	68.0 (61.9, 74.1)	4.87
Summary meta-analysis result (I-squared = 94%)				50.3 (43.9, 56.7)	100.00
95% prediction interval				21.8 to 77.8	

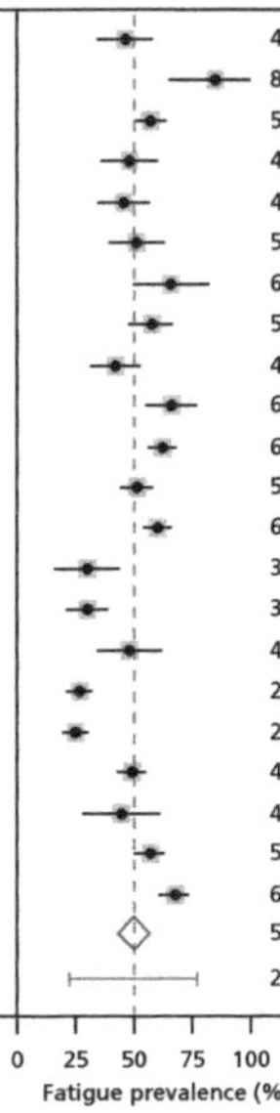

0   25   50   75   100
Fatigue prevalence (%)

Figure 9.3 Case study of heterogeneity in a meta-analysis of overall prognosis studies.
Source: data from Cumming TB, Packer M, Kramer SF, et al. The prevalence of fatigue after stroke: A systematic review and meta-analysis. International Journal of Stroke. 11(9):968-77. Copyright 2016 © SAGE.

(without showing a pooled result). When meta-analysis is performed in the face of heterogeneity, it is important to quantify and disseminate the magnitude of heterogeneity itself, for example via the estimate of τ^2 (the between-study variance) (75), or a $100(1-\alpha)\%$ prediction interval. The latter gives the potential true value (e.g. true prognostic effect, or true prognostic model performance) in a new population conditional on the meta-analysis results (76, 77). An approximate prediction interval is calculated using:

$$\hat{\mu} \pm t_{\alpha,N-2}\sqrt{\hat{\tau}^2 + \hat{\sigma}^2_\mu},$$

where $t_{\alpha,N-2}$ is the $100(1-\alpha/2)\%$ percentile of the t-distribution for N-2 degrees of freedom, N is the number of studies, $\hat{\sigma}_\mu$ is the standard error of $\hat{\mu}$, and τ is the between-study standard deviation (76). This analysis should again be undertaken on the correct scale for meta-analysis (Table 9.2), with back-transformation then used if necessary. Unfortunately, this prediction interval equation has poor coverage in situations where the percentage of the total variability due to between-study differences (I^2) is small and studies have very different sizes (65). A Bayesian approach is more natural for deriving predictive inferences, and provides the probability that the statistic of interest will be above a useful value (17, 70, 72, 76). For example, after a meta-analysis of prognostic factor studies, one may derive the probability that a factor's prognostic effect will be above some useful value (e.g. a HR > 1.5 for a binary factor, which indicates risk is increased by at least 50%), or that it improves discrimination of a model by a particular amount (e.g. increases the C statistic by 0.05 or more). Similarly, after a meta-analysis of prognostic model performance, one may calculate the probability that the C statistic for the model will be above a particular value (e.g. 0.7), or that the (mis)calibration will be acceptable, despite the presence of heterogeneity (e.g. $0.8 \leq O/E \leq 1.2$).

In the Debray et al. review of the EuroSCORE (17), a random effects meta-analysis gave a summary C statistic of 0.79 (95% CI: 0.77–0.81). However, there was considerable heterogeneity, and the approximate 95% prediction interval was 0.72–0.84. Heterogeneity was even more severe for calibration performance. The summary O/E (mean Observed risk / mean Expected risk) was 0.53, indicating that the model generally over-predicts outcome risk. Heterogeneity in calibration was severe, with an approximate 95% prediction interval of 0.19–1.46, suggesting that in some settings the score may vastly over-predict risk, but in others it may under-predict risk. Based on the meta-analysis, the probability of 'good' performance in a new setting (defined by a C statistic above 0.75 and $0.8 \leq O/E \leq 1.2$) was just 0.13, mainly due to the potentially poor and heterogeneous calibration.

9.2.7 **Examining heterogeneity**

Subgroup analyses and meta-regression can be used to examine or explore the causes of heterogeneity. A subgroup analysis performs a separate meta-analysis for categories defined by a particular characteristic, such as those with a follow-up < 1 year or ≥ 1 year, or those set in countries within Europe, the US, or elsewhere. Subgroups should be formally compared, by an estimate of their difference (with confidence interval). This is achieved using a meta-regression, which extends a standard random effects meta-analysis model by including study-level covariates (78). In addition to follow-up length and country, covariates may represent the case-mix variation (such as the standard deviation of the prognostic model's linear predictor values), the method of measurement, the cut point, the treatment, risk of bias, and other aspects that vary across studies (79, 80). For example, a meta-regression suggests that the aforementioned over-estimate of the EuroSCORE predictions tends to be largest in populations with a lower mean EuroSCORE value (low-risk populations), although the magnitude of association is rather weak (Figure 9.4).

Unfortunately, subgroup analyses and meta-regression are often problematic. There will typically be few studies per subgroup and low power to detect

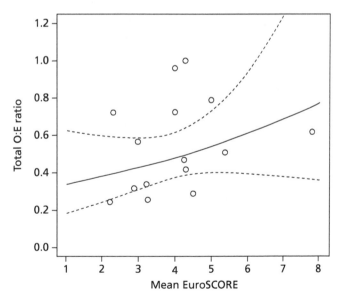

Figure 9.4 Meta-regression of the total O:E ratio (O/E) against the mean EuroSCORE value in each study.
Source: reproduced with permission from Debray, T.P., et al. A guide to systematic review and meta-analysis of prediction model performance. BMJ. 2017(356), e6460. Copyright © 2017 BMJ

genuine causes of heterogeneity. Furthermore, study-level confounding is likely, such that it is difficult to disentangle the associations for one covariate from another. For example, studies with a particular treatment may also be more likely to use a particular cut point or method of measurement, or have a particular risk of bias. Furthermore, meta-regression of study-level summaries should not be used to investigate individual-level relationships. In particular, when using multiple studies to examine predictors of treatment effect, it is tempting to perform a meta-regression of the overall treatment effect versus aggregated patient-level characteristics (e.g. mean age, proportion male). However, study-level confounding and ecological bias often make this across-study relationship very different to the true individual-level relationship of interest, which is that between the actual individual covariate value and treatment response (81). This concept is illustrated in Chapter 13.

Sensitivity analyses are important, to examine if and how conclusions change according to subjective decisions made by the systematic review team themselves, for example in regard to inclusion criteria, handling of missing data, and statistical method of model estimation. Consider again Yousef et al., who review the overall prognosis in patients with Barrett's oesophagus (8), and perform a meta-analysis of forty-seven studies and obtain a summary estimate of cancer incidence of 6.1 cases per 1000 person years. However, when restricting meta-analysis to just those eight studies considered at highest quality (defined by three criteria: study size greater than 500 person years, low likelihood of selection bias, and a robust definition of Barrett's oesophagus), the summary estimate was much lower (3.9 cases per 1000 person years), indicating that the conclusions are sensitive to the quality of included studies.

9.2.8 Small-study effects and publication bias

The term 'small-study effects' refers to a systematic difference in the results for small studies and large studies (82). Of particular concern is when small prognosis studies show larger effects (or more promising results) than larger studies. This may be a consequence of publication bias (selective publication of whole studies) or selective reporting within published articles, such that smaller studies with significant results are more likely to be published or reported in more sufficient detail, and thus included in meta-analysis, than smaller studies with non-significant results. A related concern is that smaller studies are generally at higher risk of bias than larger studies. The evidence for small-study effects is usually considered on a funnel plot, which shows the study estimates against an estimate of their precision. Its use is usually recommended only if there are ten or more studies (82). The plot should ideally show a symmetric, funnel-like shape, with results from larger studies at the centre of the funnel, with smaller studies spanning out in both directions equally. Asymmetry will arise if there are small study effects, such that the smaller studies are skewed in one particular direction (no longer symmetric around the larger studies), and this provides an indicator of potential publication bias. Statistical tests for asymmetry can be used (82), including one by Debray et al. for hazard ratios from prognostic factor studies (83).

Empirical evidence suggests that publication bias is endemic in prognosis research. For example, Kyzas et al. (45) evaluated 1575 articles on different prognostic factors for cancer, and staggeringly found that nearly all suggest significant findings, with 98.5% reporting statistically significant results or elaborating on non-significant trends. Simon concludes that: 'The literature is probably cluttered with false-positive studies that would not have been submitted or published if the results had come out differently' (84). However, small study effects may also arise due to heterogeneity, making it difficult to disentangle publication bias from the causes of heterogeneity in a single review. For example, if the smaller prognosis studies were done in populations with a wider case mix or used an analysis with fewer adjustment factors, then this may genuinely cause larger effects in such studies, rather than publication bias. Contour-enhanced funnel plots additionally show the statistical significance of individual studies. If the asymmetry suggests 'missing' studies are more likely to fall within regions of non-significance, this gives more credence to publication bias being the cause of small-study effects. A dramatic example of funnel plot asymmetry is given in Figure 9.5.

9.2.9 Reporting

As with all research studies, clear and complete reporting of prognosis reviews is essential. Most of the reporting guidelines of PRISMA and MOOSE are relevant (86, 87), and complement those for primary prognosis studies, such as REMARK and TRIPOD (88, 89).

9.3 Certainty of summarized evidence

For any meta-analysis, the interpretation of estimated summary effects should take the quality of the included studies carefully into account. In particular, researchers may choose to grade down the assurance in the summary meta-analysis results when there are concerns about bias, imprecision, between-study heterogeneity, or applicability. This process might be achieved using the Grades of Recommendation, Assessment, Development, and Evaluation (GRADE) framework, which scores the quality of evidence for obtained summary results. This was originally initiated for use in a meta-analysis of intervention studies, but has since been adopted for grading the quality of evidence of summary estimates of overall prognosis (90), addressing the same five domains: risk of

Hemingway et al. performed a systematic review to evaluate whether C-reactive protein (CRP) is a prognostic factor for fatal and nonfatal events among patients with stable coronary disease.[10] A literature search identified 1,566 articles of which 83 studies fulfilled the inclusion criteria containing a total of 61,684 patients and 6,485 outcome events. After summarising the evidence, the authors conclude that there is great concern about the quality and reliability of existing studies evaluating CRP due to an absence of pre-specified protocols, inconsistent adjustment for existing factors, poor and potentially biased reporting, and strong potential for publication bias. The latter is exemplified by a dramatically asymmetric funnel plot (below). The smaller studies (those with higher standard errors) fall mainly in the bottom right of the plot, and give substantially higher prognostic effect estimates than larger studies, and a suspiciously large proportion of the available studies gave estimates corresponding to a p-value < 0.05. Hemingway et al. conclude that their findings "explicitly challenge the statement for healthcare professionals made by the Centers for Disease Control that measuring CRP is both 'useful' and 'independent' as a marker of prognosis."[83]

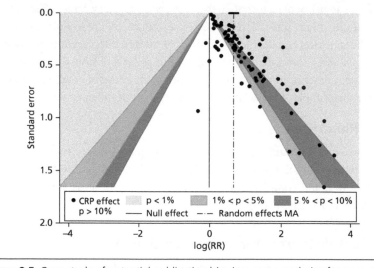

Figure 9.5 Case study of potential publication bias in a meta-analysis of prognostic factor studies, based on Hemingway et al.

Source: reproduced from Hemingway, H., et al. Evaluating the quality of research into a single prognostic biomarker: a systematic review and meta-analysis of 83 studies of C-Reactive protein in stable coronary artery disease. PLoS Medicine. 7(6), e1000286. Copyright © 2017 PLoS. Open Access.

bias (across the included studies), inconsistency, imprecision, indirectness, and publication bias. There is yet limited empirical evidence for the use of the existing domains for grading the certainty of summary estimates of prognostic factor studies, although a first attempt has been made (91), and extension to other prognosis research types is anticipated.

9.4 **Prognosis systematic reviews within Cochrane**

Systematic reviews of prognosis studies have now become a formal review type within Cochrane, alongside reviews of interventions and diagnostic tests. The Cochrane Prognosis Methods Group was formed to meet this objective. Exploratory meetings held at the Ottawa (2004), Melbourne (2005), and Dublin (2006) Cochrane Colloquia identified members interested in prognosis reviews and establishing methodology standards. At the Dublin Cochrane Colloquium (2006), participants attending an open meeting agreed unanimously to work toward the establishment of a prognosis methods group. Six convenors were identified to move this application forward and the group was formally established and registered with Cochrane in 2008, signalled by correspondence in the *Journal of Clinical Epidemiology* (2). The Cochrane prognosis methods group is inclusive and continually expanding its membership, with resources and training details available at http://methods.cochrane.org/prognosis/. Much of the guidance provided in this chapter stems from work published by the convenors and members of this group.

Due to the growing methods and demand for reviews of prognosis studies, various exemplar reviews have now been approved by Cochrane and will soon be published in the Cochrane Library. These address prognosis research types I–III. As mentioned earlier, reviews to examine subgroups or predictors of intervention effects (type IV prognosis research) can be embedded within standard reviews of interventions, for which much guidance already exists (1).

9.5 **Summary**

This chapter has highlighted the process, methodology, and guidelines for a systematic review and meta-analysis of prognosis studies, for each of the four types of prognosis research question. Our case studies illustrate how such reviews can lead to important clinical and methodological findings. We expect the number of reviews of prognosis studies to increase steadily in the coming years. In particular, given the growing demand for prognostic factors or (bio) markers, prognostic models, and predictors of treatment effect, there will be an increasing need to identify reliable and replicable (validated) prognosis findings, for which reviews and meta-analysis will be paramount. Obtaining individual participant data from a subset of higher-quality prognosis studies could enhance evidence synthesis further (Chapter 13), as could health economic modelling, to summarize the cost benefit of using prognostic information to inform healthcare decisions. A summary of the key messages of this chapter is now provided.

9.5.1 **Summary points**

- Systematic reviews and meta-analyses are needed to identify, evaluate, and summarize prognosis studies and their findings.

- They should form the cornerstone of evidence-based prognosis in healthcare and decision making, providing guidance about overall prognosis, prognostic factors, prognostic models, and predictors of treatment effect.

- Methods and guidelines are available for conducting reviews of prognosis studies and subsequent meta-analysis, for each of the four types of prognosis research question.

- A clear review objective, including the targeted population, prognostic models or factors, and outcomes of interest (including time points) need to be defined; the CHARMS and CHARMS-PF tools provide a checklist to guide this process.

- A carefully constructed search strategy is needed to identify existing prognosis research studies, and engagement with research groups may help to uncover unpublished evidence.

- A data extraction phase is needed to obtain the relevant information from each study, and the CHARMS and CHARMS-PF tools provide a checklist of items to extract. This may require contact with original study authors, as even basic information (such as numbers of events, hazard ratios, and confidence intervals) is often missing.

- The quality of identified studies should be examined using risk of bias tools, such as QUIPS (for prognostic factor research) and PROBAST (for prognostic model research). Many existing prognosis studies are at high risk of bias, for example due to selective recruitment of individuals, inappropriate statistical methods, and selective reporting.

- Meta-analysis can be used to combine key measures of interest across studies to produce an overall summary estimate (e.g. of prognostic effect of a particular factor, or predictive performance of a prognostic model). Between-study heterogeneity should always be expected, acknowledged (e.g. using random effects models), quantified (e.g. using prediction intervals), and if possible explained (e.g. using meta-regression).

- Reviews of prognostic factors are often problematic, as publication bias and selective reporting within primary studies are endemic, and heterogeneity is often large, especially in regard to the choice of cut points of the prognostic factor (and outcome), adjustment for other prognostic factors, and methods of measurement of the prognostic factor (and outcome). Availability of individual participant data may reduce these problems.

♦ Despite their potential difficulties, case studies show that prognosis reviews can inform evidence-based clinical guidelines and healthcare, including for personalized medicine, and various exemplar Cochrane reviews of prognosis studies are underway

References

1. **Higgins JPT** and **Green SB** (2011) Cochrane Handbook for Systematic Reviews of Interventions Version 5.1.0 (updated March 2011): The Cochrane Collaboration (Available from www.handbook.cochrane.org).

2. **Riley RD, Ridley G, Williams K**, et al. (2007) Prognosis research: toward evidence-based results and a Cochrane methods group. *J Clin Epidemiol* **60**(8), 863–5.

3. **Peat G, Riley RD, Croft P**, et al. (2014) Improving the transparency of prognosis research: the role of reporting, data sharing, registration, and protocols. *PLoS Med* **11**(7), e1001671.

4. **Hemingway H, Croft P, Perel P**, et al. (2013) Prognosis research strategy (PROGRESS) 1: a framework for researching clinical outcomes. *BMJ* **346**, e5595.

5. **Riley RD, Hayden JA, Steyerberg EW**, et al. (2013) Prognosis Research Strategy (PROGRESS) 2: prognostic factor research. *PLoS Med* **10**(2), e1001380.

6. **Steyerberg EW, Moons KG, van der Windt DA**, et al. (2013) Prognosis Research Strategy (PROGRESS) 3: prognostic model rescarch. *PLoS Med* **10**(2), e1001381.

7. **Hingorani AD, Windt DA, Riley RD**, et al. (2013) Prognosis research strategy (PROGRESS) 4: stratified medicine research. *BMJ* **346**, e5793.

8. **Yousef F, Cardwell C, Cantwell MM**, et al. (2008) The incidence of esophageal cancer and high-grade dysplasia in Barrett's esophagus: a systematic review and meta-analysis. *Am J Epidemiol* **168**(3), 237–49.

9. **Foroutan F, Guyatt GH, O'Brien K**, et al. (2016) Prognosis after surgical replacement with a bioprosthetic aortic valve in patients with severe symptomatic aortic stenosis: systematic review of observational studies. *BMJ* **354**, i5065.

10. **Hemingway H, Philipson P, Chen R**, et al. (2010) Evaluating the quality of research into a single prognostic biomarker: a systematic review and meta-analysis of 83 studies of C-Reactive protein in stable coronary artery disease. *PLoS Med* **7**(6), e1000286.

11. **Riley RD, Burchill SA, Abrams KR**, et al. (2003) A systematic review and evaluation of the use of tumour markers in paediatric oncology: Ewing's sarcoma and neuroblastoma. *Health Technol Assess* **7**(5), 1–162.

12. **Riley RD, Moons KGM, Snell KIE**, et al. (2018) A guide to systematic review and meta-analysis of prognostic factor studies. *BMJ* **364**:k4597.

13. **Moons KG, de Groot JA, Bouwmeester W**, et al. (2014) Critical appraisal and data extraction for systematic reviews of prediction modelling studies: the CHARMS checklist. *PLoS Med* **11**(10), e1001744.

14. **Perel P, Edwards P, Wentz R**, et al. (2006) Systematic review of prognostic models in traumatic brain injury. *BMC Med Inform Decis Mak* **6**, 38.

15. **Siregar S, Groenwold RH, de Heer F**, et al. (2012) Performance of the original EuroSCORE. *Eur J Cardiothorac Surg* **41**(4), 746–54.

16. **Warnell I, Chincholkar M, and Eccles M** (2015) Predicting perioperative mortality after oesophagectomy: a systematic review of performance and methods of multivariate models. *Br J Anaesth* **114**(1), 32–43.

17. **Debray TP, Damen JA, Snell KI,** et al. (2017) A guide to systematic review and meta-analysis of prediction model performance. *BMJ* **356**, i6460.

18. **Donegan S, Williams L, Dias S,** et al. (2015) Exploring treatment by covariate interactions using subgroup analysis and meta-regression in cochrane reviews: a review of recent practice. *PLoS One* **10**(6), e0128804.

19. **Skoetz N, Trivella M, Kreuzer KA,** et al. (2016) Prognostic models for chronic lymphocytic leukaemia: an exemplar systematic review and meta-analysis. *Cochrane Database of Systematic Reviews* (1), CD012022.

20. **Rehn M, Perel P, Blackhall K,** et al. (2011) Prognostic models for the early care of trauma patients: a systematic review. *Scand J Trauma Resusc Emerg Med* **19**, 17.

21. **Patel S, Friede T, Froud R,** et al. (2013) Systematic review of randomized controlled trials of clinical prediction rules for physical therapy in low back pain. *Spine* **38**(9), 762–69.

22. **Geersing GJ, Bouwmeester W, Zuithoff P,** et al. (2012) Search filters for finding prognostic and diagnostic prediction studies in Medline to enhance systematic reviews. *PLoS One* **7**(2), e32844.

23. **Ingui BJ and Rogers MA** (2001) Searching for clinical prediction rules in MEDLINE. *J Am Med Inform Assoc* **8**(4), 391–7.

24. **Haynes RB, McKibbon KA, Wilczynski NL,** et al. (2005) Optimal search strategies for retrieving scientifically strong studies of treatment from Medline: analytical survey. *BMJ* **330**(7501), 1179.

25. **Wong SS, Wilczynski NL, Haynes RB,** et al. (2003) Developing optimal search strategies for detecting sound clinical prediction studies in MEDLINE. *AMIA Annu Symp Proc* 728–32.

26. **Altman DG, De Stavola BL, Love SB,** et al. (1995) Review of survival analyses published in cancer journals. *Br J Cancer* **72**(2), 511–8.

27. **Riley RD, Abrams KR, Sutton AJ,** et al. (2003) Reporting of prognostic markers: current problems and development of guidelines for evidence-based practice in the future. *Br J Cancer* **88**(8), 1191–8.

28. **Rover C, Andreas S, and Friede T** (2016) Evidence synthesis for count distributions based on heterogeneous and incomplete aggregated data. *Biom J* **58**(1), 170–85.

29. **Parmar MK, Torri V, and Stewart L** (1998) Extracting summary statistics to perform meta-analyses of the published literature for survival endpoints. *Stat Med* **17**(24), 2815–34.

30. **Tierney JF, Stewart LA, Ghersi D,** et al. (2007) Practical methods for incorporating summary time-to-event data into meta-analysis. *Trials* **8**, 16.

31. **Perneger TV** (2008) Estimating the relative hazard by the ratio of logarithms of event-free proportions. *Contemporary Clinical Trials* **29**, 762–6.

32. **Collins GS, de Groot JA, Dutton S,** et al. (2014) External validation of multivariable prediction models: a systematic review of methodological conduct and reporting. *BMC Med Res Methodol* **14**, 40.

33. **Mallett S, Royston P, Waters R,** et al. (2010) Reporting performance of prognostic models in cancer: a review. *BMC Medicine* **8**, 21.

34. **Debray TP, Damen JA, Riley RD**, et al. (2018) A framework for meta-analysis of prediction model studies with binary and time-to-event outcomes. *Stat Methods Med Res.* doi: 10.1177/0962280218785504. [Epub ahead of print]

35. **Jinks RC, Royston P**, and **Parmar MK** (2015) Discrimination-based sample size calculations for multivariable prognostic models for time-to-event data. *BMC Med Res Methodol* 15, 82.

36. **Harrell FE, Jr.** (2015) *Regression Modeling Strategies: with Applications to Linear Models, Logistic and Ordinal Regression, and Survival Analysis* (second edition). New York: Springer.

37. **Pencina MJ, D'Agostino RB, Sr.**, and **Song L** (2012) Quantifying discrimination of Framingham risk functions with different survival C statistics. *Stat Med* 31(15), 1543–53.

38. **Wolbers M, Blanche P, Koller MT**, et al. (2014) Concordance for prognostic models with competing risks. *Biostatistics* 15(3), 526–39.

39. **Vickers AJ, Van Calster B**, and **Steyerberg EW** (2016) Net benefit approaches to the evaluation of prediction models, molecular markers, and diagnostic tests. *BMJ* 352, i6.

40. **Vickers AJ** and **Elkin EB** (2006) Decision curve analysis: a novel method for evaluating prediction models. *Med Decis Making* 26(6), 565–74.

41. **Wynants L, Riley RD, Timmerman D**, et al. (2018) Random-effects meta-analysis of the clinical utility of tests and prediction models. *Stat Med* (in press).

42. **Moons KG, Altman DG, Vergouwe Y**, et al. (2009) Prognosis and prognostic research: application and impact of prognostic models in clinical practice. *BMJ* 338, b606.

43. **Altman DG** and **Bland JM** (2003) Interaction revisited: the difference between two estimates. *BMJ* 326(7382), 219.

44. **Moons KGM, Wolff RF, Riley RD**, et al. (2019) PROBAST: a tool to assess risk of bias and applicability concerns of prediction model studies–explanation and elaboration. *Ann Int Med* (in press).

45. **Kyzas PA, Denaxa-Kyza D**, and **Ioannidis JP** (2007) Almost all articles on cancer prognostic markers report statistically significant results. *European Journal of Ccancer* 43(17), 2559–79.

46. **Kyzas PA, Denaxa-Kyza D**, and **Ioannidis JP** (2007) Quality of reporting of cancer prognostic marker studies: association with reported prognostic effect. *J Natl Cancer Inst* 99(3), 236–43.

47. **Kyzas PA, Loizou KT**, and **Ioannidis JP** (2005) Selective reporting biases in cancer prognostic factor studies. *J Natl Cancer Inst* 97(14), 1043–55.

48. **Mallett S, Royston P, Dutton S**, et al. (2010) Reporting methods in studies developing prognostic models in cancer: a review. *BMC Medicine* 8, 20.

49. **Collins GS, Mallett S, Omar O**, et al. (2011) Developing risk prediction models for type 2 diabetes: a systematic review of methodology and reporting. *BMC Medicine* 9, 103.

50. **Collins GS, Omar O, Shanyinde M**, et al. (2013) A systematic review finds prediction models for chronic kidney disease were poorly reported and often developed using inappropriate methods. *J Clin Epidemiol* 66(3), 268–77.

51. **Bouwmeester W, Zuithoff NP, Mallett S**, et al. (2012) Reporting and methods in clinical prediction research: a systematic review. *PLoS Med* 9(5), e1001221.

52. **Burton A** and **Altman DG** (2004) Missing covariate data within cancer prognostic studies: a review of current reporting and proposed guidelines. *Br J Cancer* **91**(1), 4–8.

53. **Hayden JA, van der Windt DA, Cartwright JL**, et al. (2013) Assessing bias in studies of prognostic factors. *Ann Intern Med* **158**(4), 280–6.

54. **Higgins JP, Altman DG, Gotzsche PC**, et al. (2011) The Cochrane Collaboration's tool for assessing risk of bias in randomized trials. *BMJ* **343**, d5928.

55. **Lagakos SW** (2006) The challenge of subgroup analyses—reporting without distorting. *N Engl J Med* **354**(16),1667–9.

56. **Sun X, Briel M, Walter SD**, et al. (2010) Is a subgroup effect believable? Updating criteria to evaluate the credibility of subgroup analyses. *BMJ* **340**, c117.

57. **Pincus T, Miles C, Froud R**, et al. (2011) Methodological criteria for the assessment of moderators in systematic reviews of randomised controlled trials: a consensus study. *BMC Med Res Methodol* **11**, 14.

58. **Riley RD, Lambert PC, Abo-Zaid G** (2010) Meta-analysis of individual participant data: rationale, conduct, and reporting. *BMJ* **340**, c221.

59. **Vergouwe Y, Moons KG**, and **Steyerberg EW** (2010) External validity of risk models: use of benchmark values to disentangle a case-mix effect from incorrect coefficients. *Am J Epidemiol* **172**(8), 971–80.

60. **Knottnerus JA** (2002) Between iatrotropic stimulus and interiatric referral: the domain of primary care research. *J Clin Epidemiol* **55**(12), 1201–6.

61. **DerSimonian R** and **Laird N** (1986) Meta-analysis in clinical trials. *Control Clin Trials* **7**(3), 177–88.

62. **Langan D, Higgins JP**, and **Simmonds M** (2015) An empirical comparison of heterogeneity variance estimators in 12,894 meta-analyses. *Res Synth Methods* **6**(2), 195–205.

63. **Cornell JE, Mulrow CD, Localio R**, et al. (2014) Random-effects meta-analysis of inconsistent effects: a time for change. *Ann Intern Med* **160**(4), 267–70.

64. **Hartung J** and **Knapp G** (2001) A refined method for the meta-analysis of controlled clinical trials with binary outcome. *Stat Med* **20**(24), 3875–89.

65. **Partlett C** and **Riley RD** (2017) Random effects meta-analysis: Coverage performance of 95% confidence and prediction intervals following REML estimation. *Stat Med* **36**, 301–17.

66. **Snell KI, Ensor J, Debray TP**, et al. (2017) Meta-analysis of prediction model performance across multiple studies: Which scale helps ensure between-study normality for the C-statistic and calibration measures? *Stat Methods Med Res* 962280217705678.

67. **Hamza TH, van Houwelingen HC**, and **Stijnen T** (2008) The binomial distribution of meta-analysis was preferred to model within-study variability. *J Clin Epidemiol* **61**(1), 41–51.

68. **Stijnen T, Hamza TH**, and **Özdemir P** (2010) Random effects meta-analysis of event outcome in the framework of the generalized linear mixed model with applications in sparse data. *Stat Med* **29**, 3046–67.

69. **Riley RD, Ahmed I, Debray TP**, et al. (2015) Summarising and validating test accuracy results across multiple studies for use in clinical practice. *Stat Med* **34**(13), 2081–103.

70. **Riley RD, Elia EG, Malin G**, et al.(2015) Multivariate meta-analysis of prognostic factor studies with multiple cut-points and/or methods of measurement. *Stat Med* **34**(17), 2481–96.

71. **Collaboration FS** (2009) Systematically missing confounders in individual participant data meta-analysis of observational cohort studies. *Stat Med* **28**(8), 1218–37.

72. **Snell KI, Hua H, Debray TP**, et al. (2016) Multivariate meta-analysis of individual participant data helped externally validate the performance and implementation of a prediction model. *J Clin Epidemiol* **69**, 40–50.

73. **Webber EM, Kauffman TL, O'Connor E**, et al. (2015) Systematic review of the predictive effect of MSI status in colorectal cancer patients undergoing 5FU-based chemotherapy. *BMC Cancer* **15**, 156.

74. **Cumming TB, Packer M, Kramer SF**, et al. (2016) The prevalence of fatigue after stroke: A systematic review and meta-analysis. *Int J Stroke* **11**(9), 968–77.

75. **Rucker G, Schwarzer G, Carpenter JR**, et al. (2008) Undue reliance on I(2) in assessing heterogeneity may mislead. *BMC Med Res Methodol* **8**, 79.

76. **Higgins JP, Thompson SG**, and **Spiegelhalter DJ** (2009) A re-evaluation of random-effects meta-analysis. *Journal of the Royal Statistical Society, Series A* **172**, 137–59.

77. **Riley RD, Higgins JP**, and **Deeks JJ** (2011) Interpretation of random effects meta-analyses. *BMJ* **342**, d549.

78. **Berkey CS, Hoaglin DC, Mosteller F**, et al. (1995) A random-effects regression model for meta-analysis. *Stat Med* **14**(4), 395–411.

79. **Riley RD, Ensor J, Snell KI**, et al. (2016) External validation of clinical prediction models using big datasets from e-health records or IPD meta-analysis: opportunities and challenges. *BMJ* **353**, i3140.

80. **Pennells L, Kaptoge S, White IR**, et al. (2014) Assessing risk prediction models using individual participant data from multiple studies. *Am J Epidemiol* **179**(5), 621–32.

81. **Berlin JA, Santanna J, Schmid CH**, et al. (2002) Individual patient versus group-level data meta-regressions for the investigation of treatment effect modifiers: ecological bias rears its ugly head. *Stat Med* **21**(3), 371–87.

82. **Sterne JAC, Sutton AJ, Ioannidis JPA**, et al. (2011) Recommendations for examining and interpreting funnel plot asymmetry in meta-analyses of randomised controlled trials. *BMJ* **342**, d4002.

83. **Debray TPA, Moons KGM**, and **Riley RD** Detecting small-study effects and funnel plot asymmetry in meta-analysis of survival data: a comparison of new and existing tests. *Research Synthesis Methods* **9**, 41–50.

84. **Simon R** (2001) Evaluating prognostic factor studies. In: **Gospodarowicz M**, ed. *Prognostic Factors in Cancer*. New York: Wiley-Liss. pp. 49–56.

85. **Pearson TA, Mensah GA, Alexander RW**, et al. (2003) Markers of inflammation and cardiovascular disease: application to clinical and public health practice: A statement for healthcare professionals from the Centers for Disease Control and Prevention and the American Heart Association. *Circulation* **107**(3), 499–511.

86. **Moher D, Liberati A, Tetzlaff J**, et al. (2009) Preferred reporting items for systematic reviews and meta-analyses: the PRISMA statement. *BMJ* **339**, b2535.

87. **Stroup DF, Berlin JA, Morton SC,** et al. (2000) Meta-analysis of observational studies in epidemiology: a proposal for reporting. Meta-analysis Of Observational Studies in Epidemiology (MOOSE) group. *JAMA* **283**(15), 2008–12.

88. **McShane LM, Altman DG, Sauerbrei W,** et al. (2005) REporting recommendations for tumour MARKer prognostic studies (REMARK). *Br J Cancer* **93**(4), 387–91.

89. **Collins GS, Reitsma JB, Altman DG,** et al. (2015) Transparent Reporting of a multivariable prediction model for Individual Prognosis Or Diagnosis (TRIPOD): The TRIPOD Statement. *Ann Intern Med* **162**, 55–63.

90. **Iorio A, Spencer FA, Falavigna M,** et al. (2015) Use of GRADE for assessment of evidence about prognosis: rating confidence in estimates of event rates in broad categories of patients. *BMJ* **350**, h870.

91. **Huguet A, Hayden JA, Stinson J,** et al. (2013) Judging the quality of evidence in reviews of prognostic factor research: adapting the GRADE framework. *Systematic Reviews* **2**, 71.

Part 4

Exemplars of prognosis research impact

Chapter 10

Prognosis research in people with low back pain

Nadine E Foster, Danielle A van der Windt, Kate M Dunn, and Peter Croft

10.1 Definition of the health condition, startpoints and endpoints

Low back pain (LBP) is common. The Global Burden of Disease Project estimated the worldwide one-month prevalence of LBP in adults at 37% in 2016. Years lived with disability by people with LBP were estimated to total 57.6 million globally, making it the leading cause of years lived with disability (1). The symptom of LBP occasionally indicates an underlying disease, such as cancer, infection, or spinal fracture ('red flag' diagnoses), which means that a person with LBP has an increased risk of premature mortality or serious complications if untreated. For most LBP sufferers, however, the symptom itself is the problem, together with the possibility of future long-term disability and its personal, financial, healthcare, and societal burden. This chapter takes the presence of LBP as the relevant startpoint for prognosis research, and considers the prognosis of individuals with LBP in different settings: healthcare, workplace, and in the general population.

Death, although unusual, can be a relevant endpoint for population studies of people with LBP because of the aforementioned small but important group with 'red flag' diagnoses, and because of the risk of complications related to some treatments, for example prescription and/or misuse of opioids, potentially leading to an increase in mortality.

The most useful endpoints in patients with LBP, however, are patient-reported outcomes such as reduction in pain severity and improvement in back-related tasks (e.g. ability to put on socks), general wellbeing, physical activity, and the ability to work and engage in social life. These endpoints are most directly obtained from validated self-completed questionnaires such as the Roland-Morris Disability Questionnaire or the Oswestry Disability Index (reviewed as outcomes for LBP trials (2, 3)). LBP prognosis research studies that use healthcare records often focus on proxy endpoints for continuing pain and disability, such as referral for surgery, change in medication, and future healthcare contacts. For example, follow-up of people with LBP in the Danish population found higher rates of healthcare use twenty years later compared with controls without LBP (4). Other record-based endpoints relevant to patients with LBP include sickness certification and disability payments. Linkage with healthcare records in population-based cohorts, or adding patient-reported outcomes to cohorts identified from healthcare databases (as in the example in Section 10.2), has added relevant endpoints to prognosis studies in people with LBP.

10.2 Overall prognosis of people with low back pain

The main application of overall prognosis studies in people with LBP has been to draw attention to the substantial variation in short-term prognosis among people with an episode of LBP and to the important minority of people who progress from a short-term episode to chronic or intermittent LBP that often persists for many years.

In the general population setting, overall prognosis can be estimated using questionnaire surveys to identify people reporting LBP, with follow-up surveys used to investigate their outcomes. Box 10.1 illustrates an overall

---

Box 10.1 Overall prognosis of people reporting occasional LBP in the general population

Setting: Stockholm, Sweden

Design: (1) cross-sectional population survey in 2006; (2) prospective cohort of people completing the follow-up in 2010.

Startpoint: self-reported 'occasional LBP' in 2006 = LBP for up to a few days on average every month during the previous six months. The prevalence of this startpoint in the study population was 35.7% (a typical figure for adult populations).

Endpoint: 'persistent troublesome LBP after four years' that reduced workability or interfered with daily activities, to some or high degree, on at least a few days per week on average during the previous six months.

Overall prognosis: 9.9% (95% CI 9.2–10.6%) of those with occasional LBP report persistent troublesome LBP four years later. This is similar to figures from other countries.

Source: data from Bohman T (2014) Does a healthy lifestyle behaviour influence the prognosis of low back pain among men and women in a general population? A population-based cohort study. *BMJ Open* (4), e005713. Copyright © 2014 BMJ Publishing Group.

prognosis study that summarizes the probability of 'persistent troublesome LBP' (endpoint) after four years, among a population-based sample of people who reported occasional LBP in a baseline survey (startpoint).

In primary care settings, healthcare records are used to identify patients with LBP. Box 10.2 concerns a systematic review showing that LBP-related disability persists in the majority of primary care attenders one year after consultation about their LBP.

The frequency and importance of work absence related to LBP means that cohorts for prognosis research in this domain are often based in occupational settings or workers' compensation systems. In a cohort of 6657 workers in Ontario, Canada, receiving at least four weeks of compensation for LBP (startpoint), 1442 (22% (95% CI 21–23%)) remained on full compensation benefits after four years (endpoint) (5).

LBP can extend across the life course. Prognosis studies often sample people at one point in the course of their condition. But a new episode of LBP may also be a recurrence or exacerbation of earlier LBP. One approach to this problem of changing or overlapping startpoints and endpoints is to separate LBP at the startpoint into short and long-term duration of their LBP ('acute' and 'persistent' LBP). When followed up, pain and disability levels in both startpoint groups tend to decline during six weeks following a healthcare

---

Box 10.2 Overall prognosis of patients presenting with non-specific LBP in primary care

Population: patients seeking primary care for LBP.

Setting: primary care.

Design: systematic review of cohort studies with at least twelve months of follow-up.

Startpoint: consultation in primary care for LBP of less than three months' duration and classified as 'non-specific' (red flag diagnoses excluded).

Endpoints: self-reported 'recovery' at twelve months: either (1) complete absence of pain, or (2) complete absence or some continuing mild pain.

Overall prognosis: the summary estimate for the proportion of patients still reporting pain one year after onset of LBP was 65% (95% CI: 54–75%).

Source: data from Itz CJ, et al. (2012) Clinical course of non-specific low back pain: a systematic review of prospective cohort studies set in primary care. *European Journal of Pain* 17(1), 5–15. Copyright © 2012 John Wiley & Sons, Inc. All rights reserved.

consultation, and then stabilize, with more people reporting moderate levels of pain and disability at twelve months' follow-up in the group with persistent pain at the startpoint (6).

10.3 **Prognostic factors for people with low back pain**

The main application of prognostic factor research in people with LBP has been to identify the wide range of characteristics (biological, psychological, and social) associated with outcomes of continuing or worsening pain and disability over time. This evidence informs the biopsychosocial approach to LBP care (7).

Physical, psychological, lifestyle, and social measures and characteristics are prognostic factors in LBP. For example, the extent of pain outside the back in people with LBP (measured by number of self-reported pain locations (8)) is associated with future back-related disability. General health and co-morbidities at the startpoint are also prognostic factors, and low physical activity is a potentially modifiable prognostic factor. Psychological factors (beliefs and attitudes regarding pain) and emotional distress (anxiety and depression) at baseline are also associated with poorer prognosis and may be modifiable. In a Dutch study (9), pain catastrophizing at baseline (e.g. I believe my LBP will last forever) was associated with persistent LBP at twelve months (odds ratio 1.7, 95% confidence interval 1.0–2.8). Adverse social factors, such as low socioeconomic status, are also associated with worse outcomes over time.

Prognostic factor studies may also lead to the definition of new startpoints for overall prognosis studies. For example, some people with LBP have a highly variable or fluctuating course of symptoms. Repeated measures of pain experience and back-related disability over time have been used to identify subgroups of people with distinct longitudinal symptom or disability trajectories, using techniques such as latent class growth analysis. Box 10.3 illustrates that these trajectories are associated with future outcomes, and a six-month 'persistent high pain' trajectory is a prognostic factor for poor outcome (pain and disability) seven years later. These trajectories help to define more dynamic startpoints and endpoints for prognosis research in people with LBP generally.

Prognostic factors identify subgroups at risk of poor outcome in people with LBP, explain variability in outcome, and may provide specific targets for treatment. Multivariable prognostic models are, however, needed to enhance prediction of outcomes in individuals with LBP, conditional on combinations of these prognostic factors.

Box 10.3 Six-month pain trajectories as prognostic factors in patients presenting with LBP in primary care

Population: 342 patients with LBP in primary care.

Setting: UK primary care.

Design: cohort study of primary care patients with LBP, followed up with self-report questionnaires.

Startpoint: patients consulting for LBP in primary care.

Prognostic factor: six-month trajectories of back pain after a primary care consultation for LBP, identified by longitudinal latent class analysis applied to participants' monthly pain self-reports.

Endpoints: (1) disability and work absence at seven-year follow-up; (2) six-month pain trajectories at seven-year follow-up, identified by longitudinal latent class analysis applied to participants' pain self-reports.

Results: six-month pain trajectories in patents after a primary care consultation for LBP were associated with disability and work outcomes and six-month LBP trajectories at seven years.

Source: data from Dunn KM, et al. (2013) Long-term trajectories of back pain: cohort study with seven-year follow-up. *BMJ Open* (3), e003838. Copyright © 2013 BMJ Publishing Group.

10.4 Prognostic models for people with low back pain

The contribution of prognostic models in LBP is to provide the basis for more effective and efficient delivery of care tailored to the outcome probabilities of an individual with LBP. This contribution is crucial for current LBP-related healthcare, given the high prevalence of LBP and the high costs and potential hazards of overinvestigation and overtreatment in people with LBP. Prognostic models, using a small number of easily assessed prognostic factors to estimate the probabilities of long-term pain, disability, or work loss in individuals with LBP, have reasonable calibration and C statistics ranging from 0.6 to 0.8. A score used in patients consulting with chronic LBP had a C statistic of 0.84 (95% CI 0.79–0.88) for persistent disabling pain four months later (10). Adding MRI scan results to an existing primary care prognostic model did not significantly or importantly change the twelve-month C statistic of 0.77 (11). Box 10.4 describes one of the few prognostic models ('PICKUP') developed according to the principles described in Chapter 7.

Box 10.4 A prognostic model for patients with acute LBP

Population: patients attending primary care with acute LBP.

Setting: Australian primary care physiotherapy, chiropractic and general practices.

Startpoint: acute LBP (less than two weeks' duration).

Endpoint: onset of chronic LBP (ongoing pain at three months after index consultation).

Design: development sample (n = 1230) 2003–2005; external validation sample (n = 1528) 2009–2013.

Prognostic factor selection: all potential prognostic factors (continuous and categorical) from the original cohort study were included in a forward stepwise logistic regression analysis, with significance set at p < 0.10, resulting in a five-item model: disability compensation; leg pain; pain intensity; depression; perceived risk of pain persistence.

Results: 30% of the development sample and 19% of the validation sample developed chronic LBP. Discrimination was modest (C statistic 0.66, 95% CI 0.63–0.69); calibration was acceptable, although better for low than high-risk groups.

Implication: use of this five-item tool to support decisions in patients with acute LBP would avoid unnecessary interventions in forty out of one hundred consulting patients with a good prognosis, as compared with a 'treat everyone' approach, but this has to be balanced against the number of false negatives (patients incorrectly assessed as having a good prognosis) who might miss out on relevant referral or treatment.

Source: data from Traeger AC, et al. (2016) Estimating the risk of chronic pain: development and validation of a prognostic model (PICKUP) for patients with acute low back pain. *PLoS Medicine* (13), e1002019. Copyright © 2013 PLoS.

Other models in common use in clinical practice and research are based on short questionnaires designed to identify prognostic factors in routine healthcare or workplace practice, and include the Orebro Musculoskeletal Pain Screening Questionnaire (12) and the STarT Back tool (13). External validation of the predictive performance of the STarT Back tool in countries other than the UK has confirmed similar predictive performance in primary care but poorer performance in secondary care settings. A systematic review suggested that no existing prognostic model for predicting outcome in individuals with LBP has clear value in secondary care and a 'treat-all-patients' approach may be better in that setting (14).

10.5 Predicting effects of treatment in people with low back pain

10.5.1 Stratified care

The Keele STarT Back tool (13) exemplifies stratified care based on prognostic sub-grouping and matched treatments. The two problems tackled by stratified care are: (1) variable outcomes between different subgroups of LBP patients and (2) small average effect estimates observed in randomized trials of treatments in LBP patients. Research suggests the use of this tool in practice leads to better patient outcomes and more efficient healthcare (15, 16).

The tool was developed (Box 10.5) to classify patients with non-specific LBP (i.e. no red flag diagnoses) into one of three prognostic groups (low, medium,

---

Box 10.5 A tool that screens for LBP prognostic indicators relevant to primary care treatment decision making

Population: adults consulting in general practice with LBP.

Setting: UK.

Startpoint: non-specific LBP (excluding people with red flags or specific spinal diagnoses).

Endpoint: back-specific disability using the Roland and Morris Disability Questionnaire (RMDQ) at six months.

Design: (1) selection of modifiable prognostic factors from literature, which were tested for predictive performance in two existing cohorts. (2) new cohort for model development (n = 131). (3) independent external validity cohort (n = 500).

Results: the tool comprises nine items covering eight physical and psychological prognostic factors, easily completed by the patient with or without healthcare professional help. Cut offs for three groups (low, medium, and high risk of persistent disabling pain) were established from the development sample, and predictive validity confirmed in the external sample: at six months' follow-up, 39 (16.7%) of patients in the low-risk group, 99 (53.2%) in the medium-risk group, and 58 (78.4%) in the high-risk group had a poor disability outcome.

or high risk of persistent disabling pain), with the high-risk group characterized by psychosocial prognostic factors. Matched treatments were defined, linked to each of the risk groups: brief low-cost intervention (advice, support to self-manage, and reassurance) for those at low risk, active course of evidence-based physiotherapy for medium risk, and a combined physical and psychological intervention that draws on cognitive behavioural approaches for high-risk patients.

Although the associations between the separate prognostic factors included in the STarT Back tool (or the tool as a whole) and treatment effect were not examined by testing treatment-predictor interactions, as described in Chapter 8, the impact of using the tool to subgroup patients and offer matched treatments was investigated in a randomized trial. Impact was measured in terms of healthcare decision making, and clinical and cost-effectiveness (16). All participants completed the tool at baseline, but only in one arm of the trial (the 'stratified care' arm) was information from the tool used to select and match treatments (17). Patients in the control arm continued to receive current best care for LBP. Impact on referral decisions is shown in Table 10.1: more patients received a referral relevant to their outcome risk in the intervention group compared to the control group. This included a lower referral rate for physiotherapy among low-risk patients in the intervention than in the control group.

Patient-reported endpoints showed significantly larger improvements in the stratified care group compared with the controls, including better LBP-related

Table 10.1 Impact of use of STarT Back prognostic tool in the intervention group (I) to guide referral by consulting physiotherapists, compared with controls (C) among whom it was not used.

	Low risk (percentage with no onward referral)		Medium risk (percentage referred on for standard physiotherapy)		High risk (percentage referred on for specialized pain management physiotherapy)	
	I	C	I	C	I	C
Percentage of patients with referral decision appropriate to their level of risk of poor outcome	93	51	98	60	100	65

Source: data from Hill JC, et al. (2011) Comparison of stratified primary care management for low back pain with current best practice (STarT Back): a randomised controlled trial. *Lancet* 378, 1560–71. Copyright © 2011 Elsevier.

disability scores at four and twelve months, less time off work, higher satisfaction with care, at lower cost. Cost reductions were achieved by a lower referral rate in low-risk patients with no adverse health consequences. Implementation in 'real life' primary care was investigated in a before and after sequential cohort study (the IMPaCT Back study) based in UK general practice and NHS physiotherapy services (18). This replicated the findings of the STarT Back randomized trial.

10.5.2 Differential treatment effect

The STarT Back and IMPaCT Back studies were not designed to develop a purely predictive prognostic model. Variables were selected because of their potential for modifiability and potential response to matched treatment, as well as for their prognostic value. The high-risk group was defined by high prevalence of psychological predictors of poor outcome. This provided a clear rationale for treatments directly addressing these prognostic factors in the 'high-risk' group, which was therefore partly defined on the potential for differential treatment response.

In a trial of a targeted intervention for workers with LBP at high risk for poor work-related outcomes (19), participants were randomized to a communication and problem-solving skills package for both worker and supervisor or to 'treatment as usual'. The intervention was effective in improving return-to-work rates. This trial was carried out in high-risk workers only, so questions remain as to whether or not the intervention might also be effective but inefficient in people at low risk (i.e. absolute risk reduction too small to justify the scale and cost) or ineffective in those at low risk (i.e. possible differential treatment effect). The investigators are pursuing these questions in future study design and interpretation.

10.6 Summary

LBP provides an example of a common syndrome where there is a lack of evidence for disease-based classification that can drive treatment decision making. Strong evidence from cohorts, however, has identified consistent prognostic factors. This has led to a prominent role for prognosis research in defining subgroups and in using this information to make treatment selection more efficient. Prognostic factors and models include a range of biological, psychological, and social factors which help to shape different treatment strategies, recommending reassurance, advice, and support to remain active (among those at low risk of poor outcomes) and cognitive-behavioural approaches to overcoming more complex barriers to recovery (for those at high risk of poor outcomes).

References

1. **GBD 2016 Disease and Injury Incidence and Prevalence Collaborators** (2017) Global, regional, and national incidence, prevalence, and years lived with disability for 328 diseases and injuries for 195 countries, 1990–2016: a systematic analysis for the Global Burden of Disease Study 2016. *Lancet* 390(10100), 1211–59.

2. **Chiarotto A, Deyo RA, Terwee CB, Buchbinder R, Corbin TP, Costa LOP**, et al. (2015) Core outcome measurement instruments for clinical trials in non-specific low back pain. *Pain* 24, 1127–42.

3. **Chiarotto A, Boers M, Deyo RA, Buchbinder R, Corbin TP, Costa LOP**, et al. (2018) Core outcome measurement instruments for clinical trials in nonspecific low back pain. *Pain* 159(3), 481–95.

4. **Hartvigsen J, Davidsen M, Sogaard K, Roos EM**, and **Hestbaek L** (2014) Self-reported musculoskeletal pain predicts long-term increase in general health care use: a population-based cohort study with 20-year follow-up. *Scand J Public Health* 42(7), 698–704.

5. **Steenstra IA, Busse JW, Tolusso D, Davilmar A, Lee H, Furlan AD**, et al. (2015) Predicting time on prolonged benefits for injured workers with acute back pain. *J Occup Rehabil* 25(2), 267–78.

6. **da C Menezes Costa L, Maher CG, Hancock MJ, McAuley JH, Herbert RD**, and **Costa LO** (2012) The prognosis of acute and persistent low-back pain: a meta-analysis. *CMAJ* 184(11), E613–24.

7. **Waddell G** (1987) Volvo award in clinical sciences. A new clinical model for the treatment of low-back pain. *Spine* 12(7), 632–44.

8. **Thomas E, Silman AJ, Croft PR, Papageorgiou AC, Jayson MI**, and **Macfarlane GJ** (1999) Predicting who develops chronic low back pain in primary care: a prospective study. *BMJ* 318(7199), 1662–7.

9. **Picavet HS, Vlaeyen JW**, and **Schouten JS** (2002) Pain catastrophizing and kinesiophobia: predictors of chronic low back pain. *Am J Epidemiol* 156(11), 1028–34.

10. **Turner JA, Shortreed SM, Saunders KW, Leresche L, Berlin JA**, and **Von Korff M** (2013) Optimizing prediction of back pain outcomes. *Pain* 154(8), 1391–401.

11. **de Schepper EI, Koes BW, Oei EH, Bierma-Zeinstra SM**, and **Luijsterburg PA** (2016) The added prognostic value of MRI findings for recovery in patients with low back pain in primary care: a 1-year follow-up cohort study. *Eur Spine J* 25(4), 1234–41.

12. **Linton SJ** and **Boersma K** (2003) Early identification of patients at risk of developing a persistent back problem: the predictive validity of the Orebro Musculoskeletal Pain Questionnaire. *Clin J Pain* 19(2), 80–6.

13. **Hill JC, Dunn KM, Lewis M, Mullis R, Main CJ, Foster NE**, et al. (2008) A primary care back pain screening tool: identifying patient subgroups for initial treatment. *Arthritis Rheum* 59(5), 632–41.

14. **Karran EL, McAuley JH, Traeger AC, Hillier SL, Grabherr L, Russek LN**, et al. (2017) Can screening instruments accurately determine poor outcome risk in adults with recent onset low back pain? A systematic review and meta-analysis. *BMC Med* 15(1), 13.

15. **Whitehurst DG, Bryan S, Lewis M, Hill J**, and **Hay EM** (2012) Exploring the cost-utility of stratified primary care management for low back pain compared with current best practice within risk-defined subgroups. *Ann Rheum Dis* 71(11), 1796–802.

16. **Hill JC, Whitehurst DG, Lewis M, Bryan S, Dunn KM, Foster NE,** et al. (2011) Comparison of stratified primary care management for low back pain with current best practice (STarT Back): a randomised controlled trial. *Lancet* **378**(9802), 1560–71.

17. **Main CJ, Sowden G, Hill JC, Watson PJ,** and **Hay EM** (2012) Integrating physical and psychological approaches to treatment in low back pain: the development and content of the STarT Back trial's 'high-risk' intervention. *Physiotherapy* **98**(2), 110–6.

18. **Foster NE, Mullis R, Hill JC, Lewis M, Whitehurst DG, Doyle C,** et al. (2014) Effect of stratified care for low back pain in family practice (IMPaCT Back): a prospective population-based sequential comparison. *Ann Fam Med* **12**(2), 102–11.

19. **Linton SJ, Boersma K, Traczyk M, Shaw W,** and **Nicholas M** (2016) Early workplace communication and problem solving to prevent back disability: results of a randomized controlled trial among high-risk workers and their supervisors. *J Occup Rehabil* **26**(2), 150–9.

Chapter 11

Prognosis research in people with coronary heart disease

Adam Timmis, Pablo Perel, and Peter Croft

11.1 Definition of the health condition, startpoints, and endpoints

The term 'coronary heart disease' (CHD), and its synonyms, 'ischaemic heart disease' and 'coronary artery disease', refer to the pathological narrowing or spasm in blood vessels supplying heart muscle. The restricted blood flow may compromise the pumping function of the heart, cause symptoms such as chest pain (classical angina), injure the heart muscle (the classical heart attack or 'acute myocardial infarction' (AMI)), and interfere with the rhythmic contraction of the heart (arrhythmias). Clinically this has many possible manifestations, from mild chest pain on exertion to sudden death, depending on the nature and extent of the underlying problem.

Symptoms, however, are not in a neat one-to-one relationship with the underlying pathology. Heart attacks can be painless. People with angina may have no evidence of arterial narrowing. The definitions of these classical syndromes of CHD, defined by symptoms and signs, have changed as new tests of cardiac function (e.g. electrocardiogram and echocardiogram), pathophysiology (e.g. measures of muscle damage) and direct imaging of the coronary arteries (angiography) have emerged. These new techniques concern the representation and visualization of underlying pathology to establish the presence of CHD (i.e. diagnosis), but also contain prognostic information that guides clinical management (1). Prognosis related to all these differing but overlapping measures has become a major driver of healthcare activity, and the investigation, classification, and selection for treatment of patients with suspected and proven CHD provide an example of stratified healthcare in action.

The startpoint for CHD prognosis studies could be people with 'coronary artery disease'. However, this already poses problems. When do the fatty streaks that commonly pattern the vascular endothelium of children constitute the start of a coronary artery disease diagnosis? Are the minor atherosclerotic irregularities identified by angiographs in many older people a valid startpoint? Is even the presence of 'coronary artery disease' too far downstream in the pathogenic cascade, given that public health professionals argue cholesterol and blood pressure screening can identify people at risk for future CHD? The choice of startpoint for prognosis research in people with 'CHD' is arbitrary, depending on the definition of CHD presence. All the potential startpoints above might be reasonable depending on the context, setting, and purpose of study.

Another issue in defining CHD startpoints for prognosis research is identifying the best source of data. Even if people with a diagnosed acute myocardial infarction are selected as the startpoint for study, different data sources will potentially contain different case mixtures of patients with an AMI. Figure 11.1 shows UK data for AMI incidence from different sources (2). Disease registries depending on voluntary or administrative action often underestimate hospital CHD admissions, and both may miss some AMI events, certainly the directly fatal ones, recorded in primary care.

In people with a new diagnosed CHD event, the immediate endpoint of concern is early death or survival (pre-hospital or up to thirty days after hospital admission pre- or post-discharge). Secondary endpoints, such as further CHD diagnoses, arrhythmias, or the need for pacemakers or implantable defibrillators, are also important, as well as subsequent complicating co-morbidity (such as stroke), disability (such as permanent work loss), and long-term survival, especially as early survival is continually improving. Long-term need for specific medications may be a marker of complications or severity and thus also serve as a patient-relevant endpoint for prognosis of patients with CHD.

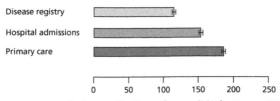

Figure 11.1 Crude incidence of acute myocardial infarction estimated using different sources and combinations of UK data from primary care (Clinical Practice Research Datalink), hospital admissions (Hospital Episode Statistics), and disease registry (MINAP, Myocardial Ischaemia National Audit Project).
Source: data from Herrett, E. et al. Completeness and diagnostic validity of recording acute myocardial infarction events in primary care, hospital care, disease registry, and national mortality records: cohort study. BMJ Clinical Research Edition. 2013(346):e2350. Copyright © 2013 BMJ

11.2 **Overall prognosis for people with coronary heart disease**

The study of overall prognosis in people with proven CHD provides information about average outcomes or endpoints (as listed in the previous section) in such people in the context of current care.

The estimated overall prognosis of people with CHD has changed in recent years. This partly relates to new startpoint definitions, created by new ways of subgrouping and classifying patients with CHD, based on the results of new tests and investigations. Moreover, treatment innovations, including anti-platelet medications, such as aspirin and clopidogrel, and procedures to re-open and restore patency to occluded coronary arteries by percutaneous and surgical techniques, have also contributed to changes in observed prognostic outcomes in patients with CHD.

Studies of CHD in the US and Europe report declining overall fatality in patients with diagnosed AMI. For example, based on linked death and disease registers, one-year case fatality among 658,110 patients aged 35–84 years, with first-time AMI in Sweden occurring between 1987 and 2010, decreased from 23.5% in 1987 to 8.5% in 2010 (3). In the same study, patients with a different startpoint (defined as 'survived for twenty-eight days after AMI') had one-year case fatality of 15.3% in 1987 compared with 7.7% in 2010. Similar figures come from Canada where, among 8493 patients admitted to hospital for AMI between 2006 and 2010, one-year disease-free survival was 79.5% (4).

Severity of the underlying pathology is estimated by the number of narrowed coronary arteries, the extent of their narrowing, and the degree of dysfunction in the left ventricle of the heart. These all have prognostic implications. People with single coronary artery disease and good heart muscle function have better long-term survival than those with widespread artery involvement. In a healthcare record study of 37,674 US veterans undergoing angiography for the first time to investigate symptoms of probable CHD, one-year mortality ranged from 1.4% among patients with no narrowed arteries to 4.3% among patients with obstruction in the main artery or all three branch vessels (5).

Type and extent of AMI in people with CHD is judged in a number of ways, including an electrocardiogram (ECG) feature known as the 'ST phase' which can be elevated (STEMI) or not (nonSTEMI)), and levels of proteins in the blood (e.g. troponin) released by cardiac muscle damage. People with nonSTEMI heart attacks and raised troponin levels have worse long-term mortality. Figure 11.2 illustrates contrasting overall prognosis, related to mortality as the outcome, in different CHD subgroups, including those diagnosed with AMI.

Studies of people with CHD across populations show contrasts in overall prognosis (6, 7) that may reflect variations in healthcare provision. Figure 11.3

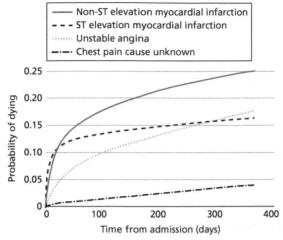

Figure 11.2 Mortality outcomes in persons with different CHD syndromes.

Source: data from Herrett, E. et al. Completeness and diagnostic validity of recording acute myocardial infarction events in primary care, hospital care, disease registry, and national mortality records: cohort study. BMJ Clinical Research Edition. 2013(346):e2350. Copyright © 2013 BMJ

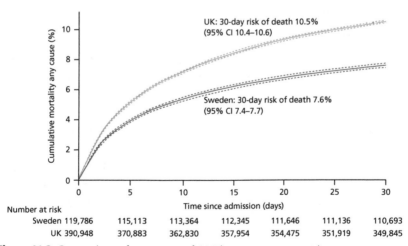

Figure 11.3 Comparison of outcomes of AMI between two countries.

Source: data from Chung, SC., et al. Comparison of hospital variation in acute myocardial infarction care and outcome between Sweden and United Kingdom: population based cohort study using nationwide clinical registries. BMJ Clinical Research Edition. 2015(351), e3913. Copyright © 2015 BMJ

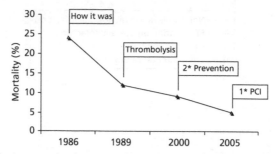

Figure 11.4 The impact of treatment innovations on CHD outcomes: data from the East London Coronary Care Unit Registry (PCI = percutaneous coronary intervention). Source: reproduced courtesy of Adam Timmis

shows a comparison of patients diagnosed with AMI in Sweden and UK. After adjustment for case mix and other confounders, persisting differences in early mortality outcomes between the two patient groups might be related to quality of healthcare in the two countries (8).

The clinical impact of widely introduced therapeutic innovations in healthcare settings can be evaluated by changes in overall prognosis endpoints across time. Figure 11.4 shows the decline in AMI case fatality with treatment changes superimposed, as recorded in one UK coronary care unit.

11.3 **Prognostic factors for people with coronary heart disease**

The study of prognostic factors in patients with CHD is important to identify new subgroups who may need different treatments and care, new targets for therapeutic development, and factors that could input into prognostic models for predicting the course of patients with diagnosed CHD. In general, older age is associated with worse prognosis, although at any age prognosis is further influenced by the presence of co-morbidities (9). Many studies suggest CHD prognosis is worse in females. In the most recent studies (3), gender differences largely disappear after adjustment for physical and mental co-morbidity differences between the genders. Co-morbidity extends to psychological distress, with persistent moderately severe depression and anxiety over at least two years post-AMI predicting four-year mortality (10).

Ethnicity is another challenging area in this domain. One study found that black people with CHD in the US had higher mortality than white people with CHD after adjustment for other factors (11). Whether this reflects structural disadvantage (neighbourhood deprivation predicts case fatality also (12)) or poor treatment is under debate. In a UK study (13), young south Asian people

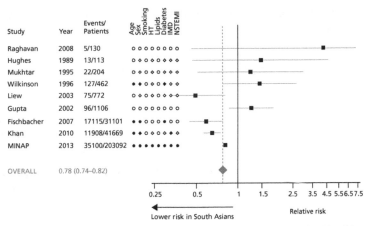

Figure 11.5 Prognosis of coronary disease in South Asians compared with white subjects: meta-analysis of 12 prognosis populations including 14 531 South Asian patients. Startpoint: acute coronary syndromes. Events: All-cause mortality except Liew and Gupta (in-hospital mortality).

Source: adapted with permission from Zaman, MJS., et al. South Asians and coronary disease: is there discordance between effects on incidence and prognosis? Heart. 99(10), 729-36. Copyright © 2013 BMJ

were at two-fold higher risk than young white people of dying in the first six months post-AMI, but this reduced substantially after adjusting for diabetes. Diabetes is more common in south Asians living in the UK than in the white population. A meta-analysis across nine different populations (Figure 11.5) concluded that south Asian people with CHD had a better outcome, measured by mortality at twelve months, than white people with CHD, once diabetes and other co-morbidities were considered (14).

The prognostic value of biomarkers in patients with CHD is the subject of much research activity. One example is lipoprotein levels at the time of diagnosis. These are associated with future CHD risk in the general adult population, but are also a prognostic factor for long-term cardiovascular-related mortality in people with diagnosed non-obstructive CHD (15). A second example is B-type natriuretic peptide, which is known to be a prognostic factor in people with heart failure but also associated with mortality in people with CHD (16). Imaging provides refined assessments of the extent of myocardial damage, and quantified changes on computerized tomographic angiography are an example of a potential prognostic factor for future major adverse cardiovascular events in people with diagnosed CHD (17). Such investigations may provide further discrimination of patients with CHD in terms of different prognosis. For example, coronary artery calcium detected on computerized tomography is a prognostic factor for worse outcomes in women with CHD.

11.4 **Prognostic models for people with coronary heart disease**

Prognostic models are increasingly important for predicting outcomes in individuals with CHD. Identifying who is at elevated risk of early death or future major cardiovascular events can be used to tailor and target treatment of patients with CHD. A number of prognostic models have been developed to inform stratified care for patients following a CHD event. Five examples illustrate different startpoints, endpoints, and applications:

1. A prognostic model to predict an individual's two-year mortality risk after discharge from hospital with acute coronary syndrome, was developed in a study from twenty-eight countries across Europe, Latin America, and Asia (18). A model with eleven predictors had a C statistic of 0.79 (95% CI = 0.78–0.81)).

2. A prognostic model to predict risk of heart failure over five years in patients after acute coronary syndrome was developed in an Australian setting (19). The model had a C statistic of 0.73; addition of biomarkers (including B-type natriuretic peptide and troponin) increased the C statistic to 0.77.

3. An easy-to-use risk prediction model for thirty-day mortality was developed using data from a randomized trial in patients with cardiogenic shock after AMI (20). Six variables were included, and the C statistic was 0.79. External validation in a different patient sample had a C statistic of 0.73.

4. A score was developed in a US population of patients awaiting coronary artery bypass surgery, based on easily available variables of history, clinical examination, and laboratory measurements, which predicted likelihood of early perioperative death or morbidity such as renal failure and brain damage, after surgery had been performed (21).

5. A prognostic model (SYNTAX II) in patients with anatomically complex CHD combined an anatomical score of severity and extent of coronary artery narrowing with seven other variables (22). The endpoint was mortality at four years. The C statistic was 0.73 (95%CI), and in external validation it was 0.72.

In general, in this field, there has been little formal validation of developed prognostic models, let alone studies of their impact on decision making, patient outcomes, and healthcare provision. The ideal studies would be randomized trials comparing outcomes after use versus no use of the model in clinical practice.

11.5 Predicting treatment effect in people with coronary heart disease

The presence of major interventions for people with CHD, such as surgery, and the rapid progress in new non-invasive techniques, such as coronary stents, has stimulated research into the possibility that different treatments may have different effects for particular patients.

An example of research into differential treatment effects in patients with CHD is provided by a meta-analysis of six randomized trials of coronary artery bypass graft (CABG) surgery versus percutaneous coronary intervention (PCI) in patients with coronary artery disease defined as unprotected left main coronary artery disease (23). All-cause mortality was similar in the two trial arms after thirty-nine months median follow-up. But there was significant interaction between the intervention and the SYNTAX prognosis score. Mortality risk in the PCI group was lower than in the CABG group among patients with low SYNTAX scores (less severe anatomical involvement) and higher than in the CABG group among patients with high SYNTAX scores, indicating a potential differential treatment effect on the basis of prognostic score. A more recent pooled analysis of individual participant data from eleven randomized trials has confirmed this differential effect, again reporting a significant interaction with SYNTAX score (24). The SYNTAX score could thus potentially be used to improve treatment decision making in patients with CHD, offering PCI to those with low SYNTAX scores and CABG to those with high scores (i.e. stratified care on the basis of differential treatment effect).

11.6 Summary

CHD provides an important example of how prognosis research is being used to inform the treatment, provision, and evaluation of healthcare in practice. Overall prognosis results have influenced subgrouping and treatment choice, and been used to judge the impact of new treatments and healthcare delivery over time and between countries. New technologies such as imaging have defined potential prognostic factors with more precision and detail, but their influence on patient outcomes has yet to be clearly established. Prognostic models are emerging in this domain, but the impact of their use in decision making and on patient outcomes remains an important topic for future prognosis research.

References

1. Lampe FC, Whincup PH, Wannamethee SG, Shaper AG, Walker M, and Ebrahim S (2000) The natural history of prevalent ischaemic heart disease in middle-aged men. *Eur Heart J* **21**(13), 1052–62.

2. Herrett E, Shah AD, Boggon R, Denaxas S, Smeeth L, van Staa T, et al. (2013) Completeness and diagnostic validity of recording acute myocardial infarction events in primary care, hospital care, disease registry, and national mortality records: cohort study. *BMJ* **346**, f2350.

3. Berg J, Bjorck L, Nielsen S, Lappas G, and Rosengren A (2017) Sex differences in survival after myocardial infarction in Sweden, 1987–2010. *Heart* **103**(20), 1625–30.

4. Tangri N, Ferguson TW, Whitlock RH, Rigatto C, Jassal DS, Kass M, et al. (2017) Long term health outcomes in patients with a history of myocardial infarction: a population based cohort study. *PLoS One* **12**(7), e0180010.

5. Maddox TM, Stanislawski MA, Grunwald GK, Bradley SM, Ho PM, Tsai TT, et al. (2014) Nonobstructive coronary artery disease and risk of myocardial infarction. *JAMA* **312**(17), 1754–63.

6. Degano IR, Salomaa V, Veronesi G, Ferrieres J, Kirchberger I, Laks T, et al. (2015) Twenty-five-year trends in myocardial infarction attack and mortality rates, and case-fatality, in six European populations. *Heart* **101**(17),1413–21.

7. Nichols M, Townsend N, Scarborough P, and Rayner M (2014) Cardiovascular disease in Europe 2014: epidemiological update. *Eur Heart J* **35**(42), 2929.

8. Chung SC, Sundstrom J, Gale CP, James S, Deanfield J, Wallentin L, et al. (2014) Comparison of hospital variation in acute myocardial infarction care and outcome between Sweden and United Kingdom: population based cohort study using nationwide clinical registries. *BMJ* **351**, h3913.

9. Barakat K, Wilkinson P, Deaner A, Fluck D, Ranjadayalan K, and Timmis A (1999) How should age affect management of acute myocardial infarction? A prospective cohort study. *Lancet* **353**(9157), 955–9.

10. Stewart RAH, Colquhoun DM, Marschner SL, Kirby AC, Simes J, Nestel PJ, et al. (2017) Persistent psychological distress and mortality in patients with stable coronary artery disease. *Heart* **103**(23), 1860–6.

11. Colantonio LD, Gamboa CM, Richman JS, Levitan EB, Soliman EZ, Howard G, et al. (2017) Black-white differences in incident fatal, nonfatal, and total coronary heart disease. *Circulation* **136**(2), 152–66.

12. Winkleby MA and Cubbin C (2003) Influence of individual and neighbourhood socioeconomic status on mortality among black, Mexican-American, and white women and men in the United States. *J Epidemiol Community Health* **57**(6), 444–52.

13. Wilkinson P, Sayer J, Laji K, Grundy C, Marchant B, Kopelman P, et al. (1996) Comparison of case fatality in south Asian and white patients after acute myocardial infarction: observational study. *BMJ* **312**(7042), 1330–3.

14. Zaman MJ, Philipson P, Chen R, Farag A, Shipley M, Marmot MG, et al. (2013) South Asians and coronary disease: is there discordance between effects on incidence and prognosis? *Heart* **99**(10), 729–36.

15. Xie H, Chen L, Liu H, Cui Y, Zhang Z, and Cui L (2017) Long-term prognostic value of lipoprotein(a) in symptomatic patients with nonobstructive coronary artery disease. *Am J Cardiol* **119**(7), 945–50.

16. **Omland T, Sabatine MS, Jablonski KA, Rice MM, Hsia J, Wergeland R**, et al. (2007) Prognostic value of B-Type natriuretic peptides in patients with stable coronary artery disease: the PEACE Trial. *J Am Coll Cardiol* **50**(3), 205–14.

17. **Ayoub C, Erthal F, Abdelsalam MA, Murad MH, Wang Z, Erwin PJ**, et al. (2017) Prognostic value of segment involvement score compared to other measures of coronary atherosclerosis by computed tomography: a systematic review and meta-analysis. *J Cardiovasc Comput Tomogr* **11**(4), 258–67.

18. **Pocock SJ, Huo Y, Van de Werf F, Newsome S, Chin CT, Vega AM**, et al. (2017) Predicting two-year mortality from discharge after acute coronary syndrome: an internationally-based risk score. *Eur Heart J Acute Cardiovasc Care* 2048872617719638.

19. **Driscoll A, Barnes EH, Blankenberg S, Colquhoun DM, Hunt D, Nestel PJ**, et al. (2017) Predictors of incident heart failure in patients after an acute coronary syndrome: the LIPID heart failure risk-prediction model. *Int J Cardiol* **248**, 361–8.

20. **Poss J, Koster J, Fuernau G, Eitel I, de Waha S, Ouarrak T**, et al. (2017) Risk stratification for patients in cardiogenic shock after acute myocardial infarction. *J Am Coll Cardiol* **69**(15), 1913–20.

21. **Higgins TL, Estafanous FG, Loop FD, Beck GJ, Blum JM**, and **Paranandi L** (1992) Stratification of morbidity and mortality outcome by preoperative risk factors in coronary artery bypass patients. A clinical severity score. *JAMA* **267**(17), 2344–8.

22. **Farooq V, van Klaveren D, Steyerberg EW, Meliga E, Vergouwe Y, Chieffo A**, et al. (2013) Anatomical and clinical characteristics to guide decision making between coronary artery bypass surgery and percutaneous coronary intervention for individual patients: development and validation of SYNTAX score II. *Lancet* **381**(9867), 639–50.

23. **Palmerini T, Serruys P, Kappetein AP, Genereux P, Riva DD, Reggiani LB**, et al. (2017) Clinical outcomes with percutaneous coronary revascularization vs coronary artery bypass grafting surgery in patients with unprotected left main coronary artery disease: a meta-analysis of six randomized trials and 4686 patients. *Am Heart J* **190**, 54–63.

24. **Head SJ, Milojevic M, Daemen J, Ahn J-M, Boersma E, Christiansen EH**, et al. (2018) Mortality after coronary artery bypass grafting versus percutaneous coronary intervention with stenting for coronary artery disease: a pooled analysis of individual patient data. *Lancet* **391**, 939–48.

Chapter 12

Prognosis research in people with traumatic bleeding

Katherine I Morley and Pablo Perel

12.1 Definition of the health condition, startpoints, and endpoints

Physical trauma is the consequence of sudden injury to the body. Such injuries are a feature of everyday life, and much trauma is trivial or brief—a transient pain, a small bruise, a superficial graze to the skin—resolving rapidly with little treatment. Trauma as a clinical problem can be defined as injuries severe enough to need healthcare, including those that result in death before healthcare is received.

The urgent task is to recognize injured people at risk of early death or irreversible damage and disability, and to initiate appropriate treatment. Immediate questions are driven by prognostic concern—in particular, is the trauma immediately life threatening? Trauma care provides an example of stratified care, captured by the concept of 'triage'—assignment of degrees of urgency for prioritizing treatment. Treating everyone the same is not an option, since most people with an injury or wound will get better. If all patients with minor injuries bypass primary care ('over-triage'), hospitals will be overwhelmed. If major trauma victims are treated locally rather than stabilized and transported for high-level care ('under-triage'), avoidable deaths may occur (1).

The broadest startpoint for prognosis studies of trauma is the presence of a trauma-related injury at the instant it occurs. Injuries may happen in a civilian (e.g. road traffic crashes) or battlefield context, both requiring decision making in a short time frame, often without access to sophisticated diagnostic tests or procedures. Even when severe injuries are first encountered in a hospital setting, this is most likely to be in an emergency department, often with limited time to access sophisticated diagnostic tests.

Classifications of trauma or injury, such as the International Classification of Diseases, commonly start with causes (e.g. traffic accidents or fall), followed by anatomical location (e.g. head, lower limb), and type of injury (e.g. fracture, bleeding). Any of these may be a startpoint for prognosis studies. In this chapter we focus on traumatic bleeding (or haemorrhage), regardless of the cause or site of the injury.

The primary endpoint of interest in patients with traumatic bleeding is usually mortality, both early and late. Prevention of early mortality is a crucial target for immediate care in these patients, and directs the initial responses of emergency services, primary care, and hospital treatment. Early mortality may focus on pre-admission deaths or deaths within hours or days of hospital admission, but in prognosis research often includes deaths up to thirty days after admission.

Sometimes combined endpoints are used, for example when survival and disability are merged as 'years lived with disability'. This is done to evaluate long-term consequences of early survival following trauma (2). In patients with severe trauma who survive, dependency status is often characterized by measures such as the Modified Oxford Handicap Scale (3). This consists of five categories: (i) no symptoms; (ii) minor symptoms; (iii) some restriction in lifestyle but independent; (iv) dependent but not requiring constant attention; (v) fully dependent requiring attention day and night (3).

12.2 Overall prognosis of people with traumatic bleeding

Estimates of overall prognosis in individuals with traumatic bleeding are important for the evaluation of current emergency care, and for monitoring progress, or lack of progress, in reducing early mortality and avoidable long-term disability associated with injury. Haagsma et al. estimated that globally 4.8 million people died within one year following traumatic injury in 2013; most of these deaths were in low and middle-income countries (4). A similar proportion of the deaths was observed before (52%) and after (48%) admission to hospital. Register-based follow-up studies provide estimates of overall prognosis in particular healthcare systems, for example 9% early mortality among 80,544 patients in the Major Trauma Outcome Study in North American hospitals between 1982 and 1987 (5). Such figures will vary with setting, time period, and type of population included.

Severe blood loss is the most common cause of early death post-trauma (6). Uncontrolled post-traumatic bleeding accounts for the most deaths within the first hour of clinical care, and more than 50% of all trauma-related deaths in civilian and military settings within the first forty-eight hours after hospital admission (6, 7). Current UK prognosis in patients with traumatic bleeding comes from a recent study across twenty-two UK hospitals (8). The startpoint was 'need for massive transfusion' (defined as four units of packed red blood cells) within twenty-four hours of admission. The mortality within the subsequent twenty-four hours was 17.9%.

These statistics on early mortality clearly indicate that identifying trauma patients with haemorrhage at high risk of death, and initiating appropriate management to improve prognosis, is a time-critical task (9). Clinical guidelines recommend that on-scene care should not exceed ten minutes and operations for visceral injuries should commence within sixty minutes of admission (10). However, despite these recommendations, uncontrolled haemorrhage due to missed diagnosis or delayed intervention remains a leading cause of preventable death in trauma patients (11).

12.3 Prognostic factors for people with traumatic bleeding

The importance of research into prognostic factors for the endpoints of individuals with traumatic bleeding relates to the concern to characterize easily measurable factors in emergency settings that are associated with these endpoints. Such knowledge could yield new targets for treatment, and contribute to prognostic models for deciding best treatment for an individual patient. These prognostic factors can be divided into four groups: patient demographic characteristics, injury characteristics, physiological variables, and biomarkers (near-patient, laboratory, or imaging tests).

Age is a strong prognostic factor for mortality in patients with traumatic bleeding, with older patients at increased risk (12, 13). Severity of injury and time from injury to treatment are also positively associated with mortality risk (12). Type of injury is a prognostic factor, for example significant injury in more than one body region ('polytrauma') is associated with higher early mortality. Some pre-existing co-morbidities, such as renal disease, are also associated with higher rates of early death. Level of consciousness assessed by the Glasgow Coma Scale (GCS) is a prognostic factor for early death after traumatic bleeding, with lower scores associated with worse outcomes (13–15).

Extent, rapidity, and persistence of blood loss are important determinants of early mortality following trauma, and various measures have been investigated because of their association with blood loss and its effects. These include simple measures of falling blood volume (low or dropping systolic blood pressure; rapid or rising heart rate (13, 14)), or of reduced oxygen delivery to body tissues and rise in their acidity (rapid or rising respiratory rate) (16). Biomarker tests provide other measures of blood loss (e.g. haemoglobin) and its metabolic consequences for body tissues (lactic acid and ratio of base-to-acid (12, 13)), and of blood-clotting capacity (e.g. fibrinogen). Other prognostic factors under investigation include blood glucose, potassium levels, inflammatory markers, and genetic components of the inflammatory response.

Some of the above prognostic factors are purely descriptive, such as age and type of injury, and others represent potential targets for intervention (e.g. markers of blood loss) as they may be on the causal pathway between traumatic bleeding and early death. No single prognostic factor is strongly predictive of mortality on its own, and combinations of factors are needed within prognostic models for more precisely estimating mortality risk in individual patients with traumatic bleeding, and as the basis for stratified care.

12.4 Prognostic models for people with traumatic bleeding

Prognostic models are important for supporting rapid decisions in individual patients with traumatic bleeding. We here describe the development and validation of a specific model. It was designed for civilian and battlefield settings across countries of differing income levels (17). Most models available at the time of the study (the first decade of the twenty-first century) depended on data collected decades previously and had methodological limitations (1). Treatments had changed, and the mean age of trauma patients in high-income countries had increased. Although most trauma-related deaths were occurring in low and middle-income countries, most prognostic models at the time were based on data from high-income countries. The new model was based on information that could be collected rapidly after injury. Its presentation needed to be straightforward and user friendly for decision making at an early stage, for example on the scene of trauma.

12.4.1 Model development

First, semi-structured interviews were conducted with potential end users of the prognostic model: paramedics, military doctors, and consultants in emergency medicine (17). These meetings informed both selection of potential predictors to be studied for inclusion in the model, and user-friendly presentation of results. Selection of potential predictors was also informed by the available literature.

The sample, on which the prognostic model was to be developed, was drawn from the Clinical Randomization of an Antifibrinolytic in Significant Haemorrhage (CRASH-2) study, a large (N = 20,207) trial recruiting from 274 hospitals in 40 countries to evaluate the effect of tranexamic acid on mortality and the need for transfusion among trauma patients with significant bleeding

(18). (Tranexamic acid is a drug used to promote clotting at the site of a haemorrhage, whilst transfusion of blood products may have paradoxical harms as well as benefits for patients with traumatic bleeding.) The trial included patients within eight hours of injury and data on outcome at hospital discharge with a high follow-up rate (99%). Data collected at hospital admission included: demographic characteristics (age and sex); characteristics of the injury (type of injury and time from injury to randomization); and physiological variables (Glasgow Coma Scale score, systolic blood pressure, heart rate, respiratory rate).

The endpoint for the prognostic model was death in hospital during four weeks after injury (n = 3076 endpoints). A multivariable logistic regression framework and backwards selection including all potential predictors was used to identify the strongest set of predictors. Glasgow Coma Scale score, systolic blood pressure, and age were the three strongest predictors. Heart rate, respiratory rate, and hours since injury were associated with mortality and also included in the final model. All these predictors of early mortality were considered measurable in patients in low and middle-income countries and in battlefield situations (19).

12.4.2 Internal validation of the model's predictive performance

Apparent calibration performance of the developed model was assessed graphically by plotting the observed outcomes in the CRASH-2 dataset against predicted probabilities of the outcome from the model, grouped in tenths of predicted risk (Figure 12.1a). The model had good apparent calibration, except in patients at very high risk, for whom the model overpredicted risk (17). Discrimination was given by an apparent C statistic of 0.836 (17). Optimism in model performance was assessed using bootstrap re-sampling with 200 samples. The optimism-adjusted C statistic was 0.835, only slightly lower than the apparent value, indicating very low optimism (overfitting) in the model developed, and reflecting the large number of patients who developed the endpoint (19).

12.4.3 External validation

External validation was evaluated using data from patients presenting between 2000 and 2008 in the Trauma Audit and Research Network (TARN), which includes 60% of hospitals receiving trauma patients in England and Wales, and some hospitals in Europe (19). This setting reflected a more complete (i.e. register-based compared with trial recruitment) sample of patients within a healthcare system compared with the development sample, but was more restricted in the number of healthcare systems represented and their geographical

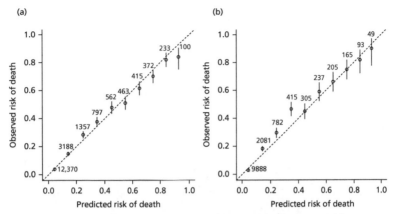

Figure 12.1 Calibration performance of the CRASH-2 prognostic model for patients with traumatic bleeding (a) internal validation using CRASH-2 trial, and (b) external validation using TARN register data.

Source: reproduced with permisson from Perel, P., et al. Predicting early death in patients with traumatic bleeding: development and validation of prognostic model. BMJ Clinical Research Edition. 2012(345), e5166. Copyright © 2012 BMJ

spread than the intended setting for model application in practice. Data in TARN are collected on patients who arrive at hospital alive and either: (1) die from injury during admission; (2) stay in hospital for longer than three days; (3) require intensive or high-dependency care or inter-hospital transfer for specialist care.

The physiological data available in TARN are identical to those in the CRASH-2 trial, except that significant haemorrhage is not defined. Consequently, only adult patients with an estimated blood loss of at least 20% were included (considered clinically comparable to CRASH-2 trial patients). The TARN data had substantially more missing predictor data than the CRASH-2 trial, so multiple imputation was used. Discrimination of the model when tested in the validation sample showed a *C* statistic of 0.88 and a good calibration (Figure 12.1b).

12.4.4 **Model presentation**

The CRASH-2 model for traumatic bleeding is made available as an online risk calculation tool (http://crash2.lshtm.ac.uk) which provides an estimated risk of death for individual patients. However, potential users also requested a simple version for bedside use. This included the three strongest predictors (Glasgow Coma Scale score, systolic blood pressure, and age), and was developed for patients within three hours of injury and stratified by economic region (Figure 12.2). This is displayed as a chart, cross tabulating the

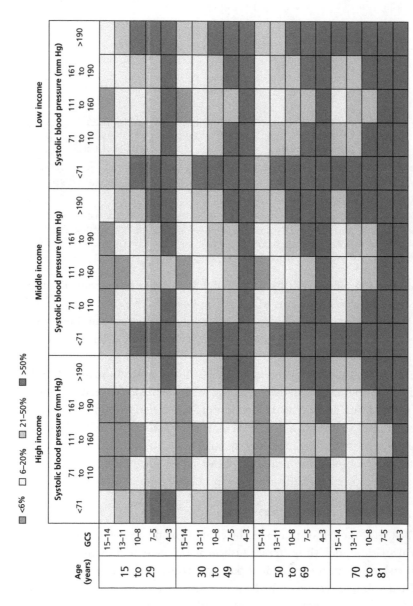

Figure 12.2 Chart to predict death up to 28 days after trauma in patient with traumatic bleeding

Source: data from Clinical randomisation of antifibrinolytic in significant haemorrhage. available at: http:// crash2.lshtm.ac.uk Copyright © 2017 london school of hygiene & tropical Medicine.

predictors, and shading each cell by probability of death by 28 days post-trauma in four groups, based on feedback from users and previous publications. There are, to date, no formal studies of the impact of the use of the model on decision making or patient outcomes.

12.5 Predicting effects of treatment in people with traumatic bleeding

The best immediate management of individuals with traumatic bleeding remains controversial because of the hazards involved. Identifying whether particular treatments benefit or harm specific patients is an important task for prognosis research in helping to tailor treatment for the individual. Here we take red blood cell (RBC) transfusion as an example.

Red blood cell (RBC) transfusion is used in the management of bleeding trauma patients, but it is a scarce and expensive intervention with potential adverse effects, including allergic reaction, transfusion-related lung injury, graft versus host disease, and infection (20). A systematic review suggested that RBC transfusion is associated with increased morbidity and mortality in critically ill patients, including trauma patients (21), so the effect of RBC transfusion may depend on baseline mortality risk.

Perel and colleagues hypothesized a beneficial effect of RBC transfusion among patients at high risk of death (poor prognosis), but a harmful effect in those patients at low risk of death (20). In the CRASH-2 trial described above, patients were randomized to tranexamic acid or placebo, but received other management, including RBC transfusion, by clinician choice. So the full CRASH-2 cohort could be used for an observational study of differential outcomes between cohort participants who did and did not receive RBC transfusion treatment. The CRASH-2 prognostic model was then used to stratify participants who were treated within three hours of injury into ten strata of increasing baseline (i.e. untreated) estimated 28-day mortality risk, each containing approximately one-tenth of the observed primary outcome. The association of RBC transfusion with deaths from all causes was then estimated within each risk stratum (Figure 12.3). In patients with a low risk, transfusion was associated with an increase in all-cause mortality compared with those who did not receive transfusion, while in patients with high predicted risk, transfusion was associated with reduced mortality compared with those not transfused.

Practical implications drawn in the original paper from this result were cautious because of the observational nature of the comparison between transfused and non-transfused participants in the CRASH-2 cohort, but suggested that

Risk category	Predicted 28-day mortality risk (%)		Deaths according to transfusion status	
			Transfusion	No transfusion
1	<6.1%		223/3479	68/5367
2	(6.1% to <10%)		242/1911	58/1651
3	(10.0% to <15.4%)		202/1260	89/851
4	(15.4% to <22.8%)		210/966	90/543
5	(22.8% to <31.3%)		195/698	101/386
6	(31.3% to <42.1%)		175/511	120/282
7	(42.1% to <53.7%)		172/360	125/227
8	(53.7% to <65.4%)		181/327	113/191
9	(65.4% to 77.8%)		176/301	120/164
10	>77.8%		155/219	140/163

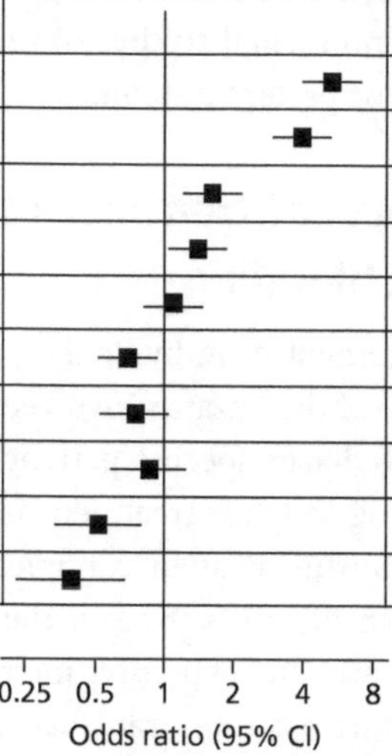

0.25 0.5 1 2 4 8
Odds ratio (95% CI)

Risk categories created with approximately an equal number of deaths in each of the 10 categories

Figure 12.3 Predicting effects of treatment: transfusion.

Source: reproduced from Perel, P., et al. Red Blood Cell Transfusion and Mortality in Trauma Patients: Risk-Stratified Analysis of an Observational Study. PLoS Medicine. 11(6):e1001664. Copyright © 2014 PLoS. Open Access.

using RBC transfusion may be hazardous in very-low-risk patients and beneficial in patients with a high mortality risk (20).

This example illustrates the challenge of interpreting research on differential treatment effects. It may indeed be that there is a different treatment effect defined by the baseline risk categories, but the observed results could alternatively represent different absolute effects arising solely from the different baseline risks. Higher baseline risks can result in different odds ratios because odds ratios are sensitive to event prevalence (22). See the related discussion in Chapter 4.

12.6 **Summary**

Traumatic bleeding represents a major threat to life. Many deaths are avoidable with timely treatment, and a major challenge for healthcare is to ensure that the most effective healthcare is delivered by the most efficient means in emergency settings. Prognosis research has a crucial role to play in monitoring the effectiveness and efficiency of current trauma care, and in providing up-to-date useful models that estimate an individual's risk of poor outcomes well enough to guide civilian and professional emergency care practice that improves outcomes. The impact of using such models on healthcare practice has yet to be fully established.

References

1. Rehn M, Perel P, Blackhall K, and Lossius HM (2011) Prognostic models for the early care of trauma patients: a systematic review. *Scand J Trauma Resusc Emerg Med* **19**(17),17.

2. Mitra B, Gabbe BJ, Kaukonen K-M, Olaussen A, Cooper DJ, and Cameron PA (2014) Long-term outcomes of patients receiving a massive transfusion after trauma. *Shock* **42**(4), 307–12.

3. Perel P, Edwards P, Shakur H, and Roberts I (2008) Use of the Oxford Handicap Scale at hospital discharge to predict Glasgow Outcome Scale at six months in patients with traumatic brain injury. *BMC Med Res Methodol* **8**(1), 72.

4. Haagsma JA, Graetz N, Bolliger I, Naghavi M, Higashi H, Mullany EC, et al. (2016) The global burden of injury: incidence, mortality, disability-adjusted life years and time trends from the Global Burden of Disease study 2013. *Inj Prev* **22**(1), 3–18.

5. Champion HR, Copes WS, Sacco WJ, Lawnick MM, and Keast SL (1990) The Major Trauma Outcome Study: establishing national norms for trauma care. *J Trauma* **30**, 1356–65.

6. Kauvar DS, Lefering R, and Wade CE (2006) Impact of hemorrhage on trauma outcome: an overview of epidemiology, clinical presentations, and therapeutic considerations. *J Trauma* **60**(6 Suppl), S3–11.

7. Sauaia AMD, Moore FAMD, Moore EEMD, Moser KSPRA, Brennan RRNMS, Read RAMD, et al. (1995) Epidemiology of trauma deaths: a reassessment. *J Trauma* **38**(2), 185–93.

8. Stanworth SJ, Davenport R, Curry N, Seeney F, Eaglestone S, Edwards A, et al. (2016) Mortality from trauma haemorrhage and opportunities for improvement in transfusion practice. *Brit J Surg* **103**(4), 357–65.

9. van der Velden MWA, Ringburg AN, Bergs EA, Steyerberg EW, Patka P, and Schipper IB (2008) Prehospital interventions: time wasted or time saved? An observational cohort study of management in initial trauma care. *Emerg Med J* **25**(7), 444–9.

10. The Royal College of Surgeons of England, British Orthopaedic Association (2000) *Better Care for the Severely Injured.* London: Royal College of Surgeons of England, British Orthopaedic Association.

11. Mabry R and McManus JG (2009) Prehospital advances in the management of severe penetrating trauma. *J Spec Oper Med* **9**(2), 93–101.

12. Lichtveld RA, Panhuizen IF, Smit RBJ, Holtslag HR, and Van Der Werken C (2007) Predictors of death in trauma patients who are alive on arrival at hospital. *Eur J Trauma Emerg Surg* **33**(1), 46–51.

13. Kondo Y, Abe T, Kohshi K, Tokuda Y, Cook EF, and Kukita I (2011) Revised trauma scoring system to predict in-hospital mortality in the emergency department: Glasgow Coma Scale, Age, and Systolic Blood Pressure score. *Crit Care* **15**(R191), 1–8.

14. **Rainer TH, Ho AMH, Yeung JHH, Cheung NK, Wong RSM, Tang N**, et al. (2011) Early risk stratification of patients with major trauma requiring massive blood transfusion. *Resuscitation* **82**(6), 724–9.

15. **Dutton RP** (2007) Current concepts in hemorrhagic shock. *Anesthesiol Clin* **25**(1), 23–34.

16. **Gale SC, Kocik JF, Creath R, Crystal JS**, and **Dombrovskiy VY** (2016) A comparison of initial lactate and initial base deficit as predictors of mortality after severe blunt trauma. *J Surg Res* **205**(2), 446–55.

17. **Perel P, Prieto-Merino D, Shakur H, Clayton T, Lecky F, Bouamra O**, et al. (2012) Predicting early death in patients with traumatic bleeding: development and validation of prognostic model. *BMJ* **345**(1), e5166–e.

18. **Roberts I, Shakur H, Coats T, Hunt B, Balogun E, Barnetson L**, et al. (2013) The CRASH-2 trial: a randomized controlled trial and economic evaluation of the effects of tranexamic acid on death, vascular occlusive events and transfusion requirement in bleeding trauma patients. *Health Technol Assess* **17**(10), 1–79.

19. **Perel P, Prieto-Merino D, Shakur H**, and **Roberts I** (2013) Development and validation of a prognostic model to predict death in patients with traumatic bleeding, and evaluation of the effect of tranexamic acid on mortality according to baseline risk: a secondary analysis of a randomised controlled trial. *Health Technol Assess* **17**(24).

20. **Perel P, Clayton T, Altman DG, Croft P, Douglas I, Hemingway H**, et al. (2014) Red blood cell transfusion and mortality in trauma patients: risk-stratified analysis of an observational study. *PLoS Med* **11**(6), e1001664–e.

21. **Marik PE** and **Corwin HL** (2008) Efficacy of red blood cell transfusion in the critically ill: a systematic review of the literature. *Crit Care Med* **36**(9), 2667–74.

22. **Shrier I** and **Pang M** (2015) Confounding, effect modification, and the odds ratio: common misinterpretations. *J Clin Epidemiol* **68**(4), 470–4.

Part 5

Novel topics in prognosis research

Chapter 13

Individual participant data meta-analysis of prognosis studies

Richard D Riley, Thomas PA Debray, and Karel GM Moons

13.1 Introduction

Chapter 9 highlighted that meta-analysis of *aggregate data* (e.g. estimates of hazard ratios, C statistics, or treatment-covariate interactions) from published prognosis research is often hampered by poor reporting and quality of the primary studies, and much heterogeneity in their design, conduct, and analysis methods (1–3). Here, we consider an alternative approach: the meta-analysis of *individual participant data* (IPD), where the raw individual-level data are obtained from primary studies or data sources, and then synthesized to answer the prognosis questions at hand (4, 5). For prognosis studies IPD would typically include participant values of (potential) prognostic factors (e.g. age, sex, treatment, biomarker values) measured at baseline (startpoint), alongside follow-up information and details of any outcomes. The IPD approach is increasingly feasible (5–7), as data sharing and open data approaches are growing in appeal (8–14). For prognosis research, this is allowing more reliable and robust evidence-based findings than previously possible using only published aggregate results. A leading example is the IMPACT (International Mission for Prognosis and Analysis of Clinical Trials) consortium, who share IPD from multiple studies to examine prognostic factors and to develop and validate prognostic models for patients with traumatic brain injury (15).

Here, we outline the key steps within an IPD meta-analysis for prognosis research.

13.2 What does an IPD meta-analysis project involve?

All IPD meta-analysis projects should consider whether ethical approval is required (10), and be registered, protocol-driven, and have a suitable statistical analysis plan for primary and secondary research questions. The stages thereafter include the identification of relevant studies or data sources; obtaining, cleaning, and harmonizing the IPD of the different studies and datasets; meta-analysis of the IPD and presentation of meta-analysis results; and consideration of implications for healthcare and further research (Box 13.1).

Box 13.1 Necessary stages of an IPD meta-analysis for prognosis research

- Define the primary and secondary prognosis research questions, and establish why an IPD meta-analysis is required (rather than a traditional meta-analysis of published aggregate data).
- Obtain ethical approval where considered necessary.
- Register the IPD project and publish a protocol, including analysis plan for primary and secondary outcomes.
- Identify relevant datasets from published and unpublished studies (preferably using a systematic review), or data sources (e.g. patient registries).
- Set-up of a collaborating group involving investigators providing IPD.
- Classify the risk of bias for each study or dataset, for example using tools such as QUIPS or PROBAST.
- Request and receive anonymized IPD from identified studies or data sources. Before receiving data, signed data sharing agreements will usually be required between the host institution and those other institutions providing IPD.
- Check and clean the IPD received, often requiring regular communication with original investigators.
- Harmonize IPD across studies and data sources (e.g. outcome definitions, coding of variables), and finalize eligible IPD for primary and secondary analyses.
- Perform statistical analyses to obtain results that address research questions, in particular, one-stage or two-stage IPD meta-analyses.
- Examine the magnitude and causes of any between-study heterogeneity.
- Perform sensitivity analyses to key assumptions.
- Examine potential biases and their impact (e.g. publication bias, unavailable IPD for some studies).
- Report and disseminate findings, including implications for healthcare and further research.

Source: reproduced courtesy of Richard D Riley.

Obtaining, cleaning, and harmonizing IPD from multiple prognosis studies or data sources may take considerable time (16). A crucial step is deciding how much IPD is needed. Potentially the most rigorous option is to adopt a systematic review approach, where *all* relevant published and unpublished studies, or indeed any relevant data sources, are identified through a transparent, systematic search on the prognosis question at hand. Then, investigators or data source holders are contacted to provide their IPD. Another option is to first establish a collaboration of research groups who agree to pool their resources to answer specific prognosis questions. For example, an IPD meta-analysis of prognostic markers in breast cancer (17) was facilitated by eighteen datasets provided by members of the Receptor and Biomarker Group within the European Organization for Research and Treatment of Cancer. It is important for such collaborations to be inclusive. In both instances, data sharing agreements are necessary between the host institution and those other institutions providing their IPD, detailing the project aims, the requirements (and timescale) for providing IPD and responding to queries, the process for disseminating results and the timescale for feedback, the publication and authorship strategy, and any financial commitments.

The quality and applicability of IPD obtained should also be examined, using risk of bias and data extraction tools (such as CHARMS, QUIPS and PROBAST (18–20), see Chapter 9), focusing on the domains relating to the participant selection, study design, and specification of startpoints, outcomes, and predictors. Where resources are limited for the IPD projects, it may be sensible to undertake these assessments in advance of IPD collection, to identify the most applicable and high-quality studies to prioritize for IPD retrieval.

Once the IPD is cleaned and harmonized, statistical methods can be used to undertake the meta-analysis. It is inappropriate to simply analyse the IPD as if all coming from a single study. A correct IPD meta-analysis preserves the clustering of patients within studies (data sources), using either a one-stage or a two-stage approach (21, 22). In the two-stage approach, the IPD are first analysed separately in each study or data source using an appropriate statistical method for the type of data being analysed; for example for continuous outcomes such as pain score a linear regression model might be fitted, or for time-to-event data such as mortality a Cox regression might be applied. This produces aggregate data for each primary study or dataset relevant to the question of interest (such as a hazard ratio estimate for a potential prognostic factor, a C statistic estimate for a prognostic model, or a treatment-covariate interaction estimate for a potential treatment effect modifier) alongside its standard error or confidence interval. These study-specific estimates are then synthesized in the second stage using a suitable model for meta-analysis of aggregate data, such as a random effects meta-analysis as outlined in Chapter 9.

In the one-stage approach, the IPD from all studies or data sources are modelled simultaneously whilst accounting for the clustering of participants within studies/data sources. This again requires a model specific to the type of data being synthesized, alongside appropriate specification of the meta-analysis assumptions (e.g. random effects to allow for between-study heterogeneity). When they make the same assumptions and use the same estimation methods, one-stage and two-stage methods usually give very similar results (23–25). PRISMA-IPD provides reporting guidelines for IPD meta-analysis of randomized trials, and most of these are also relevant for IPD meta-analysis of prognosis studies. They should, however, be considered alongside the reporting guidelines for prognosis studies: REMARK and TRIPOD (26, 27).

13.3 What are the advantages of an IPD meta-analysis for prognosis research?

Box 13.2 summarizes the potential advantages of having IPD for meta-analysis of prognosis research compared to using published aggregate data (5, 6, 28–30).

Box 13.2 Key advantages of having IPD for meta-analysis of prognosis studies compared to traditional meta-analysis of published aggregate data

- ◆ Encourages greater collaboration across researchers, and increases the opportunity to identify and incorporate unpublished studies or data sources, thereby increasing total sample size (and number of events).
- ◆ Allows communication with original study investigators to clarify aspects such as the underlying design, recruitment strategy, startpoint/outcome definitions, and follow-up.
- ◆ Allows more consistent participant inclusion and exclusion criteria across studies/datasets, and, if appropriate, reinstates individuals into the analysis who were originally excluded.
- ◆ Enables results presented in the original study publications to be verified, and may allow a more enhanced assessment of each study's risk of bias.
- ◆ Uses up-to-date follow-up information, which is potentially longer than used in the original study publications, and may address more outcomes.
- ◆ Improves the identification of data from the same participants in multiple studies or data sources.

Box 13.2 Continued

- Improves standardization of the definitions of prognostic factors and outcomes across studies or data sources.

- Allows the calculation of results (e.g. hazard ratios or calibration plots) previously not reported in sufficient detail; it may thus reduce the problem of selective within-study reporting.

- Allows the calculation of results for unpublished studies providing IPD; it may thus reduce the problem of publication bias (small-study effects).

- Allows the use of multiple imputation to deal with missing data (factors or outcomes), which is often not done in primary studies, and if desired to borrow information across datasets (e.g. in case of systematically missing variables in some datasets).

- Ability to standardize the strategy of statistical analysis across datasets and potentially improve upon the methods used in original publications, to reduce statistical heterogeneity. Notably, choice of regression model, analysis of time-to-event data, handling of continuous prognostic factors, consideration of interactions and choice of time points assessed.

- Ability to assess statistical assumptions in each dataset, such as proportional hazards in Cox regression models, and model complex relationships like time-dependent prognostic factors.

- Ability to derive prognostic factor associations adjusted for other prognostic factors, where previously only unadjusted estimates were available.

- Enables a more consistent set of adjustment factors across datasets.

- Improved ability to examine causes of heterogeneity in prognostic factor effects across individuals and across datasets.

- Improved ability to develop and validate prognostic models; to compare relative performance of different prognostic models head-to-head; to examine the need for model updating strategies (e.g. recalibration, revision, or inclusion of new predictors).

- Obtain meta-analysis results for specific subgroups of participants across datasets (e.g. those receiving a particular treatment, those with a particular biomarker level), and assess differential effects across individuals (in particular, estimate treatment-covariate interactions).

Box 13.2 Continued

- Perform advanced statistical approaches where necessary, for example competing risks analysis, joint modelling of survival and longitudinal data, and accounting for multiple (correlated) data points per individual.

- Discuss the implications of findings with the wide network of investigators involved.

Source: reproduced courtesy of Richard D. Riley, drawing on ideas in Tierney JF, et al. (2015) Individual Participant Data (IPD) meta-analyses of randomized controlled trials: guidance on their use. *PLoS Medicine* 12(7), e1001855. Copyright © 2015 PLoS; Debray TP, et al. (2015) A new framework to enhance the interpretation of external validation studies of clinical prediction models. *Journal of Clinical Epidemiology* 68(3), 279–89. Copyright © 2015 Elsevier; Ahmed I, et al. (2014) Developing and validating risk prediction models in an individual participant data meta-analysis. *BMC Medical Research Methodology* 14(3). Copyright © 2014 BMC. Open Access; Abo-Zaid G, et al. (2012) Individual participant data meta-analysis of prognostic factor studies: state of the art? *BMC Medical Research Methodology* 12(56). Copyright © 2012 BMC. Open Access; and Riley RD, et al. (2010) Meta-analysis of individual participant data: rationale, conduct, and reporting. *BMJ* 340, c221. Copyright © 2010 BMJ

13.3.1 Overall prognosis

For overall prognosis research, the notable potential advantage of IPD is to standardize the participant inclusion and exclusion criteria and outcome definitions, and thereby improve the translation and relevance of overall prognosis meta-analysis results (e.g. summary risks and rates) for specific populations and settings. For example, IPD from multiple randomized trials and observational studies enabled the IMPACT consortium to standardize summaries of the Glasgow Coma Scale at six months following a traumatic brain injury; in particular, to examine the odds of each category of the outcome scale, and avoid categorizations used in the original study publications (31). IPD also allows specific subgroups of individuals to be identified (e.g. ethnic groups, particular treatment groups), so that overall prognosis summaries can be broken down to relevant subgroups, settings, and aspects of current care (e.g. across countries or settings). For example, the IMPACT collaborators summarized the distribution of the Glasgow Coma Scale at six months for patients with and without secondary insults of hypoxia, hypotension, and hypothermia (32).

13.3.2 Prognostic factors

For prognostic factor research, particular advantages of IPD include the ability to derive adjusted prognostic factor estimates (e.g. hazard ratios); to adjust for a more consistent set of adjustment factors across studies; to analyse continuous factors on their original scale rather than using categorizations applied in the original study publication; to check whether non-linear prognostic factor associations exist; and to examine consistency of findings across datasets, studies, or settings. This leads to more meaningful meta-analysis results about prognostic factors, and thus improves their translation to improved healthcare, decision making, and research.

A notable IPD meta-analysis for prognostic factor research is by Trivella et al. (33), who obtained IPD from seventeen (published and unpublished) studies, involving a total of 3200 patients, to examine whether microvessel-density counts (a measure of angiogenesis) is a prognostic factor for disease-free or overall survival in patients with non-small-cell lung carcinoma. Across studies there were two different approaches to counting: the 'all vessels' method and the Chalkley method. A two-stage IPD meta-analysis was applied to summarize the prognostic effect of microvessel density (analysed on a continuous scale), for each measurement method separately (Figure 13.1), adjusting for age and stage of disease. There was no evidence of non-linearity in the prognostic effect. For the Chalkley method, the summary adjusted HR was 1.05 (95% CI: 1.01–1.09; $I^2 = 0\%$), suggesting that a one-count increase in microvessel density was associated with an increased rate of death. For the all vessels method, and in relation to a ten-count increase, the summary adjusted HR was 1.03 (95% CI: 0.97–1.09; $I^2 = 74\%$), providing no clear evidence of prognostic value. This contradicts the results of an earlier meta-analysis using published aggregate data which gave summary results strongly in favour of a prognostic effect. The IPD meta-analysis is more reliable as it utilizes unpublished studies, analyses microvessel density on its continuous scale, adjusts for stage and age, and considers each method of measurement separately.

13.3.3 Prognostic models

IPD from multiple studies or data sources also allows us to develop prognostic models with larger sample sizes (outcome events), which will reduce the potential for overfitting. Further, novel validation approaches can be used to examine prediction model performance in diverse settings and populations, and thus to assess the model's generalizability (34–37). In particular, irrespective of whether a new model is being developed or an existing model is being validated, IPD allows researchers to examine whether model predictions are sufficiently accurate across different locations, settings, and case mix. Ideally, such endeavour would reveal that model performance is not merely satisfactory on average, but also does consistently well across different subgroups, populations, and settings (37). If model performance is shown to be inadequate in some situations, IPD enables model updating strategies, such as recalibration of the model's intercept or shrinkage of the linear predictor, to be examined, rather than simply discarding the model outright (38). The benefit of adding a particular prognostic factor or novel biomarker to an existing model could also be considered (39).

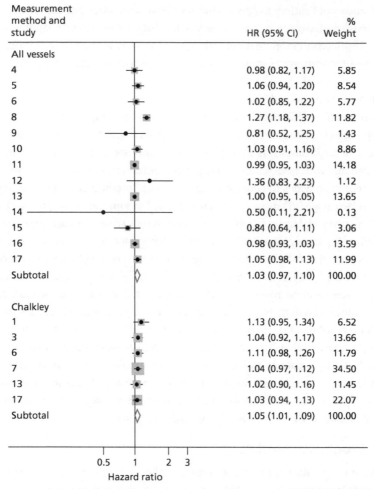

All hazard ratios (HRs) show the prognostic effect of microvessel density count adjusted for stage and age. For Chalkley the HR relates to a 1 count increase, and for all vessels the HR relates to a 10 count increase. Summary results are derived using a two-stage IPD meta-analysis. In the first stage, a multivariable Cox regression model was used to obtain a log HR estimate and its standard error for microvessel density, adjusted for stage and age (as a continuous variable). In the second stage, a random effects model was used to pool the log HR estimates. Over and above the original analysis by Trivella et al. we used the Hartung-Knapp approach to derive 95% confidence intervals.

Figure 13.1 Forest plot showing the study estimates and the meta-analysis results for the prognostic effect of micro-vessel density in regard to mortality in patients with non-small-cell lung carcinoma.

Source: data from Trivella, M., et al. Microvessel density as a prognostic factor in non-small-cell lung carcinoma: a meta-analysis of individual patient data. Lancet Oncology. 8(6):488-99. Copyright © Elsevier.

A particularly novel IPD meta-analysis approach for prognostic modelling is the 'internal-external cross-validation' framework proposed to directly address model validation and generalizability during its development (40, 41). Let us assume the IPD comes from k studies. Then, internal-external cross-validation proceeds by using IPD from all but one of the k studies for model development, with IPD from the remaining study used for external validation; this is repeated a further k-1 times, on each occasion omitting a different study to ascertain external validation performance. Each cycle should ensure an adequate sample size for model development (42–44) and the use of appropriate model derivation techniques (e.g. adjustment for optimism) (45, 46), otherwise, poor performance may simply reflect small sample sizes, overfitting, and substandard development techniques. The cross-validation process may reveal that a developed model works consistently well in all settings and populations; in that case, a final model can be developed from the complete set of IPD. However, the process may also reveal that the model has unreliable predictive performance in IPD from some settings or populations with a particular case mix (35), which signals that model updating strategies are needed to improve performance in such settings/populations, or even that IPD from some settings/populations should be removed to ensure a robust model is developed for the others (35, 38, 47).

For example, Snell et al. (36) used IPD from eight countries to externally validate a prediction model of mortality risk over time in breast cancer patients. They identified large between-country heterogeneity in overall calibration performance, as evidenced by a wide 95% prediction interval for the overall calibration in a particular country of application (0.41–1.58) (Figure 13.2a). However, consistency in calibration performance was dramatically improved after recalibration of the original baseline hazard function (Figure 13.2b), with a narrow 95% prediction interval close to 1 for the overall calibration (0.93–1.08).

13.3.4 Predictors of treatment effect

A major advantage of IPD (rather than aggregate data) from randomized or observational studies on the effects of therapeutic interventions is that it provides within-study information to estimate how patients' prognostic factors or characteristics modify (interact with) treatment effect (48, 49). Subgroups of patients with a common characteristic (e.g. same gender or co-morbidity) can be identified within IPD, and thus meta-analysis results derived specifically for them. Moreover, the *differences* in treatment effect between subgroups or prognostic factor values (treatment-covariate interactions) can be derived directly using individual-level data. For example, an IPD meta-analysis was used to identify that those breast cancer patients who are hormone receptor positive are more likely to respond to tamoxifen treatment than those who are negative (50). It also allows continuous variables to be analysed on their continuous scale, and for potential non-linear treatment-covariate interactions to be modelled.

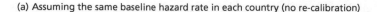

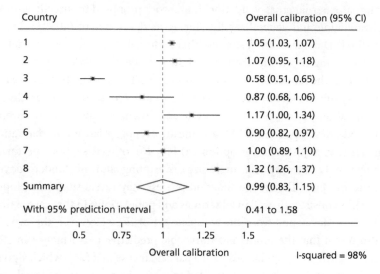

(a) Assuming the same baseline hazard rate in each country (no re-calibration)

Country	Overall calibration (95% CI)
1	1.05 (1.03, 1.07)
2	1.07 (0.95, 1.18)
3	0.58 (0.51, 0.65)
4	0.87 (0.68, 1.06)
5	1.17 (1.00, 1.34)
6	0.90 (0.82, 0.97)
7	1.00 (0.89, 1.10)
8	1.32 (1.26, 1.37)
Summary	0.99 (0.83, 1.15)
With 95% prediction interval	0.41 to 1.58

Overall calibration

I-squared = 98%

(b) Allowing a different baseline hazard rate for each country (re-calibration)

Country	Overall calibration (95% CI)
1	0.98 (0.95, 1.00)
2	1.00 (0.89, 1.11)
3	1.03 (0.96, (1.10)
4	0.99 (0.80, 1.18)
5	0.95 (0.77, 1.12)
6	0.97 (0.90, 1.04)
7	1.05 (0.95, 1.16)
8	1.04 (0.98, 1.09)
Summary	1.00 (0.97, 1.04)
With 95% prediction interval	0.93 to 1.08

Overall calibration

I-squared = 35%

*Overall calibration should ideally be 1; it provides an overall measure of the discrepancy in the magnitude of the baseline hazard and the discrepancy in the effect of the model's linear predictor.

Figure 13.2 Overall* calibration performance of a prognostic model for mortality in breast cancer patients evaluated before and after recalibration of the baseline hazard rate in each country.

Source: reproduced from Snell KI, Hua H, Debray TP, et al. Multivariate meta-analysis of individual participant data helped externally validate the performance and implementation of a prediction model. Journal of Clinical Epidemiology. 2016(69):40-50. Copyright © Elsevier. Open Access.

Without IPD, usually researchers can only perform a meta-regression to estimate how the treatment effect estimates in each study (based on all participants)
are associated with aggregated (prognostic) factor values (such as mean age,
proportion males). Such aggregate across-study associations usually have low
power, and are prone to ecological bias and study-level confounding (51, 52),
and thus may not accurately reflect individual-level associations (53). This is illustrated in Figure 13.3 through an IPD meta-analysis of ten randomized trials
in hypertension patients, examining whether sex is a predictor of response to
anti-hypertensive treatment (54). The dramatic difference in within-study (flat
dashed lines) and across-study (steep solid line) relationships is due to the latter

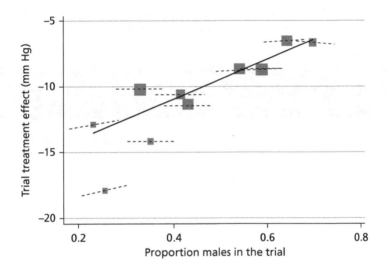

Across-trial association (from meta-regression of treatment effect versus
proportion of males) denoted by gradient of solid line (———); this suggests a
large improved effect of on average 15.10 mmHg (95% CI: 8.78 to 21.41) more
reduction in females compared to males.

Individual-level associations (treatment-sex interaction within each trial) denoted
by gradient of dashed lines (--------); on average they suggest a 0.89 mmHg
(95% CI: 0.07 to 1.30) better treatment effect for females than males, which is
small and clinically unimportant.

Each block represents one trial, and the block size is proportional to the size of
the trial.
Figure 13.3 Is blood pressure lowering treatment more effective amongst women
than men? Example from an IPD meta-analysis of ten hypertension trials showing
difference in across-trial association and individual-level association.
Source: data from Wang, JG., et al. Systolic and diastolic blood pressure lowering as determinants
of cardiovascular outcome. Hypertension. 45(5), 907-13. ©2005 American Heart Association, Inc.

having ecological bias and study-level confounding; those trials with a higher proportion of males are also systematically different in other characteristics such as age, co-morbidities, and treatment dose.

13.4 What are the challenges of an IPD meta-analysis of prognosis studies?

Though the advantages of an IPD meta-analysis for prognosis studies are exciting, it also comes with potential challenges. Abo Zaid et al. (30) and Ahmed et al. (29) previously reviewed published IPD meta-analyses of prognostic factors and prognostic models, respectively, and identified numerous logistical and methodological issues that can arise. These are summarized in Box 13.3. In particular, it often takes considerable time to collect and clean the data (55).

Box 13.3 Potential issues faced during an IPD meta-analysis of prognosis studies

- Time and resources necessary to obtain, clean, and standardize the IPD from multiple datasets.

- Costs of travel for collaborator meetings, employment of necessary expertise (e.g. health professionals, data managers, statisticians) to improve IPD provision, resolve data cleaning and standardization issues, and undertake the statistical analyses

- Obtaining ethical approval for the IPD project if considered necessary; this may include checking that primary studies have ethical approval to share their data for the purpose of the IPD project.

- Dilemma of seeking the IPD from *all* existing studies or data sources identified by a systematic review, or rather just the IPD from a subset of (convenient) yet representative (high-quality) studies.

- Identifying unpublished studies/data sources and avoiding publication bias (small-study effects) affecting the IPD obtained.

- Unavailability of IPD in some studies, and examining the impact of their absence on conclusions (potential availability bias).

- Examining a study's risk of bias (either before or after requesting/harmonizing IPD), for example using QUIPS or PROBAST, and deciding whether to restrict IPD meta-analyses (or even IPD collection) to studies at low risk of bias.

Box 13.3 Continued

- Dealing with some IPD that can be stored locally and other IPD that can only be accessed remotely (e.g. via secure servers).
- Dealing with different definitions of startpoints and outcomes across studies.
- Dealing with different timings and/or methods of measurement for a particular prognostic factor across studies.
- Dealing with different (or outdated) treatment strategies across studies, especially when a mixture of older and newer studies are combined.
- Dealing with complex statistical issues, such as:
  - partially missing values of prognostic factors and outcome data
  - completely (systematically) missing prognostic factors and outcomes in some studies
  - inconsistent coding of continuous variables across studies (e.g. some categorized and others left as continuous)
  - implementing/tailoring prognostic models in the presence of between-study heterogeneity
  - separating within-study and across-study associations when examining predictors of differential treatment response
  - examining and dealing with statistical heterogeneity

Source: reproduced courtesy of Richard D Riley.

IPD may not be obtained from all the identified studies and sources, yet, ignoring the evidence of such studies may lead to data availability bias (30, 56). Meta-analysis methods for combining IPD with aggregate data from non-IPD studies may be useful in such situations (24, 56–61). Another challenge is dealing with 'systematically missing' prognostic factors, where some factors are entirely unavailable (not recorded for any individuals) in some of the datasets. One then needs to either restrict analyses to only those prognostic factors included in all datasets, or (if considered appropriate) use advanced methods of multiple imputation to impute their values by borrowing information from datasets that do provide them (62, 63).

Finally, a critical issue in IPD meta-analyses (as in aggregate data meta-analyses) is dealing with statistical heterogeneity. In particular, if the meta-analysis reveals that a prognostic factor's effect or a prognostic model's performance is highly inconsistent across studies, summary (overall) meta-analysis results may have limited usefulness. However, this in itself is an important finding, and encourages researchers to use their IPD to identify the causes of heterogeneity and improve (tailor) prognostic results across different settings and (sub)populations, as illustrated in Box 13.3 (35, 37, 40, 41).

13.5 **Summary**

Data sharing and open access to data are increasingly becoming 'the expected norm' (8). We highlighted how IPD meta-analyses in prognosis research herald an exciting opportunity to improve, often substantially, upon systematic reviews and meta-analyses based on published aggregate data. Many challenges still remain for an IPD meta-analysis, but it is quickly becoming an achievable and essential tool for establishing evidence-based prognosis research findings.

References

1. **Riley RD, Abrams KR, Sutton AJ**, et al. (2003) Reporting of prognostic markers: current problems and development of guidelines for evidence-based practice in the future. *Br J Cancer* **88**(8), 1191–8.

2. **Holländer N** and **Sauerbrei W** (2007) On statistical approaches for the multivariable analysis of prognostic marker studies. In: **Auget J-L, Balakrishnan N, Mesbah M**, et al. (eds). *Advances in Statistical Methods for the Health Sciences*. Boston: Birkhäuser. pp. 19–38.

3. **Kyzas PA, Loizou KT**, and **Ioannidis JP** (2005) Selective reporting biases in cancer prognostic factor studies. *J Natl Cancer Inst* **97**(14), 1043–55.

4. **Stewart LA** and **Parmar MK** (1993) Meta-analysis of the literature or of individual patient data: is there a difference? *Lancet* 341.

5. **Riley RD, Lambert PC**, and **Abo-Zaid G** (2010) Meta-analysis of individual participant data: rationale, conduct, and reporting. *BMJ* **340**, c221.

6. **Debray TPA, Riley RD, Rovers MM**, et al. (2015) Individual participant data (IPD) meta-analyses of diagnostic and prognostic modeling studies: guidance on their use. *PLoS Med* **12**(10), e1001886.

7. **Simmonds M, Stewart G**, and **Stewart L** (2015) A decade of individual participant data meta-analyses: a review of current practice. *Contemp Clin Trials* **45**(Pt A), 76–83.

8. **Krumholz HM** (2015) Why data sharing should be the expected norm. *BMJ* **350**, h599.

9. **Peat G, Riley RD, Croft P**, et al. (2014) Improving the transparency of prognosis research: the role of reporting, data sharing, registration, and protocols. *PLoS Med* **11**(7), e1001671.

10. **Taichman DB, Backus J, Baethge C**, et al. (2016) Sharing clinical trial data: a proposal from the International Committee of Medical Journal Editors. *BMJ* **532**, i255.

11. **Pisani E, Aaby P, Breugelmans JG**, et al. (2016) Beyond open data: realizing the health benefits of sharing data. *BMJ* **355**, i5295.

12. **Loder E** and **Groves T** (2015) The BMJ requires data sharing on request for all trials. *BMJ* **350**, h2373.

13. **Koenig F, Slattery J, Groves T,** et al. (2015) Sharing clinical trial data on patient level: opportunities and challenges. *Biom J* **57**(1), 8–26.

14. **Groves T** (2010) BMJ policy on data sharing. *BMJ* **340**, c564.

15. **Steyerberg EW, Mushkudiani N, Perel P,** et al. (2008) Predicting outcome after traumatic brain injury: development and international validation of prognostic scores based on admission characteristics. *PLoS Medicine* **5**(8), 1251–61.

16. **Altman DG, Trivella M, Pezzella F,** et al. (2006) Systematic review of multiple studies of prognosis: the feasibility of obtaining individual patient data. In: **Auget J-L, Balakrishnan N, Mesbah M,** et al. (eds). *Advances in Statistical Methods for the Health Sciences*. Boston: Birkhäuser. pp. 3–18.

17. **Look MP, van Putten WL, Duffy MJ,** et al. (2002) Pooled analysis of prognostic impact of urokinase-type plasminogen activator and its inhibitor PAI-1 in 8377 breast cancer patients. *J Natl Cancer Inst* **94**(2), 116–28.

18. **Hayden JA, van der Windt DA, Cartwright JL,** et al. (2013) Assessing bias in studies of prognostic factors. *Ann Intern Med* **158**(4), 280–6.

19. **Moons KG, de Groot JA, Bouwmeester W,** et al. (2014) Critical appraisal and data extraction for systematic reviews of prediction modelling studies: the CHARMS checklist. *PLoS Med* **11**(10), e1001744.

20. **Moons KGM, Wolff RF, Riley RD,** et al. (2019) PROBAST: a tool to assess risk of bias and applicability concerns of prediction model studies - explanation and elaboration. Ann Int Med (in press).

21. **Simmonds MC, Higgins JPT, Stewart LA,** et al. (2005) Meta-analysis of individual patient data from randomized trials: a review of methods used in practice. *Clinical Trials* **2**, 209–17.

22. **Debray TPA, Moons KGM,** and **Abo-Zaid GMA** (2013) Individual participant data meta-analysis for a binary outcome: one-stage or two-stage? *PLoS One* **8**, e60650.

23. **Mathew T** and **Nordstrom K** (1999) On the equivalence of meta-analysis using literature and using individual patient data. *Biometrics* **55**(4), 1221–3.

24. **Riley RD, Lambert PC, Staessen JA,** et al. (2008) Meta-analysis of continuous outcomes combining individual patient data and aggregate data. *Stat Med* **27**(11), 1870–93.

25. **Burke DL, Ensor J,** and **Riley RD** (2017) Meta-analysis using individual participant data: one-stage and two-stage approaches, and why they may differ. *Stat Med* **36**(5), 855–75.

26. **McShane LM, Altman DG, Sauerbrei W,** et al. (2005) Reporting recommendations for tumour marker prognostic studies (REMARK). *Br J Cancer* **93**(4), 387–91.

27. **Collins GS, Reitsma JB, Altman DG,** et al. (2015) Transparent reporting of a multivariable prediction model for individual prognosis or diagnosis (TRIPOD): the TRIPOD Statement. *Ann Intern Med* **162**, 55–63.

28. **Tierney JF, Vale C, Riley R,** et al. (2015) Individual participant data (IPD) meta-analyses of randomized controlled trials: guidance on their use. *PLoS Med* **12**(7), e1001855.

29. **Ahmed I, Debray TP, Moons KG,** et al. (2014) Developing and validating risk prediction models in an individual participant data meta-analysis. *BMC Med Res Methodol* **14**, 3.

30. **Abo-Zaid G, Sauerbrei W,** and **Riley RD** (2012) Individual participant data meta-analysis of prognostic factor studies: state of the art? *BMC Med Res Methodol* **12**, 56.

31. **Marmarou A, Lu J, Butcher I**, et al. (2007) IMPACT database of traumatic brain injury: design and description. *J Neurotrauma* **24**(2), 239–50.

32. **McHugh GS, Engel DC, Butcher I**, et al. (2007) Prognostic value of secondary insults in traumatic brain injury: results from the IMPACT study. *J Neurotrauma* **24**(2), 287–93.

33. **Trivella M, Pezzella F, Pastorino U**, et al. (2007) Microvessel density as a prognostic factor in non-small-cell lung carcinoma: a meta-analysis of individual patient data. *Lancet Onc* **8**(6), 488–99.

34. **Van Calster B, Nieboer D, Vergouwe Y**, et al. (2016) A calibration hierarchy for risk models was defined: from utopia to empirical data. *J Clin Epidemiol* **74**, 167–76.

35. **Debray TP, Vergouwe Y, Koffijberg H**, et al. (2015) A new framework to enhance the interpretation of external validation studies of clinical prediction models. *J Clin Epidemiol* **68**(3), 279–89.

36. **Snell KI, Hua H, Debray TP**, et al. (2016) Multivariate meta-analysis of individual participant data helped externally validate the performance and implementation of a prediction model. *J Clin Epidemiol* **69**, 40–50.

37. **Riley RD, Ensor J, Snell KI**, et al. (2016) External validation of clinical prediction models using big datasets from e-health records or IPD meta-analysis: opportunities and challenges. *BMJ* **353**, i3140.

38. **Janssen KJ, Moons KG, Kalkman CJ**, et al. (2008) Updating methods improved the performance of a clinical prediction model in new patients. *J Clin Epidemiol* **61**(1), 76–86.

39. **Pennells L, Kaptoge S, White IR**, et al. (2014) Assessing risk prediction models using individual participant data from multiple studies. *Am J Epidemiol* **179**(5), 621–32.

40. **Royston P, Parmar MKB, and Sylvester R** (2004) Construction and validation of a prognostic model across several studies, with an application in superficial bladder cancer. *Stat Med* **23**, 907–26.

41. **Debray TP, Moons KG, Ahmed I**, et al. (2013) A framework for developing, implementing, and evaluating clinical prediction models in an individual participant data meta-analysis. *Stat Med* **32**(18), 3158–80.

42. **Peduzzi PN, Concato J, Kemper E**, et al. (1996) A simulation study of the number of events per variable in logistic regression analysis. *J Clin Epidemiol* **49**(12), 1373–79.

43. **Jinks RC, Royston P, and Parmar MK** (2015) Discrimination-based sample size calculations for multivariable prognostic models for time-to-event data. *BMC Med Res Methodol* **15**, 82.

44. **Ogundimu EO, Altman DG, and Collins GS** (2016) Adequate sample size for developing prediction models is not simply related to events per variable. *J Clin Epidemiol* **76**, 175–82.

45. **Steyerberg EW, Harrell FEJ, Borsboom GJ**, et al. (2001) Internal validation of predictive models: efficiency of some procedures for logistic regression analysis. *J Clin Epidemiol* **54**, 774–81.

46. **Pavlou M, Ambler G, Seaman SR**, et al. (2015) How to develop a more accurate risk prediction model when there are few events. *BMJ* **351**, h3868.

47. **Schuetz P, Koller M, Christ-Crain M**, et al. (2008) Predicting mortality with pneumonia severity scores: importance of model recalibration to local settings. *Epidemiol Infect* **136**(12), 1628–37.

48. **Thompson SG** and **Higgins JP** (2005) Treating individuals 4: can meta-analysis help target interventions at individuals most likely to benefit? *Lancet* **365**(9456), 341–6.

49. **Davey Smith G, Egger M,** and **Phillips AN** (1997) Meta-analysis. Beyond the grand mean? *BMJ* **315**(7122), 1610–14.

50. **Early Breast Cancer Trialists' Collaborative Group** (1998) Tamoxifen for early breast cancer: an overview of the randomized trials. *Lancet* **351**, 1451–67.

51. **Schmid CH, Stark PC, Berlin JA,** et al. (2004) Meta-regression detected associations between heterogeneous treatment effects and study-level, but not patient-level, factors. *J Clin Epidemiol* **57**(7), 683–97.

52. **Berlin JA, Santanna J, Schmid CH,** et al. (2002) Individual patient versus group-level data meta-regressions for the investigation of treatment effect modifiers: ecological bias rears its ugly head. *Stat Med* **21**(3), 371–87.

53. **Hua H, Burke DL, Crowther MJ,** et al. (2017) One-stage individual participant data meta-analysis models: estimation of treatment-covariate interactions must avoid ecological bias by separating out within-trial and across-trial information. *Stat Med* **36**(5), 772–89.

54. **Wang JG, Staessen JA, Franklin SS,** et al. (2005) Systolic and diastolic blood pressure lowering as determinants of cardiovascular outcome. *Hypertension* **45**(5), 907–13.

55. **Ioannidis JP, Rosenberg PS, Goedert JJ,** et al. (2002) Commentary: meta-analysis of individual participants' data in genetic epidemiology. *Am J Epidemiol* **156**(3), 204–10.

56. **Ahmed I, Sutton AJ,** and **Riley RD** (2012) Assessment of publication bias, selection bias and unavailable data in meta-analyses using individual participant data: a database survey. *BMJ* **344**, d7762.

57. **Riley RD, Simmonds MC,** and **Look MP** (2007) Evidence synthesis combining individual patient data and aggregate data: a systematic review identified current practice and possible methods. *J Clin Epidemiol* **60**(5), 431–9.

58. **Riley RD** and **Steyerberg EW** (2010) Meta-analysis of a binary outcome using individual participant data and aggregate data. *Res Synth Methods* **1**, 2–9.

59. **Debray TP, Koffijberg H, Lu D,** et al. (2012) Incorporating published univariable associations in diagnostic and prognostic modeling. *BMC Med Res Methodol* **12**, 121.

60. **Debray TP, Koffijberg H, Nieboer D,** et al. (2014) Meta-analysis and aggregation of multiple published prediction models. *Stat Med* **33**(14), 2341–62.

61. **Stewart L, Tierney J,** and **Burdett S** (2006) Do systematic reviews based on individual patient data offer a means of circumventing biases associated with trial publications? In: **Rothstein HR, Sutton AJ, Borenstein M** (eds). *Publication Bias in Meta-Analysis: Prevention, Assessment and Adjustments.* Chichester, UK: John Wiley & Sons, Ltd.

62. **Resche-Rigon M** and **White IR** (2018) Multiple imputation by chained equations for systematically and sporadically missing multilevel data. *Stat Methods Med Res* **27**(6), 1634–49.

63. **Jolani S, Debray TP, Koffijberg H,** et al. (2015) Imputation of systematically missing predictors in an individual participant data meta-analysis: a generalized approach using MICE. *Stat Med* **34**(11), 1841–63.

Chapter 14

Electronic healthcare records and prognosis research

Kelvin P Jordan and Karel GM Moons

14.1 Introduction

Prognosis studies are often conducted in cohorts specifically set up for research, drawing on self-reported information from questionnaires, standardized examinations and additional investigations at organized follow-up visits. Such pre-designed longitudinal cohort studies face a number of limitations. For example, selectivity of study participants can threaten generalisability; non-response and other types of missing data can threaten internal validity. Moreover, sampling restrictions, related to cost and duration of follow-up, often constrain such studies to measuring only prognostic factors and common outcomes over a relatively short period. Data collection may be limited to pre-specified time points during follow-up, so that events occurring in-between and changes in prognostic factors cannot be captured at the time they occur.

One approach to addressing these limitations is the use of electronic healthcare records (EHR). Information collected over time on all patients presenting in a specified healthcare setting with a particular health condition or diagnosed with a particular disorder (startpoint) is increasingly recorded electronically. Databases of such patient information are increasingly available for healthcare research. EHR databases contain healthcare records stretching over many years, with long-term follow-up on thousands or even millions of patients. Information is collected continuously as and when patients use health services, rather than at time points pre-specified by researchers in pre-designed cohorts or trials. As patients can be followed from the time of a first-recorded symptom presented to healthcare or a first diagnosis, EHR offers potential for all forms of prognosis research with all types of startpoints.

Using EHR data, however, incurs many challenges—some common to all prognosis studies, others specific to this form of data. This chapter discusses the potential for EHR in prognosis research and the challenges involved. It uses UK primary care databases for the main examples.

14.2 **Examples of EHR databases worldwide**

Many EHR databases, whether local, regional, or national, are now available to researchers globally. They will vary according to their specific purpose and the healthcare system in which they are based. For example, information from hospitals in the US, collected originally into large administrative databases for billing or insurance purposes, has been used regularly in healthcare research. One such database is the Health Care Cost and Utilization Project (HCUP), which includes the largest longitudinal hospital care data set in the US, derived from inpatient and outpatient discharge records.

In the UK, most people with a new symptom or health condition are seen, and most chronic diseases managed, by general practitioners (GPs or family doctors) in primary care, providing a gateway to the whole UK National Health Service. UK primary care databases contain electronic records of patients' morbidities (i.e. diagnoses, diseases, or symptoms) and processes of care. A number are available for research (e.g. Clinical Practice Research Datalink (CPRD), The Health Improvement Network (THIN), QResearch, and ResearchOne), with data on reasons for consultation, prescriptions, referrals, investigations, tests (e.g. X-rays, blood pressure readings), and some demographics. By 2018 there were over 2000 publications using CPRD (1). A number have been concerned with extending the ambit of prognosis research to the study of prognostic factors and development of prognostic models for estimating future risk of health outcomes in the general population. This work informs decisions in practice about intervening to prevent those outcomes. Outcomes studied in this way include cardiovascular disease (2), osteoporotic fracture (3), and venous thromboembolism (4). Similar studies have emerged from the QResearch database with endpoints including cardiovascular disease (5), fracture (6), and cancer (7, 8).

Electronic healthcare databases may be exclusive to primary or secondary care, with restricted linkage across care providers, but some, such as the Swedish Skåne County Health Care Register (SHCR), have managed to integrate primary and secondary care data for reimbursement calculations (9). Similarly, the Information System for the Development of Research in Primary Care (SIDIAP) database contains primary care data for the Catalonia region in Spain and includes linkage to hospital admissions and mortality (10). Other databases may restrict their clinical focus. For example, the Canadian Primary Care Sentinel Surveillance Network (CPCSSN) collates information from primary care providers, and was initially focused on eight chronic conditions only (11).

14.3 **General issues for prognosis studies using EHR**

Researchers using EHR need to understand the nature of routine healthcare data, how and what is recorded in the particular database used, and how recording habits vary between healthcare professionals.

14.3.1 **Defining study populations, startpoints, outcomes, and potential prognostic factors**

Morbidities and processes of care are generally recorded in EHR using coding systems. Study populations defined by the presence of a certain disease or diagnosis, as a typical startpoint for much prognosis research, can be identified by one morbidity code, or a code list, or combinations of information in an algorithm (e.g. morbidity code plus relevant prescription, or morbidity code plus results from diagnostic tests). Determining relevant codes to define the target population (startpoint) for a prognosis study within an EHR can be time consuming. EHRs may include many thousands of codes, even though many may be rarely used. Care is needed when using EHRs to ensure as complete and accurate a code list as possible.

Researchers must always consider the most appropriate definition of disease, diagnosis, symptom, syndrome, or sign, to provide the correct startpoint needed to address a specific prognosis question, and be prepared to use 'code browsers' to examine the full list of codes used in the chosen database. Using or modifying previously derived code lists is the best place to start. Published prognosis studies based on EHRs should give access to code lists, as well as clear definitions and details of how they were developed. If code lists do not exist or need modifying, then consensus exercises with clinicians and EHR researchers to develop them should be considered (12).

Endpoints for prognosis studies, as applies for all types of medical research, need to be recorded in a systematic and fully comprehensive manner in the EHR. In EHRs these generally tend to be the so-called 'harder' outcomes, such as mortality, diagnosed diseases, hospitalization, and surgery undergone, rather than events not yet routinely recorded in healthcare data, such as self-reported disability, pain, and quality of life. An assumption needs to be made that an absence of any record of a certain outcome ('hard' or other types) does indeed mean the outcome did not occur, rather than it did occur but was not measured or recorded. The assumption could be justified by, for example, evidence of completeness of recording of the outcome within a database.

Specifying the startpoint time for identifying potential prognostic factors (equivalent to the index date and sometimes called prognostic T(ime) zero, or the moment at which a prognosis is estimated) is always a key decision in prognosis research, whether pre-designed or based on EHRs. A major advantage of using EHR is that patients at a chosen startpoint are likely also to have records of previous health events over many preceding years. This means the database often contains a good representation of a person's clinical history, and allows the study of numerous potential prognostic factors. A prognosis study based on EHR can use information drawn from a specified preceding time-period before the chosen startpoint, and ensure that potential prognostic factors can be considered present at the startpoint. This preceding time-period is chosen by the researcher, and should be long enough to allow pre-existing morbidity to be identified whilst ensuring that values of time-varying prognostic factors (such as body mass index (BMI) and blood pressure) are contemporaneous with date of entry into the defined study cohort. Patients will have variable lengths of time registered on a particular database, and EHR studies often specify a minimum registration period prior to the startpoint for patients to be eligible for the study, thus ensuring a standard time for identifying pre-existing prognostic factors.

14.3.2 Missing data

Missing data on startpoint information, prognostic factors, and outcomes (endpoints) (see Chapter 4) can be a particular problem for EHR studies, notably for lifestyle information such as smoking and drinking, but also for variables such as BMI, ethnicity, cholesterol levels, blood pressure, and so-called 'soft' outcomes. There are no perfect solutions. As discussed in previous chapters, complete-case analysis, in which cases with missing data are excluded, is the approach frequently adopted in all types of prognosis research, whether pre-designed studies or those based on EHR. Alternatively a missing or unknown category (the so-called 'missing indicator' category) can be included in the analysis (13), or a crude form of imputation used (e.g. assuming people with missing data for variables such as BMI are in the 'normal' or average category). All these approaches may yield biased results in any type of medical research (14).

Multiple imputation is generally preferable (see Chapter 4) (15), although complete-case analysis may give unbiased results for outcome data missing at random (16). Much data for measures, such as potential prognostic factors, not recorded in daily practice are likely to be selectively missing. However, healthcare professionals' decisions to gather such data in daily practice (e.g. measuring additional blood values or requesting imaging) is typically based on their knowledge of other preceding information and status of the patient. If this other information has been recorded, it can be used in multiple imputation techniques to predict the most likely value of the missing variable.

Such techniques can even include details obtained after a missing prognostic factor should have been recorded (17), and so multiple imputation can now be regarded as the approach of choice for missing prognostic factor data, often combined with comparison to other approaches such as complete-case analysis (15).

14.3.3 Variation in measurement

Many recorded measurements in clinical practice are subject to random measurement error. Blood pressure measurement, for example, has been a focus of attention over the years, a standard approach in clinical practice being to obtain multiple readings from an individual patient in order to calculate their presumed average as the basis for treatment decisions. Calculation of the individual's mean value can be incorporated into definitions of startpoints and prognostic factors. Recent interest has focused on variability itself as a potential prognostic factor, applied to measures such as blood pressure (18). More problematic for EHR prognosis research is that recording and clinical practice can vary systematically between healthcare professionals. Outcomes and outcome recording may also vary by healthcare professional and by healthcare organization. Such variation and clustering can be explored, or adjusted for, in the analysis of EHR data, by using more complex modelling techniques such as mixed models (also known as random effects, multilevel, and hierarchical models) that account for clustering of patients within different clinicians and clinical settings.

14.3.4 Accounting for treatment in EHR prognosis research

Patients in routine care and thus in EHR databases are highly likely to be receiving treatment for their conditions. Variation in endpoints observed in EHR databases may of course result from baseline differences in prognostic factors (as studied in prognosis research) but also from variability in treatment received which, when effective, is itself also a prognostic factor, as discussed in detail in Chapter 7, Section 7.4. However, treatment allocation does not occur at random, and people at higher risk of a particular outcome are likely to have been preferentially selected to receive treatment. In other words, treatment decisions in daily practice are always based on preceding prognostic factors, including co-morbidities.

Overall prognosis research (i.e. type I) using EHR will automatically incorporate both treatment effectiveness and the proportions of patients treated in the particular setting and context to arrive at estimates of current average prognosis of people with a particular startpoint. Prognostic factor and prognostic model research (i.e. types II and III) have to account for the fact that those at higher risk of a poorer prognosis are more likely to be treated (see Chapter 7, Section 7.1). If the treatment is effective, then prognostic factors associated with poor outcome in untreated populations may have a paradoxically weakened or even negative association with outcome in treated EHR populations because of the association of the factors with treatment and the resulting improved prognosis (19, 20).

Another application of observational EHR data is the investigation of causal associations between treatment and outcome, that is, treatment effectiveness which also must tackle and adjust for this 'confounding-by-indication' (21). Suggested solutions include propensity score methods, instrumental variables and, for repeated events, adjusting for estimates of outcome in a prior treatment-free period ('difference-in-differences' and 'prior event rate ratio' (22)).

14.3.5 Reporting guidelines

The RECORD reporting guidelines for EHR research (23) can be used, alongside other reporting guidelines for prognosis studies such as REMARK and TRIPOD, to ensure adequate reporting of a prognosis study using EHR (see Appendix). Also the principles of analysis and reporting of individual participant data meta-analysis may be applicable to EHR studies due to inherent clustering of individuals (within practices, hospitals, regions) (see Chapter 13); these principles can be found in, for example, Debray et al. and Riley et al. (24, 25).

14.4 Opportunities and challenges of EHR research

The typical characteristics of EHR databases offer opportunities and challenges for prognosis research that may not apply to prognosis studies set outside EHR databases. This section summarizes these.

14.4.1 Size and coverage (geography and population)

Opportunities

1. Potential for more generalizable populations. Traditional predesigned cohort studies are often restricted by socio-demographic or clinical characteristics because of age restrictions, or screening out of people with, for example, severe disease or co-morbidities.
2. Avoiding problems of selective non-response and attrition during follow-up.
3. Comparisons across relevant subgroups (e.g. by age, geographical region, co-morbidity status), avoiding assumptions that prognostic factors and models are identical across such subgroups.

4. Possibility to include a large number of potential prognostic factors in the analysis, given sample sizes will often be large.

5. Study of prognosis in rarer diseases, and modelling and prediction of rarer endpoints, becomes feasible.

6. Development of prognostic models can be conducted in large samples (with large number of events per variable), and thus overfitting is of less concern.

7. Validation of prognostic models can be conducted in large sample sizes, often considerably above the minimum suggested criteria of at least 100 to 200 events.

8. Development and validation can be done using the same EHR database, for example using a derivation sample and a test sample, with the latter using a non-random sample of data from different geographic regions or general practices to cover a wide range of settings and case-mix for extensive testing of model generalisability (25). Given the overall size of the database, large sample sizes can be maintained in both development and validation cohorts, such that data splitting is not a concern.

Challenges

1. The size: 101 million consultations were recorded in CPRD between 2007 and 2014 (26). Many of these link to multiple entries for the same patients (co-morbidities, prescriptions, referrals, investigations). This poses large demands on computing resource (storage and power) and time for checking and preparing data. These issues are one driver to the development of machine learning techniques (see Chapter 16).

2. Statistically significant but small associations between prognostic factors and outcomes are likely to emerge, which may not be clinically meaningful.

3. The need to understand the characteristics of an EHR database and how these impact on study interpretation, such as the generalizability of insurance claim databases to the health of uninsured people or of local databases to national populations. More fundamentally, EHR database content is defined by people seeking healthcare. Prognostic factors and models from EHR may not be generalizable to the healthier lower-consulting general population.

4. Validity of the data—including measurement error, and differences in measurement methods and quality between clinicians and settings (see section 14.3.3).

5. Missing data (see section 14.3.2).

14.4.2 **Contemporary and historical, time-related and time-varying data**

Many EHR databases have long-term follow-up of patients.

Opportunities

1. Determination of long-term overall prognosis and long-term outcomes in studies of prognostic factors and models, because large numbers remain under observation in the same dataset for many years.
2. Comparison of short-term risk versus long-term risk of future outcomes.
3. Updating of prognostic models. The longitudinal and continuous nature of data recorded in EHR allows examination of the effect of changes in prognostic factors and models (e.g. development of a co-morbidity during follow-up after the initial baseline exposure period). Prognostic models incorporating repeated measures of potential predictors, such as blood pressure, cholesterol level or BMI, can be studied (27).
4. Analysis of repeated outcomes. Multiple occurrences of outcomes (e.g. hospital stays or repeat occurrences of acute outcomes) can be incorporated into analyses.
5. Analysis of trends over time allows investigation of possible links between population changes in prognostic factors or in disease management with population-level outcomes. For example, one analysis identified a reduction in deaths related to the painkiller co-proxamol following its withdrawal, with little evidence of increase in other analgesia-related deaths (28).

Challenges

1. Diagnosis and coding habits change. Changes may occur in the way morbidities are recorded, for example moving between use of diagnostic and symptom codes (29). Incentives such as the UK Quality and Outcomes Framework (QoF) which introduced performance-based payments for GPs may also change the way in which morbidities are recorded (30). The coding systems may also change—in the UK, primary care is changing from use of 'Read' codes to 'SNOMED CT' so mapping of code lists between coding systems is needed.
2. Stability of healthcare organizations and patients. In UK primary care, for example, practices may start contributing to a database at any time and their historic data may then be excluded or be of lower quality. Practices can choose to stop contributing. One solution is sensitivity analyses restricted to practices contributing for the whole study period. Patients can also join and

leave practices contributing to a database, and joiners and leavers may be different—younger people are more mobile, for example. However, reasons for leaving a practice may also be a study endpoint, for example older patients moving to a nursing home, which can increase the risk of attrition bias if that reason is unobserved.

3. 'Ghost' patients who have left a practice but this is not indicated on the database. One solution is to include a minimum criterion of a recorded contact within a defined recent period of time.

14.4.3 Validation and comparison across databases

There are an increasing number of EHR databases available for researchers which offer scope for external validation of prognostic models.

Opportunities

1. Validation in other EHR databases. The performance of a prognostic model, or evidence for newly determined prognostic factors, can be tested in a second database, and potentially in different populations and clinical settings with large sample sizes (25). This has happened, for example, with cardiovascular risk scores developed in the QResearch database and subsequently validated within THIN (31). Studies have also assessed risk factors in separate databases and pooled results from across databases (32).

2. International comparisons and validation. For example, comparison of myocardial infarction outcomes between countries, such as described in Chapter 11.

Challenges

1. Expense of accessing multiple EHR databases.

2. Need to organize multiple databases with different data structures.

3. Variation in recording between databases in terms of completeness, quality, procedures, and training. This may lead to heterogeneity.

4. Differences in design of EHR databases from different countries. For example, the results of a study comparing overall prognosis for women with breast cancer between European countries were controversial because methods for compiling national registries of breast cancer varied between countries (33, 34).

14.4.4. Linkages

Several databases available to researchers include linkage across data sources (e.g. primary and secondary care, disease and mortality registers).

Opportunities

1. Linkage between healthcare data sources allows investigation of outcomes as patients progress through different healthcare settings. For example, outcomes for hip and knee joint replacements for osteoarthritis performed in the UK are linked to type of surgical procedure in Hospital Episode Statistics and the UK National Joint Registry data.

2. Linkage to new data collection, such as patient self-reported data from surveys linked to EHR data with individual patient consent. Introduction of point-of-consultation templates may provide additional information on prognostic factors and outcomes, or information on assessment and management of morbidity by GPs, and collect data not routinely recorded in the EHR (35).

Challenges

1. Need for individual patient consent in some circumstances. Individual patient consent will generally be needed, for example, to link self-reported information from a survey to EHR. Linkage may not be possible for all patients contributing to a database.

2. Complexity: for practical purposes, such as costs and time, extra data may only be available for a subsample of patients. Linkage to hospital, cause of death, and neighbourhood deprivation data in national data sets such as CPRD are restricted to consenting general practices. Data formats can differ. For example, coding systems may differ between primary and secondary care databases.

14.5 **An example of an EHR-based prognosis study**

An overall prognosis study of patients consulting in UK primary and secondary health care with chest pain (36) is shown in Box 14.1 The study was an analysis of a dataset that linked hospital and primary care EHR with mortality data.

14.6 **Conclusions**

EHR are a valuable resource for prognosis research, with long follow-up on large populations unselected other than by a patient's decision to consult. Prognosis studies using EHR require clear definitions of startpoints, prognostic factors, and endpoints readily identifiable within the healthcare records. Researchers using EHR need to understand the characteristics of the data and databases, and interpret study results within the context of these characteristics. As with all prognosis research, transparency in definitions, study design, and analysis is crucial to assessing the robustness and generalizability of findings.

Box 14.1 Prognosis of undiagnosed chest pain: linked electronic healthcare record cohort study.

Aim: to determine long-term cardiovascular outcomes in patients whose chest pain was undiagnosed six months after first presentation.

Design: cohort study.

Setting: UK EHR database (CALIBER) linking primary care, secondary care, coronary register, death register.

Startpoint: adults aged > 18 years, six months after a first episode of recorded chest pain classified in medical records as undiagnosed (cause unattributed) or non-coronary diagnosis throughout the six months.

Endpoints: fatal or non-fatal cardiovascular events over five years follow-up.

Results: five-year cumulative incidence of cardiovascular events in unattributed group was 159 per 10,000 person years, compared with incidence of 101/10,000 in those diagnosed with non-coronary chest pain (adjusted hazard ratios for 0.5–1 year after presentation: 1.95, 95% confidence interval 1.66–2.31; for 1–3 years: 1.35, 1.23–1.48; for 3–5.5 years: 1.21, 1.08–1.37).

Source: data from Jordan KP, et al. (2017) Prognosis of undiagnosed chest pain: linked electronic health record cohort study. *BMJ* 357, j1194. Copyright © 2017 British Medical Journal Publishing Group.

References

1. **Medicines and Healthcare Products Regulatory Agency (GB).** Clinical Practice Research Datalink (CPRD). www.cprd.com. Accessed 15/10/2018.

2. **Rapsomaniki E, Shah A, Perel P,** et al. (2014) Prognostic models for stable coronary artery disease based on electronic health record cohort of 102,023 patients. *Eur Heart J* **35**(13), 844–52.

3. **Klop C, de Vries F, Bijlsma JW, Leufkens HG,** and **Welsing PM** (2016) Predicting the ten-year risk of hip and major osteoporotic fracture in rheumatoid arthritis and in the general population: an independent validation and update of UK FRAX without bone mineral density. *Ann Rheum Dis* **75**(12), 2095–100.

4. **Sultan AA, West J, Grainge MJ,** et al. (2016) Development and validation of risk prediction model for venous thromboembolism in postpartum women: multinational cohort study. *BMJ* **355**, i6253.

5. **Hippisley-Cox J, Coupland C,** and **Brindle P** (2017) Development and validation of QRISK3 risk prediction algorithms to estimate future risk of cardiovascular disease: prospective cohort study. *BMJ* (clinical research ed) **357**, j2099.

6. **Hippisley-Cox J** and **Coupland C** (2012) Derivation and validation of updated QFracture algorithm to predict risk of osteoporotic fracture in primary care in the United Kingdom: prospective open cohort study. *BMJ* (clinical research ed) **344**, e3427.

7. **Hippisley-Cox J** and **Coupland C** (2013) Symptoms and risk factors to identify men with suspected cancer in primary care: derivation and validation of an algorithm. *Br J Gen Pract* **63**(606), e1–10.

8. **Hippisley-Cox J** and **Coupland C** (2013) Symptoms and risk factors to identify women with suspected cancer in primary care: derivation and validation of an algorithm. *Br J Gen Pract* **63**(606), e11–21.

9. **Turkiewicz A, Petersson IF, Bjork J,** et al. (2014) Current and future impact of osteoarthritis on health care: a population-based study with projections to year 2032. *Osteoarthritis Cartilage* **22**(11), 1826–32.

10. **Garcia-Gil Mdel M, Hermosilla E, Prieto-Alhambra D,** et al. (2011) Construction and validation of a scoring system for the selection of high-quality data in a Spanish population primary care database (SIDIAP). *Inform Prim Care* **19**(3), 135–45.

11. **Garies S, Birtwhistle R, Drummond N, Queenan J,** and **Williamson T** (2017) Data Resource Profile: National electronic medical record data from the Canadian Primary Care Sentinel Surveillance Network (CPCSSN). *Int J Epidemiol* **46**(4), 1091–2f.

12. **Dave S** and **Petersen I** (2009) Creating medical and drug code lists to identify cases in primary care databases. *Pharmacoepidemiol Drug Saf* **18**(8), 704–7.

13. **Groenwold RH, White IR, Donders AR, Carpenter JR, Altman DG,** and **Moons KG** (2012) Missing covariate data in clinical research: when and when not to use the missing-indicator method for analysis. *CMAJ* **184**(11), 1265–9.

14. **Donders AR, van der Heijden GJ, Stijnen T,** and **Moons KG** (2006) Review: a gentle introduction to imputation of missing values. *J Clin Epidemiol* **59**(10), 1087–91.

15. **Janssen KJ, Donders AR, Harrell FE, Jr.,** et al. (2010) Missing covariate data in medical research: to impute is better than to ignore. *J Clin Epidemiol* **63**(7), 721–7.

16. **Groenwold RH, Donders AR, Roes KC, Harrell FE, Jr.,** and **Moons KG** (2012) Dealing with missing outcome data in randomized trials and observational studies. *Am J Epidemiol* **175**(3), 210–7.

17. **Welch CA, Petersen I, Bartlett JW,** et al. (2014) Evaluation of two-fold fully conditional specification multiple imputation for longitudinal electronic health record data. *Stat Med* **33**(21), 3725–37.

18. **Stevens SL, Wood S, Koshiaris C,** et al. (2016) Blood pressure variability and cardiovascular disease: systematic review and meta-analysis. *BMJ* (clinical research ed) **354**, i4098.

19. **Pajouheshnia R, Peelen LM, Moons KGM, Reitsma JB,** and **Groenwold RHH** (2017) Accounting for treatment use when validating a prognostic model: a simulation study. *BMC Med Res Methodol* **17**(1), 103.

20. **Groenwold RH, Moons KG, Pajouheshnia R,** et al. (2016) Explicit inclusion of treatment in prognostic modeling was recommended in observational and randomized settings. *J Clin Epidemiol* **78**, 90–100.

21. **Danaei G, Rodriguez LA, Cantero OF, Logan R,** and **Hernan MA** (2013) Observational data for comparative effectiveness research: an emulation of randomised trials of statins and primary prevention of coronary heart disease. *Stat Methods Med Res* **22**(1), 70–96.

22. **Streeter AJ, Lin NX, Crathorne L,** et al. (2017) Adjusting for unmeasured confounding in nonrandomized longitudinal studies: a methodological review. *J Clin Epidemiol* **87**, 23–34.

23. **Benchimol EI, Smeeth L, Guttmann A**, et al. (2015) The REporting of studies Conducted using Observational Routinely-collected health Data (RECORD) statement. *PLoS Med* **12**(10), e1001885.

24. **Debray TP, Riley RD, Rovers MM, Reitsma JB**, and **Moons KG** (2015) Individual participant data (IPD) meta-analyses of diagnostic and prognostic modeling studies: guidance on their use. *PLoS Med* **12**(10), e1001886.

25. **Riley RD, Ensor J, Snell KI**, et al. (2016) External validation of clinical prediction models using big datasets from e-health records or IPD meta-analysis: opportunities and challenges. *BMJ* (clinical research ed) **353**, i3140.

26. **Hobbs FDR, Bankhead C, Mukhtar T**, et al. (2016) Clinical workload in UK primary care: a retrospective analysis of 100 million consultations in England, 2007–14. *Lancet* **387**(10035), 2323–30.

27. **Paige E, Barrett J, Pennells L**, et al. (2017) Use of repeated blood pressure and cholesterol measurements to improve cardiovascular disease risk prediction: an individual-participant-data meta-analysis. *Am J Epidemiol* **186**(8), 899–907.

28. **Hawton K, Bergen H, Simkin S, Wells C, Kapur N**, and **Gunnell D** (2012) Six-year follow-up of impact of co-proxamol withdrawal in England and Wales on prescribing and deaths: time-series study. *PLoS Med* **9**(5), e1001213.

29. **Rait G, Walters K, Griffin M, Buszewicz M, Petersen I**, and **Nazareth I** (2009) Recent trends in the incidence of recorded depression in primary care. *Br J Psychiatry* **195**(6), 520–4.

30. **Calvert M, Shankar A, McManus RJ, Lester H**, and **Freemantle N** (2009) Effect of the quality and outcomes framework on diabetes care in the United Kingdom: retrospective cohort study. *BMJ* (clinical research ed) **338**, b1870.

31. **Collins GS** and **Altman DG** (2012) Predicting the ten-year risk of cardiovascular disease in the United Kingdom: independent and external validation of an updated version of QRISK2. *BMJ* (clinical research ed) **344**, e4181.

32. **Vinogradova Y, Coupland C**, and **Hippisley-Cox J** (2015) Use of combined oral contraceptives and risk of venous thromboembolism: nested case-control studies using the QResearch and CPRD databases. *BMJ* (clinical research ed) **350**, h2135.

33. **Beral V** and **Peto R** (2010) UK cancer survival statistics. *BMJ* (clinical research ed) **341**, c4112.

34. **Woods LM, Coleman MP, Lawrence G, Rashbass J, Berrino F**, and **Rachet B** (2011) Evidence against the proposition that 'UK cancer survival statistics are misleading': simulation study with National Cancer Registry data. *BMJ* (clinical research ed) **342**, d3399.

35. **Edwards JJ, Jordan KP, Peat G**, et al. (2015) Quality of care for OA: the effect of a point-of-care consultation recording template. *Rheumatology* (Oxford) **54**(5), 844–53.

36. **Jordan KP, Timmis A, Croft P**, et al. (2017) Prognosis of undiagnosed chest pain: linked electronic health record cohort study. *BMJ* (clinical research ed) **357**, j1194.

Chapter 15

Novel statistical methods for prognosis research

Michael J Crowther and Mark J Rutherford

15.1 Introduction

In Part 2 of this book, fundamental statistical methods and concepts for prognosis research were introduced. Here, we draw attention to some advanced statistical methods that are growing in their application, as they deal with more complex data arising from prognosis research studies with longer term follow-up. Specifically, we consider competing risks, multi-state models, and joint modelling, and why they are needed in prognosis research of time-to-event outcomes, to help identify prognostic factors and to develop more dynamic prognostic models.

15.2 Competing risks

15.2.1 Introduction

In prognosis research that aims to summarize, explain, or predict the risk of a particular outcome, it is important to consider the potential for competing events; these are events that occur in an individual and preclude the main outcome of interest from occurring in that individual. For example, if someone dies due to a myocardial infarction or an accident, they can no longer die due to cancer. Such competing events may be more likely to occur in certain subgroups of a study population (1). For illustration, consider the example of a *hard* time-to-event outcome of interest, such as death due to cancer, with the competing events being different causes of death. Here, an individual, i, can only die of a single cause of death, and will therefore move from a state of 'alive' to one of N absorbing states comprising different causes of death classified into N broad categorizations (e.g. cancer, cardiovascular disease, accident, etc.). This is illustrated in Figure 15.1. The first state represents patients alive, with a diagnosis of cancer. Each patient can transition to one of the N states, with the probability of being in the state 'death due to cancer' being of primary interest, but

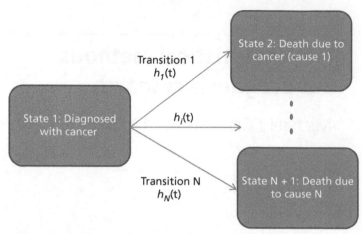

Figure 15.1 Example of competing causes of death for cancer patients.
Source: reproduced courtesy of Michael J. Crowther.

this probability also depends on transitions to other states as only one cause of death is possible for each individual. Therefore, deaths due to other causes are competing events for 'death due to cancer'.

In this situation, a typical but naïve analysis would be to censor the other causes of death at their death time, and then calculate the risk of 'death due to cancer' over time based on a non-parametric estimate (i.e. 1- Kaplan-Meier $S(t)$) or one derived from a 'cause-specific' (here, death due to cancer) survival modelling approach. This will overestimate the actual chance of dying of cancer, as it ignores the fact that other causes of death can preclude death due to cancer and thus prevent the event of 'death due to cancer' from ever occurring. In other words, the analysis assumes that cancer patients can only ever die of cancer or stay alive, which is not realistic (2). Therefore, alternative approaches are needed to properly account for the competing events.

15.2.2 **Cumulative incidence functions that account for competing events**

A prognostic model to predict the risk of outcomes other than all-cause mortality is likely to encounter competing events, and therefore prognosis researchers may need to account for this when developing or validating prognostic models. This is especially important for prognostic models in elderly or frail populations, where deaths due to other causes are common and thus have a stronger influence on the absolute probability of an outcome. To address this, the researcher should obtain the cumulative incidence function for the outcome of interest, which relates to the cumulative proportion of participants who will experience that outcome (over time) after accounting for other competing events (1, 3). The sum of the cumulative incidence functions for the main outcome (here, death due to cancer) and each competing event will total the all-cause event probability (here, all-cause mortality risk).

15.2.2.1 Multiple cause-specific models

In order to partition the all-cause mortality contributions into component parts, one approach is to model the contribution to each cause-specific hazard separately before calculating the cumulative incidence functions (1, 4). This approach has the advantage that the prognostic factor effects (i.e. hazard ratios for included variables in the model) are well defined, and correspond to their impact on increasing or decreasing mortality due to a specific cause. However, it is necessary to model multiple cause-specific models to understand the impact on the cumulative incidence functions.

15.2.2.2 Modelling excess mortality

An approach often used in cancer patient survival is to model excess mortality (5–7), rather than a cancer-specific mortality model, and a model for other causes of death. The approach is motivated by concerns over misclassification of cause of death for these patients, particularly in the elderly (8, 9). Here, the excess mortality model is a surrogate for the cancer-specific mortality model, and the other-cause mortality is estimated from population life tables rather than being modelled directly in the cancer patients. This relies on the life-table data being a suitable proxy for the cohort under study should they have not been diagnosed with cancer (10). It is vital that the life-table data is stratified by key factors that jointly influence other-cause and cancer mortality; typically this includes age, sex, calendar year, and sometimes deprivation information. Similar calculations can be carried out to obtain the cause-specific cumulative incidence functions when adopting this approach (11).

15.2.2.3 Modelling the cumulative incidence function directly

An alternative approach is to directly model how the effects of (potential) prognostic factors impact on the cumulative incidence functions by relating these to subdistribution hazard functions. An example of this is the Fine and Gray approach (12). This approach needs extra care in specifying which prognostic factor effects are important; a factor that may impact a competing cause alone (such as severity of heart disease on cardiovascular mortality) may still reduce the cumulative incidence function for cancer (13, 14). There have been recommendations that both cause-specific and subdistribution hazard ratios should be reported when analysing data with competing risks in order to obtain the whole picture (15). In both regression approaches, care should be taken to evaluate the suitability of the proportionality assumption of the hazards.

15.2.3 **Example**

We now take an example of 2982 patients with primary breast cancer, where we have information on the time to relapse and the time to death. All patients begin in the initial post-surgery state, which is defined as the time of primary surgery. We simply use a death indicator with two competing causes—those that have died following a relapse (classified as a cancer death), and those that have not (classified as an 'other cause' death). This is an over simplification and just for example purposes—a more detailed approach to this dataset will be considered in the following sections. Our example for the analysis of the breast cancer is a simplified version of Figure 15.1, with two potential transitions to death states: death due to cancer or death due to other causes.

We adopt the approach of estimating two cause-specific hazard models using flexible parametric survival models (see Chapter 3) (16), and combining those hazards to estimate the cumulative incidence functions (17), which provide the probabilities of being in each state as a function of time. Focusing on those aged seventy-five and with a tumour size in the middle category, Figure 15.2 compares the approach of estimating the risk of death due to cancer from a

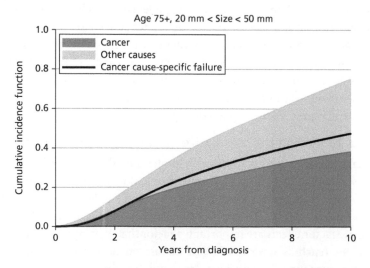

Figure 15.2 Comparison of the naïve estimate of cancer-specific mortality (labelled 'failure') (1- Kaplan-Meier *S(t)*) and the stacked cumulative incidence functions (probability of experiencing event of interest by time *t*).
Source: reproduced courtesy of Michael J. Crowther.

naïve analysis (i.e. using 1- Kaplan-Meier *S(t)* from the cancer cause-specific approach) to that when appropriately accounting for the competing events. The total height of the shaded area represents the all-cause probability of death for those aged seventy-five and with a tumour size in the middle category. We can partition this all-cause area into the two competing causes by stacking the cancer-specific and other-cause cumulative incidence functions on top of one another. The black line represents the naïve estimate of the cause-specific failure, when discounting the competing mortality from other causes. This is obviously an over estimate of the actual real-world probability of dying of cancer, because those over seventy-five will have a considerable mortality contribution from other causes.

Figure 15.3 compares the cumulative incidence functions across age groups, again for the middle tumour size category. The prognostic effect of age on cancer-specific mortality is not strong; the ten-year risk of death due to cancer is about 0.4 across the different age groups. However, there is a prognostic effect of age on the other causes of mortality, and this leads to differences in the four panels in the overall (all-cause) mortality risk (e.g. about 0.8 in the age > 75 panel, and about 0.4 in the age < 45 panel). There is not a direct relationship between the parameter estimates for the prognostic factors in the cancer-specific hazard regression and the corresponding cancer-specific cumulative incidence

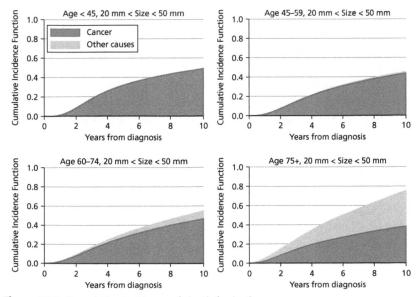

Figure 15.3 Cumulative incidence of death for both causes across age-groups.
Source: reproduced courtesy of Michael J. Crowther.

functions. However, this analysis approach allows the partitioning of the all-cause probability of death into component parts.

15.2.4 **Calibration and discrimination**

As with all prognostic models, after model development it is important for external validation in a new dataset, to consider how well outcome risk predictions from the model calibrate with observed outcome risks in new individuals. An added issue in the competing risks setting is that the risk of the competing causes may well vary in an external dataset, meaning that the estimated probabilities may vary even when the cause-specific rates for the disease of interest may be well calibrated. Wolbers et al. argue that standard calibration and discrimination statistics applicable to Cox regression can be adapted to Fine and Gray regression in the competing risks setting (18). Gerds et al. echo that, as in other prognostic model situations, calibration in the competing risks setting is an important consideration above and beyond simply reporting discrimination, and highlight approaches to estimate calibration measures in a competing risks setting using either the Fine and Gray, or cause-specific modelling approaches (19).

15.3 **Multi-state survival analysis**

15.3.1 **Introduction**

In this section we consider multi-state survival models, which are the natural extension to the competing risks models shown in the previous section. In other words, both a single time-to-event analysis, and a competing risks analysis are special cases of a multi-state survival model.

A patient's journey along a disease pathway can be highly complex, and can be impacted by recurrences of the same disease, co-morbidities, and interventions, to name a few. To disentangle such complex profiles, we need multi-state survival models (1). These enable us to investigate diverse aspects of prognosis and tease apart the impact of prognostic factors at all stages. Crucially, we can then attempt to communicate risk profiles in ways understandable to both patient and clinician, through easily interpretable measures (such as the impact on life expectancy, postponable deaths, survival probabilities). With the improved availability of linked electronic health records, it is imperative that we have appropriate methods to utilize these exciting resources, which enable us to answer multi-faceted questions.

The motivation generally comes from wanting to accommodate intermediate events, such as a relapse, which would be an event that occurs between diagnosis and death, and which obviously impacts prognosis. Not only is the occurrence of such an event important, but also the time at which it may occur. A multi-state model is governed by a transition matrix, that defines possible transitions between any two states of interest. We now introduce the general concepts of multi-state models, focusing on a simple illness-death setting to demonstrate the potential of modelling the full trajectory of a disease, and the clinically useful predictions that we can obtain.

15.3.2 Transition probabilities and hazards/intensities

Multi-state survival models can be described by two main quantities, the *transition probability* and the *transition hazard*. The transition probability represents the probability of being in state b at time t, given that a patient was in state a at time s, and conditional on the past trajectory until time s. A *Markov* multi-state model makes the following simplification that the transition probability is only dependent on which disease state a patient is currently in, not where they have been before. This is an assumption often made, which of course should be formally assessed.

The transition intensity/hazard's definition follows naturally from the cause-specific hazard from a competing risks analysis described above, where we now have the instantaneous probability of moving to state b given you are currently in state a. Although rather complex in appearance, this boils down to a collection of standard survival models between any two states, governing the multi-state model.

15.3.3 Modelling time to relapse and death in patients with primary breast cancer using a multi-state model

We now extend the analysis shown in the competing risks setting (Section 15.1.3) to accommodate the intermediate event of breast cancer relapse. All patients begin in the initial post-surgery state, which is defined as the time of primary surgery, and can then move to a relapse state, or a dead state, and can also die after relapse. This is the commonly known illness-death model, shown in Figure 15.4.

Of the 2982 patients starting in the post-surgery state, 1518 of them went on to experience a relapse, 195 died without relapse, and 1075 died after experiencing a relapse. Prognostic factors of interest include age at primary surgery, tumour size (three classes; ≤ 20 mm, 20–50 mm, > 50 mm), number of positive nodes, progesterone level (fmol/l), and whether patients were on hormonal therapy (binary, yes/no). Note that ideally tumour size would be analysed as a continuous variable, but the data were received in a

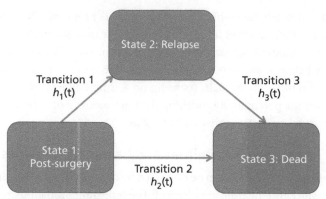

Figure 15.4 Illness-death model for the primary breast cancer example.
Source: reproduced courtesy of Michael J. Crowther.

categorized format. In all analyses we use a transformation of progesterone level ($\ln(pgr+1)$), as has been done previously (16). To each transition, we applied a flexible parametric survival model with the cumulative hazard modelled using restricted cubic splines (see Chapter 3), with best fitting models having three degrees of freedom for transitions 1 and 3, and one degree of freedom for transition 2.

We can now incorporate potential prognostic factors into each of the selected transition-specific models. We include all available factors in each of the models, and assess the proportional hazards assumption. To do this we can fit a Cox model to each transition separately and use the Schoenfeld residuals to test for non-proportionality (20), or directly include an interaction with a function of time. For transition 1, we found statistically significant ($p < 0.05$) evidence against the null hypothesis of proportionality, for tumour size (both levels, ref: ≤ 20 mm), and progesterone level. For transition 2, evidence of non-proportionality was not found for any prognostic factors. For transition 3, we found evidence of non-proportionality in progesterone level only. For simplicity, we did not investigate interactions or non-linear trends in prognostic factor effects, but this is straightforward as described in Chapters 3 and 4. We also assumed prognostic factor effects were distinct in each transition, although this assumption could be relaxed if considered appropriate.

Given our fitted multi-state model, we can now obtain predicted transition probabilities for any pattern of prognostic factor values. We illustrate this in Figure 15.5, showing transition probabilities for a patient aged fifty-four, with a transformed progesterone level of 3, and in each of the tumour size groups,

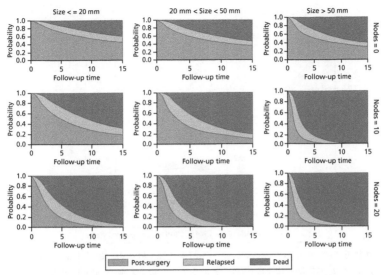

Figure 15.5 Probability of being in each state for a patient aged 54, with progesterone level (transformed scale) of 3 and no hormonal therapy, varying across tumour size and number of positive nodes.
Source: reproduced courtesy of Michael J. Crowther.

with varying number of positive nodes (0,10,20), and assuming no hormonal therapy. As tumour size increases, and number of positive nodes increase, we can see the increased probability of death across follow-up. The transition probabilities shown in Figure 15.5 also represent what is known as *state occupation probabilities*, as they are calculated assuming the patient starts in state 1 at time $s = 0$, providing clinically interpretable probabilities of being in each state as a function of time.

Stacked transition probability plots, such as Figure 15.5, are an extremely useful way of showing how risk evolves over time; however, uncertainty in the estimates cannot be easily portrayed. In Figure 15.6, we show the predicted transition probabilities from the left panel of Figure 15.5, now with associated confidence intervals.

Figures 15.5 and 15.6 exemplify the ease of obtaining patient-specific, clinically useful, predictions from a fully parametric, flexible, multi-state model. We can also illustrate the impact of different prognostic factor values by calculating differences or ratios in transition probabilities (21).

We can also predict the *restricted mean time spent in each state*, or *length of stay* in each transient state (i.e. a state that can be left), given a specific set of prognostic factor values, such as that shown in Figure 15.7. Figure 15.7 shows

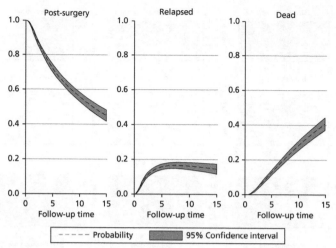

Figure 15.6 Probability of being in each state for a patient aged 54, size ≤20 mm, with progesterone level (transformed scale) of 3 and no hormonal therapy, and associated confidence intervals.
Source: reproduced courtesy of Michael J. Crowther.

that after fifteen years, a patient who was aged 54 at time of surgery, with progesterone level of 3 and in the smallest tumour size group, is predicted to spend approximately ten years in the post-surgery and relapse-free state, and two years in the relapse state.

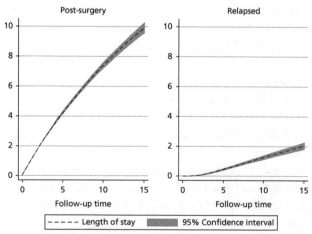

Figure 15.7 Length of stay in each state for a patient aged 54, size ≤20 mm, with progesterone level (transformed scale) of 3, and the smallest tumour size, with associated confidence intervals.
Source: reproduced courtesy of Michael J. Crowther.

15.4 **Joint modelling and dynamic prediction**

15.4.1 **Introduction**

Previous chapters have mainly focused on conducting prognosis research from one particular startpoint of interest, such as diagnosis of disease or post-surgery.

However, many diseases are complex processes which change and evolve with time, and therefore prognosis research is needed at multiple points on the disease pathway and healthcare process. For example, in the previous section we looked at how patients can move between states, and how predictions can be made conditional on the current state. Similarly, we may be interested in making individualized outcome risk predictions conditional on time, and making so-called dynamic predictions based on up-to-date prognostic factor information. To address this, we now consider how to make updated predictions over time, incorporating multiple measurements of prognostic factors to improve prediction. We consider joint modelling, allowing us to model both a longitudinal (repeatedly measured) prognostic factor and a survival outcome, in a unified framework to produce a dynamic prognostic model.

Longitudinal data of a prognostic factor, such as repeated measures of systolic blood pressure (SBP) or prostate specific antigen (PSA), are routinely collected when patients are diagnosed with conditions such as cardiovascular disease or prostate cancer. Alongside such longitudinal values, we have survival outcomes such as time to relapse or death. In such settings, the two processes often have an underlying association, for example, repeated measurements of PSA have been used to predict recurrence of prostate cancer through a *dynamic prognostic model* (22). Cluster of Differentiation 4 (CD4) counts have also been used extensively to predict time to progression to Acquired Immune Deficiency Syndrome (AIDS) in Human Immunodeficiency Virus (HIV) infected patients (23, 24). The key question here is, how do *changes* in a repeatedly measured prognostic factor impact the time to an event of interest; in other words, is the trajectory of the repeated measures itself a prognostic factor for future outcomes?

This problem can also be viewed from a different perspective. Longitudinal studies, which measure factors repeatedly over time, are often affected by drop-out. When this drop-out is associated with the underlying prognostic factor values, then the missingness process can be considered missing not at random, and will affect conclusions if ignored in the longitudinal analysis (25). Naïvely removing such patients that dropped out through a complete-case analysis can have severe consequences on results, as explained in Chapter 4. If this element of the data-generating mechanism is combined with the inherent clustering structure of the longitudinal prognostic factor data, with measurements nested within patients, then it requires a complex model framework to attempt to disentangle the various elements of the generating biological processes (26).

Recent arguments have been made that much more importance should be placed on attempting to evaluate patients' perspectives in clinical research (27). Within cancer or cardiovascular trials, such commonly available outcomes as quality of life (QOL), measured repeatedly, are often considered as supplementary information and not utilized to their full extent. The joint analysis of QOL and survival is a particular area which can benefit from a joint modelling approach, where the death can act as an informative drop-out process, especially when the two processes are strongly associated (28, 29).

15.4.2 The joint model framework

In essence, a joint model consists of two component submodels that share one or more parameters: a model for the trajectory of longitudinal prognostic factors measurements, and a model for the outcome occurrence. The form of joint model which has dominated the literature assumes that the association between the longitudinal prognostic factor values and the time-to-event is characterized by shared random effects (30), and it is this approach which we describe. Naïve approaches, such as only using baseline information, or including a prognostic factor as a time-varying covariate in a standard survival model can cause biased results (31).

15.4.2.1 Longitudinal submodel

In this submodel, the response is the value of the prognostic factor, with multiple values recorded over time per individual, and the aim is to model this as a function of time. As a prognostic factor is inherently measured intermittently, and usually with error, we can utilize a linear mixed effects framework, to estimate the true underlying, and complete, subject-specific trajectory function for the prognostic factor values (32). As this is a standard linear mixed effects model, we can still use standard tools for model flexibility, such as splines or fractional polynomials, to capture complex trends in the prognostic factor over time. Through this formulation, we now have a model representing the true unobserved prognostic factor values over time, essentially removing the measurement error at any time point t, not just the time that measurements were recorded, tailored to individual patients due to the random effects. We can then relate this longitudinal trajectory of prognostic factor values (or components of it, such as their rate of change) directly to the risk of the outcome of interest, by incorporating it within the survival submodel.

15.4.2.2 Survival submodel

Essentially, any survival model can be used within a joint model, but here we concentrate on parametric models, such as a Weibull. From our longitudinal submodel, we can now link our true unobserved patient-specific longitudinal trajectory, to the hazard rate of the outcome of interest. For example, we could investigate the association between the hazard of death at time t and the value of the prognostic factor at the same time t. This is known as the current value formulation, which gives us a hazard ratio for a one unit increase in our factor, at time t. Therefore the prognostic effect of the factor is explicitly linked to time t, which enables the factor's prognostic effect to be examined at multiple times (rather than just at a single startpoint). Similarly, outcome risk predictions can then be made at time t and conditional on an individual's trajectory of prognostic factor values up to time t. There are many other ways to link the two processes, many of which are discussed by Rizopoulos and Ghosh (33), but clinical guidance should drive the selection of association structure.

15.4.3 **Joint modelling of serum bilirubin and time to death in patients with primary biliary cirrhosis**

To illustrate the joint modelling approach, we investigate the association between repeatedly measured serum bilirubin and risk of death in a dataset of 312 patients with primary biliary cirrhosis (PBC), from Murtaugh et al. (34), where 158 patients were randomized to receive D-penicillamine, with 154 assigned to a placebo. Serum bilirubin was measured repeatedly at intermittent time points. Due to right skewness, in all analyses we work with ln (serum bilirubin).

In the longitudinal submodel, we model ln (serum bilirubin) as the continuous biomarker (prognostic factor) response with a random intercept and slope, and an interaction between time and treatment group. In the survival submodel, we model the time to death with a Weibull proportional hazards model, adjusting for treatment group. The two submodels are linked using the current value formulation described in the previous section, which enables the prognostic effect of the underlying biomarker value at time t to be estimated.

In the longitudinal submodel, we find no differential treatment effect on serum bilirubin over time. In the survival submodel, we observe a non-statistically significant direct treatment effect on survival, with log hazard ratio of 0.041 (95% CI: -0.312–0.393). However, of key interest for prognosis research, we find a strong positive association between the current value of the serum bilirubin and the mortality rate, with a hazard ratio for a one unit increase in the value of the time-dependent biomarker of 3.46 (95% CI: 2.88–4.15), indicating a higher value of serum bilirubin is associated with a larger risk of death.

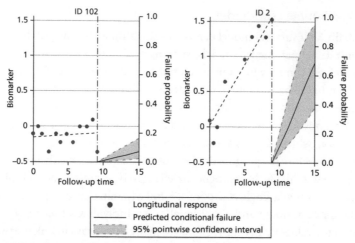

Figure 15.8 Patient-specific predicted probability of death (labelled 'failure probability') conditional on serum bilirubin ('biomarker') profiles over time. Source: reproduced courtesy of Michael J. Crowther.

A further benefit of fitting such a joint model within a shared parameter framework is the ability to tailor predictions at the individual level. For example, we may wish to predict a patient's survival conditional on a set of observed longitudinal measurements (33). We show this in Figure 15.8 for two patients with varying biomarker profiles. When new measurements of serum bilirubin are taken, these predictions can be *dynamically* updated, providing an effective patient monitoring tool.

15.5 Software

The permeation of new methods into the applied literature is partly driven by availability of user-friendly, well-documented, software packages. The methods described and applied in this chapter are all implemented in Stata, including the user-written packages multistate and stjm (21, 35). There are also a variety of other packages available, such as in R (30), including flexsurv and mstate for multi-state modelling (36, 37), JM and joineR for joint modelling (38).

15.6 Summary

This chapter has illustrated how modern advances in statistical methodology allow complex relationships and intricate prognosis pathways to be modelled, in order to examine prognostic factors and, in particular, to develop dynamic prognostic models for time-to-event outcomes.

Competing risks and multi-state models are becoming commonly used techniques. Their importance is now beginning to be understood in broadening fields of study. In particular, as the growth in access to electronic health databases continues, we can attempt to answer detailed and complex research questions, which require more complex yet appropriate statistical techniques. The ability to incorporate multi-morbidities, for example, which given the ageing population will only grow in importance, is crucial to fully understand disease pathways.

Joint modelling has been a rapidly evolving field of biostatistical research in recent years, and offers a convenient framework to address a wide variety of issues in many disease areas. Generally, computational challenges have hindered the widespread application of joint models, but with the ever-increasing availability of software packages, this is beginning to reduce. The ability to dynamically update prognostic models will play an important role in future years, as focus moves to actively capturing more high frequency prognostic information.

For brevity in our examples we did not examine or adjust for overfitting when developing the prognostic models. However, penalization and shrinkage approaches are also important for making absolute risk predictions from competing risks, multi-state, and joint models (39), for the reasons described for prognostic models generally in Chapters 4 and 7.

References

1. **Putter H, Fiocco M, and Geskus RB** (2007) Tutorial in biostatistics: competing risks and multi-state models. *Stat Med* 26(11), 2389–430.
2. **Andersen PK, Geskus RB, de Witte T**, et al. (2012) Competing risks in epidemiology: possibilities and pitfalls. *International J Epidemiol* 41(3), 861–70.
3. **Andersen PK and Keiding N** (2012) Interpretability and importance of functionals in competing risks and multistate models. *Stat Med* 31(11–12), 1074–88.
4. **Prentice RL, Kalbfleisch JD, Peterson Jr AV**, et al. (1978) The analysis of failure times in the presence of competing risks. *Biometrics* 34(4), 541–54.
5. **Esteve J, Benhamou E, Croasdale M**, et al. (1990) Relative survival and the estimation of net survival: elements for further discussion. *Stat Med* 9(5), 529–38.
6. **Dickman PW, Sloggett A, Hills M**, et al. (2004) Regression models for relative survival. *Stat Med* 23(1), 51–64.
7. **Nelson CP, Lambert PC, Squire IB**, et al. (2007) Flexible parametric models for relative survival, with application in coronary heart disease. *Stat Med* 26(30), 5486–98.
8. **Flanders WD** (1992) Inaccuracies of death certificate information. *Epidemiology* 3(1), 3–5.
9. **Schaffar R, Rapiti E, Rachet B**, et al. (2013) Accuracy of cause of death data routinely recorded in a population-based cancer registry: impact on cause-specific survival and validation using the Geneva Cancer Registry. *BMC Cancer* 13(1), 609.

10. **Dickman PW** and **Adami H-O** (2006) Interpreting trends in cancer patient survival. *J Int Med* **260**(2), 103–17.

11. **Lambert PC, Dickman PW, Weston CL**, et al. (2010) Estimating the cure fraction in population-based cancer studies by using finite mixture models. *J Royal Statistic Soc: Series C (Applied Statistics)* **59**(1), 35–55.

12. **Fine JP** and **Gray RJ** (1999) A proportional hazards model for the subdistribution of a competing risk. *J Amer Statist Assoc* **94**(446), 496–509.

13. **Lambert PC, Wilkes SR**, and **Crowther MJ** (2017) Flexible parametric modelling of the cause-specific cumulative incidence function. *Stat Med* **36**(9), 1429–46.

14. **Mozumder SI, Rutherford MJ, Lambert PC**, et al. (2017) A flexible parametric competing-risks model using a direct likelihood approach for the cause-specific cumulative incidence function. *Stata Journal* **17**(2), 462–89.

15. **Latouche A, Allignol A, Beyersmann J**, et al. (2013) A competing risks analysis should report results on all cause-specific hazards and cumulative incidence functions. *J Clin Epidemiol* **66**(6), 648–53.

16. **Royston P** and **Lambert PC** (2011) *Flexible Parametric Survival Analysis Using Stata: Beyond the Cox Model*. College Station, TX, US: Stata Press.

17. **Hinchliffe SR** and **Lambert PC** (2013) Flexible parametric modelling of cause-specific hazards to estimate cumulative incidence functions. *BMC Med Res Methodol* **13**(1), 13.

18. **Wolbers M, Koller MT, Witteman JCM**, et al. (2009) Prognostic models with competing risks: methods and application to coronary risk prediction. *Epidemiology* **20**(4), 555–61.

19. **Gerds TA, Andersen PK**, and **Kattan MW** (2014) Calibration plots for risk prediction models in the presence of competing risks. *Stat Med* **33**(18), 3191–203.

20. **Schoenfeld D** (1982) Partial residuals for the proportional hazards regression model. *Biometrika* **69**(1), 239–41.

21. **Crowther MJ** and **Lambert PC** (2017) Parametric multistate survival models: flexible modelling allowing transition-specific distributions with application to estimating clinically useful measures of effect differences. *Stat Med* **36**(29), 4719–42.

22. **Proust-Lima C** and **Taylor JMG** (2009) Development and validation of a dynamic prognostic tool for prostate cancer recurrence using repeated measures of post-treatment PSA: a joint modeling approach. *Biostatistics* **10**(3), 535–49.

23. **Wang Y** and **Taylor JMG** (2001) Jointly modeling longitudinal and event time data with application to acquired immunodeficiency syndrome. *J Amer Statist Assoc* **96**(455), 895–905.

24. **Wolbers M, Babiker A, Sabin C**, et al. (2010) Pretreatment CD4 cell slope and progression to AIDS or death in HIV-infected patients initiating antiretroviral therapy—the CASCADE collaboration: a collaboration of 23 cohort studies. *PLoS Med* **7**(2), e1000239.

25. **McArdle JJ, Small BJ, Bäckman L**, et al. (2005) Longitudinal models of growth and survival applied to the early detection of Alzheimer's disease. *J Geriatr Psychiatry Neurol* **18**(4), 234–41.

26. **Diggle PJ, Sousa I**, and **Chetwynd AG** (2008) Joint modelling of repeated measurements and time-to-event outcomes: the fourth Armitage lecture. *Stat Med* **27**(16), 2981–98.

27. **Gould AL, Boye ME, Crowther MJ,** et al. (2015) Joint modeling of survival and longitudinal non-survival data: current methods and issues. Report of the DIA Bayesian joint modeling working group. *Stat Med* **34**(14), 2181–95.

28. **Billingham LJ** and **Abrams KR** (2002) Simultaneous analysis of quality of life and survival data. *Stat Methods Med Res* **11**(1), 25–48.

29. **Ibrahim JG, Chu H,** and **Chen LM** (2010) Basic concepts and methods for joint models of longitudinal and survival data. *J Clin Oncol* **28**(16), 2796–801.

30. **Rizopoulos D** (2012) *Joint Models for Longitudinal and Time-to-Event Data With Applications in R.* London: Chapman & Hall.

31. **Sweeting MJ** and **Thompson SG** (2011) Joint modelling of longitudinal and time-to-event data with application to predicting abdominal aortic aneurysm growth and rupture. *Biom J* **53**(5), 750–63.

32. **Diggle P, Heagerty P, Liang K-Y,** et al. (2002) *Analysis of Longitudinal Data* (second edition). New York: Oxford University Press.

33. **Rizopoulos D** and **Ghosh P** (2011) A Bayesian semiparametric multivariate joint model for multiple longitudinal outcomes and a time-to-event. *Stat Med* **30**(12), 1366–80.

34. **Murtaugh P, Dickson E, Van Dam GM, M,** et al. (1994) Primary biliary cirrhosis: prediction of short-term survival based on repeated patient visits. *Hepatology* **20**, 126–34.

35. **Crowther MJ, Abrams KR,** and **Lambert PC** (2013) Joint modeling of longitudinal and survival data. *Stata J* **13**(1), 165–84.

36. **Jackson C** (2016) flexsurv: a platform for parametric survival modeling in R. *J Statistical Software* **70**(1), 1–33.

37. **de Wreede LC, Fiocco M, Putter H** (2011) mstate: an R package for the analysis of competing risks and multi-state models. *J Statistical Software* **38**(7), 30.

38. **Philipson P, Sousa I, Diggle P,** et al. (2012) *joineR–Joint Modelling of Repeated Measurements and Time-to-Event Data.* Comprehensive R Archive Network, United Kingdom.

39. **Sennhenn-Reulen H** and **Kneib T** (2016) Structured fusion lasso penalized multi-state models. *Stat Med* **35**(25), 4637–59.

Chapter 16

Machine learning in prognosis research

Mihaela van der Schaar and
Harry Hemingway

16.1 Introduction

Chapters 3–9 detailed the major concepts and fundamental methods of primary prognosis research. Chapters 13 and 14 highlighted the potential for IPD meta-analyses and large healthcare database studies to facilitate prognosis research using combined, big datasets. This increases the opportunity to develop, validate, and update prognostic models, to evaluate the effect of differences in healthcare on prognosis (e.g. over time and across regions), and to identify predictors of treatment effect. The analysis of 'Big Data' to improve prognosis research is made possible by the capacity of modern computers to handle large databases and to perform the necessary statistical analyses in a computationally feasible time.

A new element in the story has emerged with the potential to enhance prognosis research through a set of techniques known as 'machine learning' (ML). These methods place at the forefront the capacity to learn from large and complex data about the pathways, predictors, and trajectories of health outcomes in particular individuals. They reflect the wider drive for introducing a new component of 'data science' into daily life, where data-driven modelling is embedded and automated within powerful computers to manage and analyse large amounts of data. It has become familiar in such fields as weather forecasting and personalized consumer advertising, where streams of data are continuously growing and directly available to inform individuals and guide their decision making. It is therefore inevitable that machine-driven techniques have entered healthcare research, including prognosis research. Thirty per cent of the entire world's stored data is in health and healthcare (1). The more data that becomes available for analysis, the more attractive it becomes to explore the added value of machine-learning-based approaches that directly use the scale of big data to unlock new prognostic insights, as compared to more traditional methods.

There are unique opportunities and challenges in the application of ML and artificial intelligence (AI) to healthcare, summarized and debated in papers

(2–4). ML and AI have proved successful in various areas of healthcare, such as pattern recognition (e.g. outperforming dermatologists in recognizing skin cancer (5) and ophthalmologists in reading retinal images (6); natural language processing for online patient surveys (7); and early warning systems (8)). This chapter aims to introduce the key concepts behind ML techniques in the context of each of the four prognosis research types, explain where it may enhance prognosis research, and highlight potential challenges in its application. The chapter is not intended to provide in-depth methodological details, but does reference sources of more detailed accounts.

16.2 ML versus traditional approaches to prognosis research

16.2.1 The fundamental novelty of ML approaches to prognosis research

ML encompasses the methods, processes, and systems to extract and apply knowledge or insights from data. It offers an alternative to traditional analyses as a response to the growing diversity of large-scale data, increasingly available in real time, and the growing diversity of potential research questions (including all four prognosis research types, and beyond). It is supported by a diversity of research disciplines (including computer science, engineering, mathematics, and software development, as well as conventional biostatistics and clinical disciplines).

ML derives algorithms that can learn from data and can allow the data full freedom, for example, to follow a pragmatic approach in developing a prognostic model. Rather than choosing in advance the factors deemed to be important for model development, ML models allow the data to reveal which features are important for which predictions. This may involve 'unsupervised learning' from the structure of unlabelled data which contains no pre-specified or a priori classification, or 'supervised learning' using labelled training data to develop a model which can then be applied to new samples.

The most common machine learning models—classification and regression trees—build on the familiar idea of decision trees. Classification and regression trees successively partition the space of features (e.g. the characteristics of patients) in order to create clusters/subsets over which the labels/outcomes (e.g. survival) are as homogeneous as possible. Some of the most successful machine learning methods have been built as ensembles of such classification and regression trees (9, 10). These methods may also be combined with traditional statistical approaches for estimating association with endpoints such as Cox regression (11).

ML is also innovating and departing from conventional decision tree methods. For example, one novel approach (11) constructs a tree of subsets of the feature space, and associates a predictive model—determined by training one of a given family of models (regressions such as Cox or logistic, or other types) on an endogenously determined training set—to each node of the tree. The resulting construction is called a tree of predictors (ToPs). Unlike classification and regression trees, ToPs is not creating clusters or subsets over which labels and outcomes are more homogeneous, but rather subsets that have predictors which are the same. While classification and regression trees create successive splits of the feature space to maximize homogeneity of each split with respect to labels, ToPs creates such splits to maximize predictive accuracy of each split with respect to a constructed predictive model. It discovers the most relevant features (covariates), uses available features to best advantage, and is adaptable to changes in clinical practice.

Yoon and colleagues (11) used this approach to develop a novel ML algorithm for survival prediction in cardiac transplantation and tested its performance on the database of all patients who were registered for cardiac transplantation in the US during 1985–2015. The application of ToPs in this paper resulted in better discrimination performance than application of existing clinical risk scoring methods. For instance, ToPs achieved a C statistic of 0.660 for three-month survival post-transplantation compared with a C statistic of 0.587 observed with the best clinical risk scoring method (RSS). In comparison to RSS, holding specificity at 80.0%, ToPs correctly predicted three-year survival for 2442 (14.0%) more patients (of 17,441 who actually survived); holding sensitivity at 80.0%, ToPs correctly predicted three-year mortality for 694 (13.0%) more patients (of 5339 who did not survive).

This is one of an emerging number of examples of ML-derived prognostic models that suggest aspects of performance are improved compared with traditionally derived models. More work is needed on formal comparisons of ML and traditional models across all measures of performance, and of the relative merits of their application and usefulness in practice. However, the example indicates the potential for ML methods to improve outcome prediction, and hence decision making, across diseases and clinical specialities. This has far-reaching implications for clinical practice.

ML has found application in each of the four prognosis research types discussed in earlier chapters, as illustrated in Table 16.1. There are developments in the statistical analytic methods to deliver ML prognosis research outputs that are unique to ML (see Table 16.1), but many that also overlap with those of traditional approaches.

Table 16.1 Relevance of ML methods to the four prognosis research types. The challenges listed in the table are challenges that traditional techniques are also tackling. The methods listed are some of the alternative techniques utilized by ML.

Prognosis research type	Challenges where ML can add insights	Examples of methods used for, or relevant to, machine-learning approaches
Type 1: overall prognosis	Understanding disease trajectories, including missing data and non-standard observation intervals	Markov/hidden Markov models, neural networks
Type II: prognostic factor	Discovering new disease sub-phenotypes associated with outcome	Unsupervised clustering
Type III: prognostic models	Obtaining prognostic predictions, particularly where: • datasets are large • data are real time and local • a large number of prognostic models is needed • competing risks are present	Classification and regression trees Survival analysis with competing risk Bayesian non-parametrics Ensemble methods Neural networks
Type 4: predictors of treatment effect	Individualized treatment effects; causal inference	Multi-task learning Representation learning

Source: reproduced courtesy of Mihaela van der Schaar.

Table 16.2 Potential advantages and disadvantages of ML for prognosis research.

Potential advantages	Potential disadvantages
Fewer or no assumptions, so wider sources of data (such as text) and less structured data can be used	Interpretability
Large numbers of predictors can be included	Need to ensure models do not overfit
Local data sources can be optimally used to generate prognostic models	Need to ensure models do not overfit
Analysis can be automated	Ethics and governance challenges
Prognostic models can be self-learning and more easily updated using routine care data in real time when integrated into clinical data systems	Avoidance of the necessary research to investigate whether the models still suffice (in terms of impact and patient benefit) or require updating with the new data

Source: reproduced courtesy of Mihaela van der Schaar.

16.2.2 **What are the potential advantages and disadvantages of ML for prognosis research?**

Potential advantages of ML compared with traditional approaches are listed in Table 16.2, together with the corresponding potential disadvantages.

Many of the methodological problems involved in applying these new techniques to prognosis questions are the same as those for the traditional techniques. The application of ML methods to improve prognosis in healthcare practice is at an early stage of evaluation, and the process of, for example, prognostic model development, validation, and impact measurement, is as vital for prognosis research in this new field as it is for traditional analysis approaches (4).

16.2.3 **The issue of interpretability**

Interpretability or face value has for years been an important feature of developed prediction models destined for use in healthcare practice (12). If the output is a calculated probability of a particular outcome, such as predicted five-year survival in a woman diagnosed with breast cancer, then concerns about public understanding of that risk are identical, regardless of the approach that has been used to deliver it (see Chapters 5 and 7). However, the action needed to deliver that score may vary in complexity. Some prognostic models are so simple they can be calculated in a clinician's head (e.g. CHADSVASC score for risk of stroke in atrial fibrillation (13)); others, a little more complicated, can be calculated by hand (e.g. Framingham risk (14)); others may need a computer to calculate, but both input and output are understood by clinicians and readily explained to patients. ML algorithms, however, pose additional challenges to interpretability, relevant to use in clinical practice:

1. They may represent a 'black box', that is, the specific model equation or what the algorithm is doing in broad terms are insufficiently transparent. Finding ways of explaining algorithms so they are interpretable for care providers, patients, and public, is important for accountability in decision making.

2. ML algorithms may be complex, and putting into words multiple non-linear effects and interactions is not straightforward. For example predicting an individual's need for surgery in patients admitted to hospital with acute lower gastro-intestinal bleeding with a neural network model was more accurate than a regression-based bedside tool, but less user-friendly for urgent decisions (15). This problem is not unique to ML and affects traditional approaches to complex data also.

16.3 **Potential application of data science and ML to the four prognosis research types**

This section is designed to show how current ML approaches relate to the framework of four types of prognosis study.

16.3.1 **Prognosis research type 1: overall prognosis**

Challenging areas of overall prognosis research to which ML can contribute include incorporation of time spent in different health states, analysis of competing risks for survival, and new approaches to missing data:

1. Stationary models of the disease process, with startpoints and endpoints measured at single points in time, often do not address the full prognostic story, especially in people with chronic health conditions (see Chapter 5). ML has the potential to incorporate dynamic trajectories of disease, including not only the patients' current state but also time spent within the state, that is, the 'sojourn time' (8, 16).

2. ML promises to transform current disease taxonomy by helping to identify new disease subgroups or clusters, based on differences in expected course or prognosis. This opens up the possibility of new data-driven phenotypes based on extensive sources and types of data. For example the cardiac transplantation study discussed above (11) identified various clusters with contrasting outcomes.

3. ML is being used to examine alternatives to multiple imputation approaches for handling missing data, including nonparametric methods of imputation and application of neural networks (16, 17). It introduces the idea of being able to infer true disease states from the data even when they are not directly observed or recorded by the care provider, and hence to estimate overall prognosis of people with those states.

16.3.2 **Prognosis research type 2: prognostic factor studies**

Genetic variability is a major target for prognostic factor discovery using ML methods. For example, the DNA chromatin component of the nuclei of tumour cells varies in the state of its structural organization. ML algorithms analysed the chromatin organization in 461,000 images of tumour cell nuclei from 390 patients treated for colorectal cancer stage 1 or II (the training data) and a marker of chromatin heterogeneity was derived (18); traditional statistical approaches were then used to investigate its potential as a prognostic factor for survival. Patients with chromatin heterogeneous tumours had worse cancer-specific survival after adjustment for other prognostic factors (HR 1.7, 95% CI 1.1–2.5) than patients with chromatin homogenous tumours, and this was externally validated in six other independent cohorts of cancer patients.

Competing survival risks are increasingly important as multi-morbidity becomes more common. Survival analysis does not necessarily account for these (but see Chapter 15). ML approaches, drawing on flexible nonparametric Bayesian survival analyses as alternatives to parametric-based traditional methods, have the potential to learn a 'shared representation' of patients' survival times with respect to multiple co-morbidities or to the complex interactions between covariates and survival times in conditions such as cardiovascular disease with heterogeneous phenotypes (19–21).

16.3.3 **Prognosis study type 3: prognostic model studies**

ML has been used to create dynamic prognostic models by exploiting observations over time (time-series data) to describe the course of illness as a series of health states. In doing so, ML has addressed two challenges. The first is to integrate different types of time-series data (e.g. vital signs, laboratory tests, imaging) that are observed with different frequencies. The second is that the true clinical state of the patient may be hidden and not directly observed, meaning transitions between clinical states may also not be observed and so the true clinical state and the transition between states must be inferred (8). Once 'learned', such models can be used for diagnosis (inference of the current state of the patient) and prognosis (forecast of the future state of the patient). All of this can be done dynamically: as new data arrives, the model can update both the diagnosis and the prognosis and so issue dynamic predictions. Traditional analysis also addresses these possibilities (see especially Chapter 15), but ML offers an alternative approach. Box 16.1

Box 16.1 Risk estimation for transfer to intensive care among individual patients admitted to general wards of hospitals

Aim: to develop an ML-based prognostic model for early prediction of clinical deterioration in hospitalized individuals on general wards, in order to inform timely admission to an intensive care unit (ICU).

Population and startpoint: retrospective study of 6321 patients admitted to the Ronald Reagan Medical Center (UCLA) between March 2013 and February 2016.

Endpoint: clinical deterioration defined as admission to the ICU during an initial stay on the general ward.

Methods: a machine-learning approach constructed a hidden semi-Markov model using thirty-eight clinical variables to predict in-hospital clinical deterioration. The model automatically discovered six clusters (subtypes) of clinical deterioration patterns and a separate prognostic model was fitted for each cluster.

Results: the C statistic for the overall model was 0.85.

Source: data from Alaa AM, et al. (2018) Personalized risk scoring for critical care prognosis using mixtures of Gaussian processes. *IEEE Transactions on Biomedical Engineering* 65(1), 207–18. Copyright © 2018 IEEE.

Box 16.2 ML for prediction of all-cause mortality in patients with suspected coronary artery disease: a five-year multicentre prospective registry analysis

Aim: to use all the information available on patients undergoing investigation for suspected coronary artery disease to develop a prognostic model for all-cause mortality.

Population and startpoint: 10,030 patients undergoing coronary computed tomographic angiography (CCTA) for suspected coronary artery disease, who were placed on an international multicentre registry of persons having this investigation.

Endpoint: five-year all-cause mortality.

Methods: twenty-five clinical parameters and forty-four angiographic details were incorporated into a database to which ML methods (automated feature selection, model building using an ensemble algorithm, and stratified cross validation) were applied.

Results: ML prediction had a C statistic of 0.70 for predicting all-cause mortality.

Source: data from Motwani M, et al. (2016) Machine learning for prediction of all-cause mortality in patients with suspected coronary artery disease: a 5-year multicentre prospective registry analysis. *European Heart Journal* 38(7), 500–507. Copyright © 2016 OUP.

illustrates how such time-series models have been applied to early prediction of clinical deterioration of patients hospitalized in general wards.

Box 16.2 illustrates an ML approach to predicting mortality within patients undergoing computerized tomographic (CT) angiography for suspected CHD (22).

16.3.4 Prognosis research type 4: predicting individualized treatment effects

ML offers the potential for observational data to address treatment questions where trial evidence will never exist (e.g. effects of multiple treatment combinations) and for generating evidence to select the best treatments for individual patients based on predictors of treatment effects. The success of ML programmes for playing chess and Go depended on the fact that whenever a decision—a particular move or sequence of moves, for instance—led to failure/loss, it was possible to go back and try a different decision. In medicine it is not possible to go back and undo a particular surgery or choose a different drug—counterfactuals do not exist and cannot be generated. Large-scale

Box 16.3 Cross-trial prediction of treatment outcome in depression: a ML approach

Aim: to develop an algorithm to predict response to antidepressant treatment

Study population and startpoint: 4041 patients with depression recruited to a sequence of randomized controlled trials of treatments, recruitment to each trial depending on response at each stage.

Potential predictors of treatment effect: 164 patient-report variables.

Endpoint: remission of depression.

Methods: ML methods applied to clinical trial data and using potential predictors identified in the study population. External validation in a separate independent trial population.

Results: twenty-five variables were most predictive of treatment outcome from 164 patient-reportable variables, and were used to train the model. The model was internally cross validated and externally validated. The model predicted outcomes in a combined escitalopram-buprorion treatment group, but not in a combined venlafaxine-mirtazapine group, suggesting specificity of the model to underlying mechanisms.

Source: data from Chekroud AM, et al. (2016) Cross-trial prediction of treatment outcome in depression: a machine learning approach. *Lancet Psychiatry* 3(3), 243–50. Copyright © 2016 Elsevier.

routine healthcare datasets contain covariate patterns of all patients, including treatments received and outcomes experienced, but never the outcomes of individuals if they had received different treatments or none at all.

This makes predicting individual treatment effects using non-RCT data challenging. One approach taken by ML research into predicting treatment effects is similar to the approach of traditional methods outlined in Chapter 8. Box 16.3 illustrates this. The database in this example was taken from a single study which incorporated several randomized controlled trials of treatment alternatives used in sequence for patients who failed to respond to their previously allocated treatment at each stage.

Alternative approaches taken by ML frame the estimation of individualized treatment effects as a multi-task learning problem (23) or as a biased imputation problem (24). Preliminary results using these approaches suggest they may improve performance.

16.4 **The need for evaluation**

While strong claims are made for AI and ML, there needs to be a framework for their rigorous evaluation in prognosis research. In much the same way that nearly all of 1575 cancer prognostic biomarker papers were positive (25), nearly all ML publications in the biomedical literature are also positive. Familiar themes concerning the need for scientific rigour and for evidence of usefulness in practice, which have surfaced throughout this book, are applicable to the new approaches, including:

♦ Replicability and external validity

♦ Capacity for implementation

♦ Evaluation of impact on decision making and subsequent patient outcomes

♦ Interpretability of the prognostic models

♦ Accountability and privacy

16.5 **Big data and the future of prognosis research**

The hope for all the chapters in Section 5 is that harnessing the power of computers to the large and rapidly expanding banks of healthcare data and to both traditional and novel analytic techniques will discover new prognostic factors and models and deliver improved predictions of outcome and treatment effects in individual patients. The ambition is that human intuition, experience, and biases could be complemented, or even replaced, by data-driven, objective systematic analysis, discovery, and prediction.

New challenges and new questions that will be posed for prognosis research include:

♦ Can the current disease taxonomy in healthcare eventually be replaced with one that reflects disease mechanisms and patient prognosis matched to optimally effective, efficient, and safer interventions?

♦ Can ways be found to fully exploit the large and ever-expanding universe of personal health-relevant information (including 'omics' and treatment data) and identify novel prognostic factors and predictors of treatment effect?

♦ How accurate can prediction of future outcomes in individuals become, and could healthcare eventually answer the individual patient's question, 'what about me?' by delivering real-time personalized prognosis in clinical practice on the whole patient, updated over time, and analogous to a test result, in order to react optimally to immediate real-world, real-time clinical problems?

16.5.1 **An example of future potential: ML and the emergence of an 'actionable genome'**

A driver for ML and 'prognosis-based medicine' is the rapid growth in genomic information. The combination of genome sequence data with 'phenome-sequence' data (captured, for example over repeated encounters in the electronic health record, agnostic to any one disease) is increasingly available on a large scale for research (e.g. national biobank cohorts such as UK Biobank (26)) and care (e.g. the 100,000 genomes project (27)). It is predicted that by 2020 there will be twenty million people in the world with whole genome sequencing data (three billion base pairs).

The single test to reveal a patient's whole genome sequence may lead to many different clinical actions expected to alter prognosis. Many otherwise healthy individuals have genetic variants on which clinical action could be taken ('actionable' data). This introduces another domain and scale of information to prognosis research, and a new tranche of data to contribute to stratified care and to understanding the prognosis of individuals with common and rare variants in the three billion base pairs. Strong prognosis research methods will be needed to investigate the prognostic value of such information for action to improve patient outcomes (see Chapter 8) and the added value it brings to prognostic models (see Chapter 7). For example:

+ In the general adult population 3.5% may have actionable variants for single gene disorders such as breast cancer susceptibility (BRCA1) and familial hypercholesterolaemia.

+ Twenty per cent of the general population have a higher blood pressure by 10 mmHg that is genetically determined and independent of any pharmacological blood pressure reduction.

+ Twenty diseases have polygenic risk scores, some of which outperform outcome prediction based on existing prognostic models, and which might lead to different clinical decisions at different ages (28), such as younger age for individuals to start statins.

16.5.2 **Bringing it all together: the vision of precision medicine, precision health, and 'AI health systems'**

The ultimate goal of prognosis research is a personalized disease atlas which provides disease trajectories, outcome prediction, screening policies, and treatment plans (see Figure 16.1 for an example, and Lim and Van der Schaar (29) for additional examples). This is in stark contrast to current healthcare practice where many decisions are formed for one disease at a time (rather than learning from the complexity of multiple conditions) and at a single

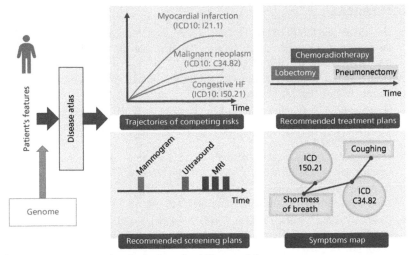

Figure 16.1 An Example of a Personalised Disease Atlas.
Source: reproduced courtesy of Mihaela van der Schaar.

time point (rather than considering the optimal sequence over time). A clinician treating a specific patient will be able to invoke this atlas, which describes a course of illness tailored to that individual and how various risks for the patient may evolve over time. The availability of such an atlas would enable a more profound understanding of diseases, their interrelationships, and their evolution in different patients, ultimately leading to new medical discoveries.

16.6 **Summary**

The emerging developments in data science, including AI and ML, will have a growing impact on prognosis research. Conversations are needed between ML and traditional approaches. On the one hand, there is ML's capacity to incorporate many more variables from large, linked datasets, including routine healthcare and the human genome, for identifying prognostic factors and in prognostic model building, particularly for creating dynamic up-to-date prognostic models for the individual. On the other hand, there is the need to prioritize core research tasks, such as demonstrating generalizability and calibration. One challenge will be to integrate the new methods with the rest of prognosis research, directly compare the new methods with traditional approaches, and define their complementary roles. Evidence is needed about the impact of the new methods on healthcare practice, and their usefulness and applicability for decision making and improving patient outcomes.

References

1. **Huesch MD** and **Mosher TJ** (2017) *Using it or Losing it? The Case for Data Scientists Inside Health Care*. Online. Available: https://catalyst.nejm.org/case-data-scientists-inside-health-care/ (Accessed 5 August 2018).

2. **Cabitza F, Rasoini R,** and **Gensini GF** (2017) Unintended consequences of machine learning in medicine. *JAMA* **318**, 517–18.

3. **Sheikhtaheri A, Sadoughi F,** and **Hashemi Dehaghi Z** (2014) Developing and using expert systems and neural networks in medicine: a review on benefits and challenges. *J Med Syst* **38**, 110.

4. **Obermeyer Z** and **Emanuel EJ** (2016) Predicting the future—Big Data, machine learning, and clinical medicine. *N Engl J Med* **375**, 1216–19.

5. **Esteva A, Kuprel B, Novoa RA,** et al. (2017) Dermatologist-level classification of skin cancer with deep neural networks. *Nature* **542**, 115–18.

6. **Gulshan V, Peng L, Coram M,** et al. (2016) Development and validation of a deep learning algorithm for detection of diabetic retinopathy in retinal fundus photographs. *JAMA* **316**, 2402–10.

7. **Ranard BL, Werner RM, Antanavicius T,** et al. (2016) Yelp reviews of hospital care can supplement and inform traditional surveys of the patient experience of care. *Health Aff (Millwood)* **35**, 697–705.

8. **Alaa AM** and **van der Schaar M** (2018). A hidden absorbing semi-Markov model for informatively censored temporal data: learning and inference. http://arxiv.org/pdf/1612.06007v2. 1–56.

9. **Douschan P, Kovacs G, Avian A,** et al. (2017) Mild elevation of pulmonary arterial pressure as a predictor of mortality. *Am J Respir Crit Care Med* **197**, 509–516.

10. **Yoon J, Zame WR,** and **Van Der Schaar M** (2018) ToPs: ensemble learning with Trees of Predictors. *IEEE Transactions on Signal Processing (TSP).*

11. **Yoon J, Zame WR, Banerjee A,** et al. (2018) Personalized survival predictions via Trees of Predictors: an application to cardiac transplantation. *PLoS One* **13**(3), e0194985.

12. **Altman DG** and **Royston P** (2000) What do we mean by validating a prognostic model? *Stat Med* **19**, 453–73.

13. **Lip GY, Frison L, Halperin JL,** and **Lane DA** (2010) Identifying patients at high risk for stroke despite anticoagulation: a comparison of contemporary stroke risk stratification schemes in an anticoagulated atrial fibrillation cohort. *Stroke* **41**, 2731–8.

14. **D'Agostino RB Sr, Vasan RS, Pencina MJ,** et al. (2008) General cardiovascular risk profile for use in primary care: the Framingham Heart Study. *Circulation* **117**, 743–53.

15. **Loftus TJ, Brakenridge SC, Croft CA,** et al. (2017) Neural network prediction of severe lower intestinal bleeding and the need for surgical intervention. *J Surg Res* **212**, 4247.

16. **Alaa AM, Hu S,** and **van der Schaar M** (2017) Learning from clinical judgements: semi-Markov-modulated marked Hawkes processes for risk prognosis. *Proceedings of Machine Learning Research.* **70**, 1–16.

17. **Yoon J, Zame WR,** and **van der Schaar M** (2018) Deep sensing: active sensing using multi-directional recurrent neural networks. *International Conference on Learning Representations* Vancouver, Canada. https://openreview.net/pdf?id=r1SnX5xCb. 1–19.

18. **Kleppe A, Albregtsen F, Vlatkovic L,** et al. (2018) Chromatin organisation and cancer prognosis: a pan-cancer study. *Lancet Oncol* **19**, 356–69.

19. **Alaa AM** and **van der Schaar M** (2017) Deep multi-task Gaussian processes for survival analysis with competing risks. Published as a conference paper at the thirty-first Conference on Neural Information Processing Systems, Long Beach, CA, USA. https://papers.nips.cc/paper/6827-deep-multi-task-gaussian-processes-for-survival-analysis-with-competing-risks.pdf: 1–9.

20. **Lee C, Zame WR, Yoon J**, and **van der Schaar M** (2018) DeepHit: A deep learning approach to survival analysis with competing risks. Published as a conference paper from the thirty-second Association for the Advancement of Artificial Intelligence Conference on Artificial Intelligence, New Orleans, Louisiana, US. https://www.aaai.org/ocs/index.php/AAAI/AAAI18/. 2314-2321.

21. **Bellot A** and **van der Schaar M** (2018) A hierarchical Bayesian model for personalized survival predictions. *IEEE J Biomed Health Inform*. 2 May. doi: 10.1109/JBHI.2018.2832599 (Epub ahead of print).

22. **Motwani M, Dey D, Berman DS**, et al. (2017) Machine learning for prediction of all-cause mortality in patients with suspected coronary artery disease: a five-year multicentre prospective registry analysis. *Eur Heart J* **38**, 500–507.

23. **Alaa AM, Yoon J**, and **Van Der Schaar M** (2018) Personalized risk scoring for critical care prognosis using mixtures of Gaussian processes. *IEEE Trans Biomed Eng* **65**, 207–218.

24. **Yoon J, Jordon M**, and **van der Schaar M** (2018) GAIN: missing data imputation using generative adversarial nets. Thirty-fifth International Conference on Machine Learning, Stockholm, Sweden. *Proceedings of Machine Learning* **80**, 1–10.

25. **Kyzas PA, Denaxa-Kyza D**, and **Ioannidis JP** (2007) Almost all articles on cancer prognostic markers report statistically significant results. *Eur J Cancer* **43**, 2559–79.

26. **Cox NJ** (2017) Reaching for the next branch on the biobank tree of knowledge. *Nat Genet* **49**, 1295–6.

27. **Gov.uk** (2012) *DNA tests to revolutionise fight against cancer and help 100,000 NHS patients*. Available: https://www.gov.uk/government/news/dna-tests-to-revolutionise-fight-against-cancer-and-help-100000-nhs-patients (Accessed 5 August 2018).

28. **Abraham G, Havulinna AS, Bhalala OG**, et al. (2016) Genomic prediction of coronary heart disease. *Eur Heart J* **37**, 3267–78.

29. **Lim B** and **van der Schaar M** (2018) *Disease-Atlas: Navigating Disease Trajectories with Deep Learning*. https://arxiv.org/abs/1803.10254v3 (stat.ML). 1–20. Published as Proceedings of the third Machine Learning for Healthcare Conference.

Appendix

Web resources

This textbook has a dedicated website (http://www.prognosisresearch.com/) where you can locate updates and continuing commentary on the book and its contents.

The Cochrane Methods prognosis group has a website (https://methods.cochrane.org/prognosis/).

Courses

The annual International Summer School organised by the Centre for Prognosis Research at Keele University, United Kingdom, and various annual courses of the Julius Center for Health Sciences and Primary Care at Utrecht University, The Netherlands, are specifically designed to align with the content of this textbook. For details of this and other relevant courses run by authors of this book, please visit www.prognosisresearch.com and www.msc-epidemiology.nl.

Complementary material

Two textbooks of major relevance are:

Steyerberg EW (2009) *Clinical Prediction Models: a Practical Approach to Development, Validation and Updating.* New York: Springer.

Harrell FE, Jr. (2015) *Regression Modeling Strategies: with Applications to Linear Models, Logistic and Ordinal Regression, and Survival Analysis* (second edition). New York: Springer.

Throughout the book we have discussed guidelines for prognosis studies. Key sources include:

Hayden JA, van der Windt DA, Cartwright JL, et al (2013) Assessing bias in studies of prognostic factors. *Ann Intern Med* **158**(4), 280–6.

McShane LM, Altman DG, Sauerbrei W, et al. (2005) Reporting recommendations for tumor marker prognostic studies (REMARK). *J Natl Cancer Inst* **97**(16), 1180–4.

Collins GS, Reitsma JB, Altman DG, et al. (2015) Transparent Reporting of a multivariable prediction model for Individual Prognosis Or Diagnosis (TRIPOD): The TRIPOD Statement. *Ann Intern Med* **162**, 55–63.

Moons KG, Altman DG, Reitsma JB, et al. (2015) Transparent Reporting of a multivariable prediction model for Individual Prognosis Or Diagnosis (TRIPOD): explanation and elaboration. *Ann Intern Med* **162**(1), W1–73.

Wolff RF, Riley RD, Whiting PF, et al. (2019) PROBAST: a tool to assess the risk of bias and applicability of prediction model studies. *Ann Int Med* (in press).

Moons KGM, Wolff RF, Riley RD, et al. (2019) PROBAST: a tool to assess risk of bias and applicability concerns of prediction model studies - explanation and elaboration. Ann Int Med (in press).

Index

Notes: Tables, figures and boxes are indicated by an italic *t, f,* and *b* following the page number.